Clinical Interviews for Children and Adolescents

The Guilford Practical Intervention in the Schools Series

Kenneth W. Merrell, Founding Editor
T. Chris Riley-Tillman, Series Editor

www.guilford.com/practical

This series presents the most reader-friendly resources available in key areas of evidence-based practice in school settings. Practitioners will find trustworthy guides on effective behavioral, mental health, and academic interventions, and assessment and measurement approaches. Covering all aspects of planning, implementing, and evaluating high-quality services for students, books in the series are carefully crafted for everyday utility. Features include ready-to-use reproducibles, lay-flat binding to facilitate photocopying, appealing visual elements, and an oversized format. Recent titles have companion Web pages where purchasers can download and print the reproducible materials.

RECENT VOLUMES

Clinical Interviews for Children and Adolescents

Assessment to Intervention

SECOND EDITION

STEPHANIE H. McCONAUGHY

THE GUILFORD PRESS
New York   London

To my husband, Stewart, who shares my passion for understanding
other people's perspectives and communicating effectively,
and my son, David, who was my most enjoyable interviewee

© 2013 The Guilford Press
A Division of Guilford Publications, Inc.
72 Spring Street, New York, NY 10012
www.guilford.com

Printed in the United States of America

This book is printed on acid-free paper.

Last digit is print number: 9 8 7 6 5 4 3 2

Library of Congress Cataloging-in-Publication Data

McConaughy, Stephanie H.
   Clinical interviews for children and adolescents: assessment to intervention /
Stephanie H. McConaughy. — Second edition.
      pages   cm. — (The Guilford practical intervention in the school series)
   Includes bibliographical references and index.
   ISBN 978-1-4625-0841-9 (pbk.: alk. paper)
   1. Interviewing in child psychiatry.   2. Interviewing in adolescent psychiatry.   I. Title.
   RJ503.6.M329   2013
   616.8900835—dc23
                                                                        2012051194

About the Author

Stephanie H. McConaughy, PhD, is Research Professor Emerita of Psychiatry and Psychology at the University of Vermont. She specializes in research and assessment of children's behavioral, emotional, and learning problems and is a member of the research team that developed the Achenbach System of Empirically Based Assessment (ASEBA). Dr. McConaughy is the author of over 60 journal articles and chapters and 8 books and assessment manuals. She is a Vermont licensed practicing psychologist and school psychologist and a nationally certified school psychologist. She has served on the editorial boards of professional journals in psychology and school psychology and was an associate editor of the *School Psychology Review*. Dr. McConaughy's research has been funded by the U.S. Department of Education, the National Institute on Disability and Rehabilitation Research, the National Institute of Child Health and Human Development, the National Institute of Mental Health, the Spencer Foundation, and the W. T. Grant Foundation.

Preface

People love to talk about themselves. Children are no exception. Yet, without even thinking, adults often hinder children from speaking for themselves. Ask a child a question in the presence of a parent or another familiar adult and watch what happens. As the child starts to speak, the adult jumps in to explain what the child thinks or feels, and then continues with his or her own view of the matter. Other times, when children do manage to express their views, adults counter with their own versions of what happened and how children *should* think or feel. This is captured poignantly in Cat Stevens's lament in the song "Father and Son" from *Tea for the Tillerman:* "From the moment I could talk, I was ordered to listen. . . ." In my practice as a psychologist and researcher, I have met many children like that son struggling to be heard. These are the ones we call "rebellious, oppositional, depressed, withdrawn, inattentive, shy, uncommunicative. . . ." Add your own words.

Learning children's viewpoints is an essential feature of good clinical assessment. I hope this book will enhance readers' professional skills for hearing what troubled children have to say and for integrating their perspectives with those of their parents, teachers, and other significant adults. To provide a broad focus, this book discusses clinical interviewing within the framework of multimethod assessment. Readers are encouraged to use other assessment methods along with clinical interviews to obtain a comprehensive picture of children's functioning. To illustrate interviewing strategies, I have included case examples and interview segments based on research and clinical experience with many children. All of the names used in these cases are pseudonyms, and details of case material have been altered to protect confidentiality.

Since the first edition of this book was published in 2005, several new developments in psychology and education have arisen, prompting the writing of this second edition. First was increased attention to the plight of children who are victims or perpetrators of bullying. In the past, it was common for parents, as well as teachers, to dismiss bullying and being bullied as a normal part of growing up. However, a growing research literature has shown that bullying is not part of normal development and that it can produce serious and lasting harm. Several highly publicized suicides have also raised awareness of the dire consequences of bullying. As a result, many adults are paying closer attention to bullying as an important social problem that warrants intervention and prevention. This second edition reviews relevant research to provide an empirical basis for interviewing children, parents, and teachers about bullying and victimization and provides guidelines and sample interview questions to address these issues. It also discusses the social problems that confront gay, lesbian, bisexual, and transgender youth who are frequent targets of bullying.

A second development was the increasing multicultural and linguistic diversity of the U.S. population and the challenges this presents for communication and understanding. According to the 2009–2010 U.S. Census, 30–45% of the population identified themselves as non-White, and 18% spoke a language other than English in the home. Sensitivity to cultural and linguistic differences is essential for effective communication with children and their parents. In this second edition I have greatly expanded the discussion of multicultural issues and provided guidelines for interviewing children and parents from diverse cultural and linguistic backgrounds.

A third development was the fast-growing use of digital technology for social communication. As noted in Chapter 4, Pew Internet studies in 2010 and 2011 showed that over 70% of American adolescents owned a cell phone, over 80% accessed social networking sites, and over 90% used the Internet. Digital communication has many positive aspects, but it has also given rise to new social hazards, including "cyberbullying" and "sexting" (transmission of sexually explicit material via cell phones and the Internet). This second edition discusses research and legal issues regarding potential social problems in digital communication and how to address such problems in clinical interviews.

Finally, to facilitate assessment of children's school and social functioning, this second edition includes a new reproducible Semistructured Student Interview (McConaughy, 2012; Appendix 3.1), which covers children's activities and interests, school functioning, peer relations, feelings, and experiences of bullying or victimization. Questions about bullying and victimization have also been added to the interview protocols for parents and teachers. As was done in the first edition, this second edition also discusses the Semistructured Clinical Interview for Children and Adolescents (SCICA; McConaughy & Achenbach, 2001), which is a more comprehensive child clinical interview for assessing children's family relations as well as school and social functioning.

In my research and the creation of this book, I have benefited from the help and advice of many colleagues. I am grateful for the support of the late Kenneth W. Merrell, Founding Editor of The Guilford Practical Intervention in the Schools Series, who encouraged me to write both editions of this book. I, along with many in our field, mourn the loss of a valuable friend and colleague. I am grateful to Natalie Graham, Editor, at The Guilford Press, who provided editorial advice and support for this second edition, and to Guilford's editorial staff for their efforts in producing this work. I am also grateful to David Miller and William Halikias for their special chapters on assessment of suicide risk and risk for violence.

I thank my colleague Thomas Achenbach at the University of Vermont, who has been a friend and my closest collaborator in over three decades of research on empirically based assessment of children's emotional and behavioral problems. Our research to develop the SCICA provided the foundation for much of the theory and interviewing strategies described in this book. Our research efforts have been supported by the University of Vermont Research Center for Children, Youth, and Families (RCCYF); the National Institute of Child Health and Human Development; the National Institute of Mental Health; the National Institute on Disability and Rehabilitation Research (U.S. Department of Education); the Spencer Foundation; and the W. T. Grant Foundation. For their insightful comments on drafts of chapters for the first edition, I am grateful to Cynthia LaRiviere, Leslie Rescorla, James Tallmadge, and Robert Volpe. I am also grateful to Guilford's reviewers for their suggestions for this second edition. I thank Rachel Berubé at the RCCYF for her help in locating many of the resource materials for this book.

I am very grateful to the hundreds of children who shared their thoughts and feelings in clinical interviews, along with the many parents, teachers, guidance counselors, principals, and special educators who contributed to my research and clinical work. This book represents much of what I have learned from them as a researcher, clinician, and caring adult.

I have tried to write the text in a manner that makes theories and interviewing techniques easy to understand and apply. Research reviews in the chapters are intended to provide empirical bases for assessment and intervention planning. The appendices include reproducible forms for student, parent, and teacher interviews and other assessment protocols. I hope that this book will meet the needs of many practitioners, including school psychologists, child and adolescent clinical psychologists, child psychiatrists, social workers, guidance counselors, special educators, behavioral specialists, and other mental health practitioners who interact with children, parents, and school staff. Graduate students in training programs for the above fields should also find this book helpful for learning the complexities of clinical interviewing.

Contents

List of Figures, Tables, Boxes, and Appendices

FIGURES

TABLES

BOXES

APPENDICES

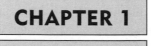

CHAPTER 1

Clinical Interviews in the Context of Multimethod Assessment

Clinical interviewing has long held a venerable position in psychological assessment. The importance of clinical interviews is reflected in the following quotes from several authors writing for clinical and school-based practitioners:

> Interviewing is a hallmark of assessment processes and perhaps the most common method used to obtain information to evaluate individuals. (Busse & Beaver, 2000, p. 235)

> Interviews are critical for obtaining information, appreciating children's unique perspectives, and establishing rapport. (La Greca, 1990, p. 4)

> Whether one is meeting informally with the teacher of a referred student, conducting a problem identification interview with a parent, or undertaking a diagnostic interview with a child or adolescent, interviewing is a widely used and valuable assessment method. (Merrell, 2008a, p. 133)

In a survey of American Psychological Association (APA) members, clinical interviews were ranked first as the most frequently used of 38 listed assessment procedures (Watkins, Campbell, Nieberding, & Hallmark, 1995). Ninety-three percent of the 412 respondents said that they "always" or "frequently" use clinical interviews, versus only 5% who "never" use them. The respondents to this survey included clinicians who work with adults and children. (For brevity, I use the term *children* to include adolescents, unless the focus of discussion is pertinent only to adolescents.) In a survey of the members of the National Association of School Psychologists (NASP), over 70% of 123 respondents reported that they used child, teacher .and parent interviews for behavioral–social–emotional assessments (Stinnett, Havey, & Oehler-Stinnett, 1994). The respondents reported using interviews more frequently than other procedures, including rating scales, self-report inventories, and projective techniques. They also ranked interviews and behavioral observations as more important than self-reports and projective techniques.

This book discusses clinical interviews with children, parents, and teachers for purposes of assessment and intervention planning. It is intended to be a practical guide and resource for school psychologists, child and adolescent clinical psychologists, school mental health and social workers, guidance counselors, special educators, school behavioral specialists, and trainees in those fields. Many of the interviewing formats and strategies discussed can also be employed by child psychiatrists and other mental health practitioners who evaluate and treat children outside of schools. Appendices for specific chapters provide reproducible interview forms and other relevant materials that practitioners can copy and use.

It is assumed that practitioners who use this book and its materials will have received appropriate professional training in clinical interviewing, as well as in the theory and methodology of standardized psychological assessment. Practitioners are also expected to adhere to the ethical codes of their professional associations, such as the APA, NASP, the American Psychiatric Association, the American Counseling Association (ACA), or the National Association of Social Workers (NASW).

This chapter lays the foundation for discussing clinical interviews in the context of a multimethod approach to assessment and intervention planning. The next section provides a brief historical perspective on clinical interviewing, followed by sections discussing the nature of clinical interviews and the working assumptions that underlie the use of clinical interviews as components of multimethod assessment. Subsequent chapters focus on specific techniques for conducting clinical interviews with children, parents, and teachers, as well as assessment procedures that can be used in conjunction with interviews.

HISTORICAL PERSPECTIVE ON CLINICAL INTERVIEWING

Clinical interviews can serve multiple educational and mental health purposes, including (1) providing initial clinical assessments of children's problems; (2) making psychiatric diagnoses; (3) designing school-based interventions and other mental health treatments; (4) evaluating the effectiveness of current services; and (5) screening for at-risk status, such as risk for suicide, risk for violence, or more general risk for emotional, behavioral, or learning problems (Sattler, 1998).

> **Clinical interviews are widely used for assessing children's problems and planning interventions.**

School psychologists, in particular, often conduct interviews with children, parents, and teachers as part of a comprehensive assessment to determine whether a child exhibits "emotional disturbance" (ED), as defined by the Individuals with Disabilities Education Act (1990, 1997, 2004; hereafter termed *IDEA* 2004). The information obtained from children, parents, and teachers in interviews can be particularly helpful for assessing ED, as well as for planning appropriate school interventions and mental health services for children with ED. Clinical psychologists and psychiatrists also rely heavily on clinical interviews with parents and children to make psychiatric diagnoses, as defined by the *Diagnostic and Statistical Manual of Mental Disorders, Fifth Edition* (DSM-5; American Psychiatric Association, 2013) and its precursor, the *Diagnostic and Statistical Manual of Mental Disorders, Fourth Edition, Text Revision* (DSM-IV-TR; American Psychiatric Association, 2000). Interviews with children, parents, and teachers are equally important in school-based behavioral assessment and problem-solving consultation for behavioral and academic problems (e.g., Beaver & Busse, 2000; Kratochwill, Elliott, & Callan-Stoiber, 2002; McConaughy & Ritter, in press; Shapiro, 2011; Sheridan, Kratochwill, & Bergan, 1996; Zins & Erchul, 2002).

Historically, clinical interviews have been a central feature of what has been termed *traditional assessment* of children's emotional and behavioral problems (Hughes & Baker, 1990; Kratochwill & Shapiro, 2000; Shapiro & Kratochwill, 2000). This term has been used to encompass diverse paradigms, including medical diagnostic, psychodynamic, psychometric, and personality assessments. Early contributors to behavioral assessment made clear distinctions between their approach and what they called *traditional assessment* (e.g., Hartmann, Roper, & Bradford, 1979). Traditional assessment was said to focus primarily on underlying states or personality traits in the individual as causes of behavior. Medical approaches also focused on physical states, diseases, or disorders in the individual as probable causes of behavior. By contrast, *behavioral assessment* focused on observable, discreet, problem behaviors and contingent events in the environment that reinforced and maintained those behaviors, without any assumptions about underlying causes in the individual, such as personality traits or disorders.

Traditional assessment has also been described as *nomothetic*, because it compared an individual's functioning with groups of other individuals (e.g., normative samples). Behavioral assessment, by contrast, was considered to be *idiographic*, because it focused on target behaviors of individuals without comparisons to other people or groups (Stanger, 2003; Shapiro & Kratochwill, 2000). Traditional approaches to assessment relied more heavily on clinical interviewing, self-report forms, and tests, whereas behavioral assessment relied on direct observation of current behaviors in naturalistic settings.

As behavioral assessment developed and matured, it began to broaden its focus and assumptions to encompass diverse methods. As a result, distinctions between traditional and behavioral assessment have become less clear-cut. In fact, as Stanger (2003) pointed out, "to contrast behavioral and traditional assessment approaches [now], one must necessarily create a false dichotomy between them" (p. 4). Instead, advocates of modern behavioral assessment argue that it is more helpful to consider methods of behavioral assessment along a continuum of direct to indirect approaches (Mash & Hunsley, 2007; Merrell, 2008a; Shapiro & Kratochwill, 2000; Stanger, 2003). Interviews and self-reports are considered more indirect methods of assessment because, presumably, interviewees report behaviors that have occurred in the past. Observations in naturalistic settings are considered more direct methods of assessment because they focus on current behaviors.

Within the context of modern behavioral assessment, clinical interviews are now valued as much as they have been valued in traditional assessment:

> "Behavioral assessment" is no longer synonymous with the direct observation of behavior; rather it refers to the use of multiple methods to assess a greatly expanded range of person and situation variables that empirical investigators have found to be important to the development, maintenance, and treatment of childhood disorders. . . . In such a broad-based assessment scheme, parent, child, and family interviews are essential components of the behavioral assessment of childhood disorders. (Hughes & Baker, 1990, p. 108)

Later chapters of this book present formats for conducting clinical interviews with children, parents, and teachers. These interviews combine aspects of traditional and behavioral forms of assessment in order to understand children's current functioning and to develop interventions, when needed. The interview topics include children's school functioning, social relations, family relations, home situation, and relevant developmental and educational history, as well as behavioral descriptions of children's current problems and competencies. The interview formats assume that practitioners will also use other assessment procedures, including tests, questionnaires, and standardized rating scales. Practitioners can use clinical interviews to obtain data that are not easily obtained by the other methods they plan to use. Interview formats are also tailored to the type of information that can best be provided by each particular informant: the child, the parent, and the teacher. The challenge for practitioners is to integrate interview data with other data to formulate a comprehensive picture of the child and to plan needed interventions.

THE NATURE OF CLINICAL INTERVIEWS

As we begin our discussion of clinical interviews, it is important to be clear about what they are and are not. Hughes and Baker (1990) defined clinical interviews with children as follows: "The child interview is a face-to-face interaction of bidirectional influence, entered into for the purpose of assessing aspects of the child's functioning that have relevance to planning, implementing, or evaluating treatment" (p. 4). This definition is a good one because it captures the basic elements of a clinical interview: a one-on-one interaction, with the dual goals of assessment and intervention planning. A similar definition can be applied to clinical interviews with parents and teachers. Merrell (2008a) also pointed out that the term *clinical* in this context refers to a purpose rather than a place. Clinical interviewing can be conducted in many different settings, including schools, clinics, hospitals, homes, and detention centers. Thus, Merrell stated, "The purpose reflected in the word *clinical* is to gather specific information regarding behavioral, social, and emotional functioning, particularly regarding deficits or problems in functioning that may be occurring in any of these places" (p. 134).

> A clinical interview involves face-to-face interaction between the interviewer and interviewee to gather information about a person's behavioral, social, and emotional functioning.

Clinical interviews, as defined above, are different from ordinary conversation. Whereas there are many linguistic parameters for good communication, ordinary conversation is usually a relatively informal, spontaneous verbal interchange between two people on some topic of mutual interest. As Sattler (1998) pointed out, clinical interviews differ from ordinary conversation in the following ways:

- The clinical interview usually takes place during a formally arranged meeting.
- The clinical interview has a specific purpose.
- The interviewer chooses the topics or broad content of the discussion.
- The interviewer and interviewee have a defined relationship—the interviewer asks questions, the interviewee responds to the questions.
- The interviewer keeps attuned to aspects of the interaction—the interviewee's affect, behavior, and style—as well as to the content of discussion.
- The interviewer uses questioning techniques and other strategies to direct the flow of conversation.
- The interviewer accepts the interviewee's expressions of feelings and factual information without casting judgment on them.
- The interviewer sometimes makes explicit what might be left unstated in ordinary conversation.
- The interviewer follows guidelines for confidentiality and disclosure of information.

Clinical interviews are also different from interviewing during psychotherapy. Sattler (1998) used the term *clinical assessment interview* to distinguish this type of interviewing from psychotherapeutic interviews. A major goal of clinical assessment interviews is to obtain information. The information is then used to evaluate an individual's emotional and behavioral functioning and to decide whether interventions are warranted, and if so, which types. The goals of psychotherapeutic interviews, by contrast, are usually to relieve emotional stress, foster insight, and promote changes in behavior or affect that can lead to improvements in an individual's life situation. This book focuses only on clinical assessment interviews, though some of the interview topics and strategies discussed may be equally applicable to psychotherapy situations.

Sattler (1998) also noted that the goals of clinical assessment interviews are different from those of forensic and survey interviews. Forensic interviews are designed to investigate specific questions about an individual or family and to provide expert opinions for a legal decision. Examples are forensic interviews for child custody disputes, termination of parental rights, and investigations of child abuse and neglect. Survey interviews are designed to collect data relevant to specific questions or variables of interest to a researcher. Examples are epidemiological surveys on the prevalence of different disorders or diseases. This book does not discuss forensic or survey interviews. Chapters 9 and 10 discuss clinical interviews that focus specifically on two special issues faced by school-based practitioners and mental health clinicians: assessing suicide risk (danger to self) and assessing potential for violence or threats of violence (danger to others). Interviews for evaluating child sexual and physical abuse are not covered in detail because these types of interviews are more typically conducted by professionals who specialize in social service or criminal investigations.

WORKING ASSUMPTIONS OF CLINICAL INTERVIEWS

When done well, clinical interviews can be rich sources of information about a child. However, in some forms of traditional assessment, interview data have been given more weight than data from other assessment methods. The sole use of structured diagnostic interviews for making psychiatric diagnoses is a good example of overreliance on interview data (McConaughy, 2000b, 2003). In early forms of behavioral assessment, the opposite was true: Direct observations were deemed more important than any other assessment method, including interviews (Shapiro & Kratochwill, 2000). With this history in mind, our discussion of clinical interviewing rests on several important working assumptions.

Need for Multiple Data Sources

The first assumption is: *There is no gold standard for assessing children's functioning.* Instead, it is assumed that comprehensive child assessment requires data from other sources in addition to interviews. Other data sources include direct observations in classrooms and other group situations, standardized parent and teacher rating scales, youth self-reports, background questionnaires, tests, and other procedures, as appropriate. Accordingly, it is helpful to keep in mind the following good advice from Shapiro and Kratochwill (2000):

> It is especially important to recognize that data collected from one method are not inherently better than data collected from others. That is, data obtained through an indirect method from

a parent (such as a rating scale) are not "less true" than data obtained by directly observing a student within a natural setting. Likewise, data collected through interviews with the student are not inherently more accurate than those collected through direct observation. . . . The key to good assessment is to find conceptual links and relationships between methods and modalities of assessment. Each form of behavioral assessment contributes unique elements to solving the assessment puzzle. (p. 13)

Situational Variability

A second assumption is: *Children's behavior is likely to vary across situations and relationships.* In behavioral assessment endeavors, it is assumed that environmental conditions influence children's behavior (Shapiro & Kratochwill, 2000; Stanger, 2003). Because environmental conditions can vary across situations, children's behavior is likely to vary from one situation to the next. Children's behavior is also likely to vary in the context of relationships with different adults, such as parents

> **Children's behavior often varies across situations and relationships with different people.**

versus teachers. Situational variations in behavior can lead to hypotheses about factors that maintain certain behaviors—for example, increased or decreased adult attention, presence or absence of peers, rewards or punishments (Stanger, 2003).

At the same time, certain patterns of children's behavior may remain consistent across different situations and relationships. Research has shown, for example, that aggressive behavior tends to be relatively stable across situations and over time (Achenbach & McConaughy, 1997; Stanger, Achenbach, & Verhulst, 1997). Good assessment requires identifying patterns of children's behavior that vary across situations and relationships as well as patterns that remain consistent, despite changes in situations and relationships.

Limited Cross-Informant Agreement

A third assumption is a corollary to the second: *There is likely to be only low-to-moderate agreement between informants who are in different situations or different relationships with the same child.* The limitation on agreement between different informants was demonstrated in meta-analytic study by Achenbach, McConaughy, and Howell (1987). Aggregating findings across 119 studies, Achenbach and colleagues found significant but modest correlations for ratings of children's behavior by different informants under different conditions. The results showed an average correlation of only .28 between ratings of children's behavior by parents versus teachers, parents

> **Research has demonstrated only low to moderate agreement between different types of informants regarding children's behavioral and emotional functioning.**

versus mental health workers, or teachers versus mental health workers. This low correlation contrasted with an average correlation of .60 between informants from similar situations or relationships with the child (e.g., pairs of parents, pairs of teachers, pairs of mental health workers, or two observers in the same situation).

Low agreement between informants does not mean that one is right and the other is wrong, or that one has a "truer" picture of a child than does the other. Parents may know more than teachers about many aspects of their child's functioning simply because parents spend more time with the child and they have a special, unique relationship with him/her. Still, teachers may know more than parents about other aspects of functioning, such as the child's approach to academic tasks or ability to relate to peers, because of the special circumstances of school versus home. Mental health professionals may also learn more than parents and teachers about certain aspects of functioning, such as the child's feelings, attitudes, and coping styles, because of the special circumstances surrounding assessment or therapy.

It is possible, of course, that a particular informant may be biased or may deliberately falsify reports for personal gain. Later chapters address this issue. However, when there is no evidence of prevarication or intentional misrepresentation in informants' reports, you should assume that *each different informant contributes valid information that represents one part of a bigger picture of the child*. Differences in people's perceptions of the child can be as informative as similarities in perceptions. Moreover, research has shown that qualitative differences in reports from different informants (e.g., child vs. parent) can provide important information for predicting children's responses to treatment and their behavioral outcomes over time (De Los Reyes, 2011). The challenge is to put all the different pieces of information together to form a meaningful picture of the child's functioning under the given circumstances. By examining similarities and differences in informants' perceptions, you can identify important clues to factors affecting the child's behavior in different situations and relationships. These clues, in turn, can lead to intervention strategies that are best suited to particular circumstances and relationships.

Variations in Interview Structure and Content

A fourth assumption is: *The structure and content of clinical interviews should vary in relation to the informant and the goals of the interview*. Later chapters in this book present formats for semistructured clinical interviews with children, parents, and teachers. As indicated above, each informant provides a unique perspective on the nature and circumstances affecting a child's functioning. By interviewing children, you can learn their views of their problems and competencies; their desires, fears, and coping strategies; and their reactions to the circumstances and relationships affecting their behavior. You can also directly observe children's behavior, affect, and coping strategies during the interview. By interviewing parents, you can learn their views about their child's problems and competencies, the child's developmental and medical history, family circumstances, and the parents' reactions to their child's behavior. Parent interviews can also provide clues about parents' own psychological functioning and coping strategies. By interviewing teachers, you can learn their views of a child's problems, competencies, and academic performance. You can also learn about teachers' instructional strategies, school interventions for academic and behavioral problems, and forms of special help or services that have been provided.

INTERVIEW CONTENT AND QUESTIONING STRATEGIES

Clinical interviews need to be tailored to particular informants. Accordingly, the content and questioning strategies should be shaped by the kind of informant to be interviewed and the kind of information sought, as outlined in Table 1.1. Later chapters discuss interview content and questioning strategies in detail for each kind of informant. As Table 1.1 shows, the clinical interviews presented in this book combine aspects of traditional and behavioral interviewing techniques. Inter-

TABLE 1.1. Content and Questioning Strategies for Child, Parent, and Teacher Interviews

Questioning strategies	Informant and interview content		
	Child interview	Parent interview	Teacher interview
Semistructured questions	Activities and interests School and homework Friendships and peer relations Home situation and family relations Self-awareness and feelings Adolescent issues	Social functioning School functioning Medical and developmental history Family relations and home situation Child's strengths and interests	Academic performance Teaching strategies Child's strengths and interests
Structured questions		Symptoms and criteria for psychiatric disorders	
Behavior-specific questions	Child's view of problems	Concerns about the child Behavioral and emotional problems	Concerns about the child School behavior problems
Problem-solving questions	Feasibility of interventions	Feasibility of interventions Initial goals and plans	Feasibility of school interventions Special help/services Initial goals and plans

viewers can use *semistructured questions* to query children, parents, and teachers about many different aspects of children's functioning, including children's activities and interests, school and social functioning, and family relations. If parents have completed questionnaires about their child's

> **Semistructured questions are open-ended and flexible to simulate a natural flow of conversation.**

developmental and medical history prior to the interview, interviewers can examine that information and then ask questions about aspects of the child's history that are likely to affect current behavior. The format of semistructured questions is relatively open-ended and flexible to simulate a natural flow of conversation. Semistructured questions generally do not elicit "yes" or "no" answers, but instead encourage interviewees to express their views, opinions, and feelings about specific topics. *Probe questions* can then be used to obtain more detailed information.

Structured questions are appropriate for querying parents about symptoms and criteria for psychiatric disorders. Structured diagnostic interviews have a standardized set of questions and probes focusing on specific problems relevant for diagnoses. Several structured diagnostic interviews have been developed for research and mental health assessments. An example is the National Institute of Mental Health's Diagnostic Interview Schedule for Children—Version IV (NIMH DISC-IV; Shaffer, Fisher, Lucas, Dulcan, & Schwab-Stone, 2000). The DISC-IV (and most other structured diagnostic interviews) have formats for parents and older children. Few have formats for interviewing teachers.

Because of their length and detail, structured diagnostic interviews are usually not feasible for school-based assessments or even many clinic-based assessments. However, school practitioners and mental health clinicians may still want to use structured questions with parents to determine whether a child meets criteria for certain common psychiatric diagnoses. One example is attention-deficit/hyperactivity disorder (ADHD), which can provide support for special education services under IDEA 2004, or for classroom accommodations through a Section 504 plan under the Rehabilitation Act of 1973 (Rehabilitation Act, 1973). Many children with ADHD are treated by pediatricians, child psychiatrists, and mental health practitioners outside of school. Children with diagnoses of depression or anxiety can also benefit from school-based interventions as well as mental health treatment (Merrell, 2008b).

Interviewers can use *behavior-specific questions* to query parents and teachers regarding their current concerns about the child. These questions are narrower in scope than semistructured questions because the focus is on a limited number of specific problem areas (Beaver & Busse, 2000). Behavior-specific questions comprise the initial phases of behavioral assessment and consultation, wherein the main purposes are (1) to identify and define problems of concern to parents and teachers (problem identification), and (2) to examine antecedents and consequences that surround the identified problems (problem analysis). Interviewers can also use behavior-specific questions to query children about their views of particular problems and their understanding of the circumstances around the problems.

> **Behavior-specific questions focus on a limited number of specific problems and are narrower than semistructured questions.**

Problem-solving questions focus on parents' and teachers' current concerns, with the goal of developing interventions for identified problems (Beaver & Busse, 2000). In behavioral consultation, problem-solving questions usually comprise later stages of plan implementation and evaluation. However, in initial clinical interviews, practitioners can use problem-solving questions to explore and gauge parents' and teachers' receptivity to different

> **Problem-solving questions focus on current concerns and possible interventions for identified problems.**

kinds of interventions prior to implementing any interventions. For example, some parents or teachers may have negative feelings about certain types of interventions (e.g., medication treatments or structured behavior contracts), but may be willing to try other alternatives. Interviewers can also use problem-solving questions to explore children's views of different interventions and to find out which approaches are acceptable or not acceptable to them.

INTERVIEWS AS COMPONENTS OF MULTIMETHOD ASSESSMENT

The working assumptions discussed in the previous section bring us to the following conclusion: *Interviews are best viewed as components of a multimethod approach to assessment of children's functioning.* Many authors have stressed the importance of multimethod assessment of children (e.g., Achenbach & McConaughy, 1997; Kratochwill & Shapiro, 2000; Mash & Hunsley, 2007; Merrell, 2008a; McConaughy & Ritter, in press; Sattler, 1998; Shapiro & Kratochwill, 2000; Stanger, 2003). However, the need for multiple data sources cannot be overstated. Interviews, like other assessment procedures, have their advantages and disadvantages. Advantages include flexibility, opportunity to observe the interviewee under structured conditions, and opportunity to establish rapport and trust toward creating a therapeutic alliance (Merrell, 2008a). By interviewing children, parents, and teachers, practitioners can also explore details of children's problems and circumstances from different points of view.

One disadvantage is that the flexibility of interviews also makes them vulnerable to low reliability and inconsistencies or misinformation across informants (Merrell, 2008a). For example, children may not report certain types of behavior, such as attention problems or aggressive behavior. Instead of using child interviews to assess the presence of these types of problems, it might be better to rely more on parent and teacher interviews, standardized parent and teacher rating scales, and direct observations. Another disadvantage is that interviews require more time than other assessment procedures. For example, parent and teacher interviews may not be as efficient, or as reliable, as standardized rating scales for assessing a wide range of potential problems. Parent and teacher interviews are also less efficient than questionnaires for obtaining details of a child's medical, developmental, and educational history. By contrast, parent and teacher interviews are good for clarifying concerns about specific current problems and for learning how parents and teachers react to identified problems. Parent and teacher interviews can also provide insights into children's strengths and competencies and the feasibility of different intervention options.

To reap the benefits of clinical interviews while avoiding their disadvantages, practitioners are encouraged to combine interviews routinely with other assessment procedures (Mash & Hunsley, 2007; McConaughy, 2000a, 2000b, 2003). To illustrate such a multimethod approach, Table 1.2

> In multimethod assessment, clinical interviews are used with other assessment methods, including questionnaires, standardized tests, rating scales, self-report scales, and/or direct observations.

outlines examples of data sources for five different assessment axes described by Achenbach and McConaughy (1997): I. parent reports; II. teacher reports; III. cognitive assessment; IV. physical assessment; and V. direct assessment of the child. Axes I and II include parent and teacher interviews, along with standardized rating scales, background questionnaires, and historical and educational records. Axis V includes the child clinical interview, along with standardized self-reports, direct observations in settings such as classrooms and playgrounds, standardized personality tests, and other direct assessment procedures. Axis III covers cognitive assessment, including standardized ability and intelligence tests, standardized achievement tests, curriculum-based assessment, and tests of perceptual–motor skills and speech and language. Observations during test sessions are also important Axis III data sources. Axis IV covers aspects of physical assessment, such as medical and neurological exams, illnesses, injuries, disabilities, hospitalizations, and medications. For comprehensive assessment, information relevant to all five axes in Table 1.2 should be considered. However, you may not need to obtain data from all five axes for all children.

The Achenbach System of Empirically Based Assessment (ASEBA) is an example of a family of standardized instruments specifically designed to fit the multimethod model outlined in Table 1.2. For school-age children, the ASEBA includes the Child Behavior Checklist for Ages 6–18 (CBCL/6–18) for obtaining parents' ratings of their children's competencies and problems; the Teacher's Report Form (TRF) for obtaining teachers' ratings of academic performance, adaptive functioning, and school problems; and the Youth Self-Report (YSR) for obtaining youth self-ratings of competencies and problems (Achenbach & Rescorla, 2001). The ASEBA also includes the Semistructured Clinical Interview for Children and Adolescents (SCICA; McConaughy & Achenbach, 2001) for interviewing children ages 6–18; the Test Observation Form (TOF; McConaughy & Achenbach, 2004b) for obtaining test examiners' ratings of children's problems during test sessions; and the Direct Observation Form (DOF; McConaughy & Achenbach, 2009) for conducting obser-

TABLE 1.2. Data Sources for Multimethod Assessment

I. Parent reports	II. Teacher reports	III. Cognitive assessment	IV. Physical assessment	V. Direct assessment of the child
Parent interview	Teacher interview	Standardized ability and intelligence tests	Medical exams	Child clinical interview
Standardized parent rating scales	Standardized teacher rating scales	Standardized achievement tests	Neurological exams	Observations during child clinical interview
Background questionnaires	Background questionnaires	Observations during test sessions	Illnesses, injuries, and disabilities	Standardized self-reports
Historical records	Educational records	Curriculum-based assessment	Hospitalizations	Direct observations in classroom, playground, and other settings
		Perceptual–motor tests	Medications	Personality tests
		Speech and language tests		

vations of children in school classrooms, playgrounds, and other group settings. Other ASEBA instruments are designed for preschool children (Achenbach & Rescorla, 2000), adults ages 18–59 (Achenbach & Rescorla, 2003), and older adults ages 60–90+ (Achenbach, Newhouse, & Rescorla, 2004).

The Behavior Assessment System for Children—Second Edition (BASC-2; Reynolds & Kamphaus, 2004) is another example of a family of standardized instruments for multimethod assessment of school-age children and college students. The BASC-2 includes instruments for obtaining parent and teacher ratings of children's problems and adaptive skills, youth self-reports, and structured observations in school settings. It also provides a structured questionnaire for obtaining parents' reports of children's developmental histories. Subsequent chapters discuss how practitioners can conduct child, parent, and teacher clinical interviews in ways that dovetail with other data sources so as to maximize the best of what interviews have to offer.

CASE EXAMPLES

Throughout this book we visit and revisit case examples that illustrate the kind of information that can be derived from clinical interviews with children, parents, and teachers. As indicated in the preface, the cases are based on research and clinical experience with many children. The names of the children, parents, and teachers are all pseudonyms and details of the case material have been altered to protect confidentiality. The following synopses introduce five of these cases.

Andy Lockwood, Age 7

Andy Lockwood was repeating first grade because of social immaturity and below-grade-level academic performance. His previous first-grade teacher had complained that he was boisterous and noisy and took forever to get anything done. At the end of that year, Andy was far behind other children in basic reading and math skills. Andy's current first-grade teacher voiced similar concerns. She said he was disruptive in class, failed to complete assigned work, and was still achieving far below other children in her class. Andy's mother agreed that he was an active child, but thought that he was typical of boys his age. She suspected that the teachers did not like Andy and were too rigid in their expectations about behavior. Ms. Lockwood also questioned whether Andy understood directions for assignments, because her attempts to help him with homework often led to tears and arguments. After several phone calls from the current teacher, Andy's mother started to worry that his second year in first grade would be no better than his first year. So she agreed to an evaluation of his learning, behavioral, and emotional functioning. The evaluation was carried out by the school psychologist and special education staff.

Bruce Garcia, Age 9

Bruce Garcia had been receiving speech and language services since age 4. When he was in third grade, the school multidisciplinary team requested a psychological evaluation as part of his 3-year reevaluation. Bruce's teacher complained that his school performance was erratic, and he seemed disorganized and confused. She also worried that Bruce had trouble fitting into peer groups because of his "odd" behavior. Bruce's mother was concerned that he seemed socially withdrawn at home and had difficulty paying attention to schoolwork. Bruce's school district had a contract with a nearby psychiatric outpatient clinic for school-based mental health and consultation services. The school multidisciplinary team referred Bruce to the clinic for a psychological evaluation of his social–emotional functioning and cognitive ability.

Catherine Holcomb, Age 11

Catherine was the younger of two children living with her mother. Catherine's father had died when she was 7 years old, and her mother had not remarried. Catherine's fifth-grade teacher was concerned because she seemed inattentive in class, was erratic in completing assignments, and was having difficulty in reading and written work. Catherine also seemed socially withdrawn and had few friends in school. Catherine's teacher voiced her concerns to Ms. Holcomb and the school psychologist. Ms. Holcomb then agreed to a school-based evaluation to assess Catherine's emotional functioning and to check for possible learning disabilities.

Karl Bryant, Age 12

Karl's sixth-grade teacher referred him for an evaluation because of behavior problems in school. She reported that Karl got into fights, had problems getting along with other students, and frequently violated school rules. Because Karl did not complete assignments, he was failing in several subjects. With permission from Karl's mother, the school multidisciplinary team conducted an evaluation to determine whether Karl qualified for special education services due to a learning disability and/or emotional disturbance. Karl's mother also wanted advice on how to manage his behavior at home.

Kelsey Watson, Age 14

Kelsey was in the custody of the state social service agency due to unmanageable behavior at home and episodes of running away. She lived in a residential group home and was enrolled in eighth grade in the local school district. She continued to have occasional home visits with her mother, who lived in a different town. Despite a history of behavioral and emotional problems and under-achievement, Kelsey had never received any special services in school. Therefore, the multidisci-plinary team in her new school referred her for a psychoeducational evaluation to determine if she were eligible for services. They also wanted recommendations for coping with potential behavior problems at school.

In each of the above cases, clinical interviews were conducted with the child, the child's parents or guardians and teachers. Parents or guardians, and teachers completed standardized rating scales to proved normative assessments of the child's competencies and behavioral and emotional problems. Catherine, Karl, and Kelsey completed standardized self-reports of their competencies and behavioral and emotional functioning. Standardized tests of cognitive ability, achievement, speech/language, and perceptual–motor functioning were also administered, as needed.

STRUCTURE OF THIS BOOK

After we discuss interviewing strategies in Chapter 2, you will learn more about each of the five case examples in subsequent chapters. Chapters 3, 4, and 5 discuss topics covered in child clinical interviews. These chapters include segments of clinical interviews with one or more of the children in the case examples. An appendix for Chapter 3 provides a reproducible protocol for a Semistruc-tured Student Interview (McConaughy, 2012). The interview protocol is modeled on the SCICA, but limited to topics most relevant for evaluations of children's academic and social functioning in schools. Chapter 6 discusses parent interviews; appendices for Chapter 6 provide a reproduc-ible protocol for a Semistructured Parent Interview (McConaughy, 2004a) plus a reproducible background questionnaire concerning the child's developmental history and family circumstances. Chapter 7 discusses teacher interviews, with an appendix that provides a reproducible protocol for a Semistructured Teacher Interview (McConaughy, 2004b). Chapter 8 discusses interpretations of clinical interviews for intervention planning, returning to the five case examples to illustrate how you can integrate interview data with other assessment data to develop intervention plans.

Chapters 9 and 10 address two special issues for clinical interviewing. In Chapter 9, David Miller describes procedures for assessing risk for suicide (danger to self). In Chapter 10, William Halikias describes school-based risk assessments of violence or threats of violence (danger to oth-ers). As scholars and licensed practicing psychologists, Drs. Miller and Halikias both have special expertise in their respective topic areas.

CHAPTER 2

Strategies for Child Clinical Interviews

As indicated in Chapter 1, most experts agree that interviewing the child is an essential component of multimethod clinical assessment (e.g., Merrell, 2008a; Sattler, 1998; Hughes & Baker, 1990). This chapter discusses strategies for conducting child clinical interviews, with an emphasis on the use of semistructured interviewing. Interviewers can use semistructured questions to cover a wide variety of topics, while adapting questioning strategies to fit children's developmental levels and interaction styles. Interviewers can also use behavior-specific questions to assess children's understanding of antecedents and consequences of specific problems, as well as problem-solving questions to explore children's views of potential interventions.

PURPOSES OF CHILD CLINICAL INTERVIEWS

Within the context of multimethod assessment, child clinical interviews are especially useful for the following purposes:

- To establish rapport and mutual respect between the interviewer and the child.
- To learn the child's perspective on his/her functioning.
- To identify which of the child's current problems would be appropriate targets for interventions.
- To identify the child's strengths and competencies that can be marshaled to bolster interventions.
- To assess the child's view of different intervention options.
- To directly observe the child's behavior, affect, and interaction style.

Although clinical interviews differ from ordinary conversations, you can still use strategies that make interviews seem more conversational and comfortable for interviewees. For example, you can ask questions in ways that encourage interviewees to express their opinions and feelings without fear of negative reactions or challenges to their viewpoints. You can also pace the flow of questions and answers in ways that encourage more talk from the interviewee than from the interviewer. These strategies are especially important when interviewing children. Many children will shut down if they feel they are being interrogated or lectured. Children can also lose interest if they have to listen more than talk and if the interview feels like a drill session or fact-finding investigation. Using professional jargon can also undermine your clinical interviews, because children may not understand it.

Good clinical interviewing requires focusing on key areas of concern, while also remaining sensitive to interviewees' reactions to the interview process. As Sattler (1998) stated, "Clinical assessment interviewing . . . even more than other assessment techniques . . . places a premium on your personal skills, such as your ability to communicate effectively and your ability to establish a meaningful relationship" (p. 3). At first, clinical interviewing may seem more like a mysterious art than an acquired skill. As Merrell (2008a) pointed out, the popular media and public beliefs have fostered distorted impressions of the power of mental health clinicians and clinical interviewing. As an example, Merrell cited the frequent experience in which complete strangers suspect that psychologists or psychiatrists are "analyzing" them or reading their minds when they are simply making ordinary conversation. Although clinical interviewing is not, as Merrell noted, "a mystical conduit to the inner life of the person being interviewed," you can use various interviewing strategies to facilitate good communication and assessment.

The guidelines in this chapter draw from other authors who have discussed techniques for interviewing children (Garbarino & Scott, 1989; Hughes & Baker, 1990; La Greca, 1990; Merrell, 2008a, 2008b; Sattler, 1998), as well as from my own work (McConaughy, 2000a, 2000b, 2003; McConaughy & Achenbach, 1994, 2001). The first sections are devoted to general issues concerning the setting, interviewer appearance, and limits of confidentiality. The next sections discuss considerations and questioning strategies for interviewing children at three broad developmental levels. Although it is beyond the scope of this book to provide in-depth discussions of children's cognitive and social–emotional development, these latter sections highlight key issues relevant to conducting developmentally sensitive clinical interviews. Additional sections cover strategies for alternating verbal and nonverbal communication, dealing with lying, and concluding the interview. Another section is devoted to special considerations for interviewing culturally and linguistically diverse children and parents.

SETTING AND INTERVIEWER APPEARANCE

Child clinical interviews should be conducted in a private location with only the child and interviewer present, unless there is a good reason for another person to be there. Finding an appropriate space can sometimes be a challenge for school-based practitioners who do not have their own offices. Nevertheless, it is important to insist on a place that affords privacy and comfort for the interviewer and interviewee.

Before interviewing young children, or overactive or aggressive children, take time to childproof the room by clearing desks and tables of loose items that are not needed for the interview, as well as potentially risky items, such as letter openers, scissors, pins, and electric pencil sharpeners. Toys and other props for the interview should be kept out of sight or out of reach until they are needed. It is also good to remove family pictures and personal mementos because they may distract children who are curious about the interviewer's personal life.

If possible, the room should have a relaxed, neutral atmosphere, with comfortable chairs and a table. Children under age 6 may be more comfortable sitting on cushions or mats on the floor, with the interviewer more or less on the same level. Older children can usually sit in a comfortable chair for their size, with the interviewer sitting in a similar chair. As a general rule, avoid sitting behind a desk or table across from the child, because this arrangement makes the interviewer look too much like an authority figure and creates a test-like atmosphere. Instead, you can sit at a diagonal corner of a table near the child. This arrangement allows you to take notes easily, while not creating a barrier between you and the child. The child can also use the table for writing or drawing, and can leave the chair occasionally, if needed. Adolescents should also be interviewed in a relaxed, neutral setting—preferably one without a childish decor. Whenever possible, avoid conducting child clinical interviews in offices of authority figures, such as the principal's office, or in spaces where disciplinary procedures are carried out, such as detention or time-out rooms.

Interviewers also need to be mindful of how their personal appearance may affect rapport with children. As a general rule, dress in professional attire congruent with community standards and the local environment. Dressing too casually may create the false impression that the interview is to be a play session or an informal conversation. Very casual dress can also undermine your "professional authority" to ask sensitive questions. On the other hand, if you dress in very formal business-type attire, children might view you as unapproachable or too stiff. In clinic settings, avoid wearing a white coat or other attire that makes you look like a medical doctor, because this can raise fears in children. If you use the term *doctor* in your title, tell young children that you are a "talking doctor" and that you do not give shots. In some special circumstances, it might be good to match the gender of the interviewer and the child to facilitate communication—for example, when interviewing children about sexual abuse or sexual orientation.

DISCUSSING PURPOSE AND CONFIDENTIALITY WITH CHILDREN

After personal introductions, explain the purpose of the interview and the limits of confidentiality. A good way to start is to ask children why they think they are being interviewed. Young children may have been told that they are going to play games. Other children may think that they are going to be tested. Some older children may think that they are being interviewed because certain adults think that they are crazy or stupid. Others may think that they will be punished for some wrongdoing. It is important to clear up any such misconceptions at the beginning of the interview.

Begin the child interview by explaining its purpose and the limits of confidentiality in a succinct and friendly manner.

Next, explain the limits of confidentiality in a clear and succinct manner, using language appropriate for the child's developmental level. An example is the following standard introduction to the SCICA (McConaughy & Achenbach, 2001):

"We are going to spend some time talking and doing things together, so that I can get to know you and learn about what you like and don't like. This is a private talk. I won't tell your parents or your teachers what you say unless you tell me it is OK. The only thing I would have to tell is if you said you were going to hurt yourself, hurt someone else, or someone has hurt you." (p. 1)

The SCICA introduction clearly states the standard limits of confidentiality in language that most children should understand. In particular, the child needs to understand that confidentiality may be breached if you suspect that he/she may be a danger to him/herself or a danger to others, or if you suspect that the child has been abused or is in danger of being abused. After such an introduction, you can ask the child if he/she understood what you said or has any questions. You should also inform the child of other circumstances that might limit guarantees of strict confidentiality. For example, inform the child of follow-up discussions that will occur with parents and/or teachers, or written reports that will include interview information. To alleviate concerns about reports to other parties, you can tell the child that at the end of the interview, you will talk with him/her about what to say to other people. For example, you might say:

"I am going to write a report about what I learn in our talk today. I will also be meeting with your parents and teachers on another day to talk about what I learned about you. At the end of this talk, we can discuss what I will say and how to say it. Do you understand?"

Sometimes you may want to tape-record the interview. When this is the case, you can say, "We are going to record our talk on this tape recorder to help remember our time together." The audiotape should be stored in a safe location and erased after you have finished your written reports or have finished your clinical work with the child. Keep all introductory remarks, including reviews of confidentiality issues, as nontechnical and brief as possible. At the end of the interview, you can summarize key issues and talk about what will be disclosed to others, as discussed in a later section.

DEVELOPMENTAL CONSIDERATIONS
FOR CHILD INTERVIEWS

Good clinical interviews with children require sensitivity to their communication skills and their levels of cognitive and social–emotional development. Although many interview topics may be appropriate for children of all ages, interviewers will still need to adapt their style of questioning to fit the child's developmental level. Table 2.1 presents some basic considerations for interviewing children who are 3–5 years old (early childhood), 6–11 years old (middle childhood), and 12–18 years old (adolescence). These ages approximate broad developmental levels. Appropriate adjustments are also needed for children who are below or above the average range of cognitive functioning. Table 2.1 outlines aspects of cognitive functioning, social–emotional functioning, and peer interactions that you can consider when framing questions and interpreting responses for children at each developmental level.

Table 2.2 outlines general "dos" and "don'ts" for interviewing children at each of the three developmental levels summarized in Table 2.1. Table 2.2 is organized in a hierarchical fashion, such that interviewing strategies listed for one level of development may also be appropriate for the next higher level of development. For example, open-ended questions can be used with children in early childhood as well as middle childhood and adolescence. Following the child's lead in the conversation is a good strategy for all ages. The next sections discuss these developmental considerations and interviewing strategies in more detail.

TABLE 2.1. Developmental Considerations for Interviewing Children

Period	Cognitive functioning	Social–emotional functioning	Typical peer interactions
Early childhood (ages 3–5)	Focus on only one feature at a time (preoperational stage) Easily confused between appearance and reality Difficulty recalling specific information accurately (limited memory development) Difficulty sustaining conversation	Difficulty understanding the viewpoint of another person (egocentric) Right or wrong based on consequences (preconventional moral reasoning) Limited verbal ability to describe emotions Can sustain a play task Can engage in reciprocal play sequences	Shared play activities Fantasy play Short interactions Frequent squabbles Unstable friendships Rough-and-tumble play Aggressive peers are generally disliked Reciprocal peers are generally liked
Middle childhood (ages 6–11)	Able to reason logically about tangible objects and actual events (concrete operations stage) Increased capacity for verbal communication	Can think about what another person is thinking (recursive thinking) Right or wrong based on rules and social conventions (conventional moral reasoning) Understands and complies with rules of a game Develops a sense of self-competence Can regulate affect in competition	Structured board games, group games, and team sports with complex rules Squabbles about rules Stable best friendships, usually with same-sex peers Aggressive or socially withdrawn peers are generally disliked Friendly, helpful, and supportive peers are liked Peer status defined by classroom group or structured activities
Adolescence (ages 12–18)	Able to reason abstractly and hypothetically (formal operations stage) Can engage in systematic problem solving Additional increases in verbal communication	Can take a third-person point of view (thinking about thinking) Right or wrong based on individual principles of conscience or ideals (postconventional moral reasoning) Identity confusion and experimentation High emotional intensity and lability Social awareness and self-consciousness Peer group acceptance extremely important	"Hanging out" and communicating with peers (e.g., talking, sending notes, phone calls, e-mail) Intimate self-disclosure, especially for girls Squabbles about relationship issues (e.g., gossip, secrets, loyalty issues) Romantic partners Aggressive and antisocial peers are generally disliked Cooperative, helpful, and competent peers are generally liked Peer status defined by norms for various groups, cliques, or clubs

Note. Adapted from Merrell (2008a). Copyright 2008 by Lawrence Erlbaum Associates. Adapted by permission.

TABLE 2.2. Developmentally Sensitive Interviewing Strategies

Period	Interviewing dos	Interviewing don'ts
Early childhood (ages 3–5)	Sit at the child's level (e.g., on a mat on the floor or a small chair) Limit the length and complexity of questions Use open-ended questions about specific and familiar situations Use toys, props, and manipulatives Use the child's terms and phrases Use people's names instead of pronouns Use extenders to encourage more child talk Allow ample time for the child to respond	Do not attempt to maintain total control of the interview Avoid embedded phrases or clauses Avoid questions that can be answered "yes" or "no" Do not follow every response with another question
Middle childhood (ages 6–11)	Take time to establish rapport Listen with empathy Solicit and restate feelings Follow the child's lead in conversation Use open-ended questions and probes Sometimes provide multiple-choice options as probes Talk about familiar settings and activities Provide contextual cues (e.g., pictures, verbal examples) Rephrase or simplify questions when the child has misunderstood or not responded Use direct requests to transition to new topics or tasks	Refrain from making judgmental comments Avoid too many factual questions Avoid too much direct questioning Avoid constant eye contact Avoid abstract questions Avoid questions with obvious right or wrong answers Avoid rhetorical questions Avoid "why" questions about motives
Adolescence (ages 12–18)	Be clear about limits of confidentiality Show respect Solicit and listen to adolescents' points of view and feelings Be prepared for emotional lability and stress Ask for possible alternative ways to solve a problem Pursue any indications of suicidal risk	Avoid psychological terms Avoid making judgments based solely on adult norms

Note. Adapted from McConaughy and Achenbach (1994). Copyright 1994 by Stephanie H. McConaughy and Thomas M. Achenbach. Adapted by permission.

Developmental Characteristics of Early Childhood

Young children can be particularly difficult to interview because of their limited communication and cognitive skills, as summarized in the second column of Table 2.1. Piaget and other developmental psychologists have characterized early childhood as "preoperational" because 3- to 5-year-olds lack the ability to perform the logical operations of the next stage (Ginsburg & Opper, 1969). Children in the preoperational stage tend to focus on only one feature or attribute of an object or situation, and they are easily confused by distinctions between appearance and reality. Puppets and cartoon characters can facilitate communication with young children. An example is the request of one 3-year-old girl to her father: "Daddy, put Beaver on your hand, and he will talk." When her father brought out the puppet, she engaged in a lively conversation with Beaver. Puppets can be especially useful when interviewing young children about social problems and potential abuse. Because of their limited memory skills, young children also have difficulty recalling specific information accurately, and may provide incomplete accounts of past events. They also have difficulty sustaining long conversations.

In terms of social–emotional functioning, summarized in the third column of Table 2.1, 3- to 5-year-olds tend to be "egocentric" because they have difficulty understanding another person's point of view or taking the perspective of another person. Egocentrism is also a classic characteristic of children with autism. Because of their difficulty understanding other people's perspectives, it is often not useful to ask young children how they think the other person felt in a problem situation or what the other person might have been thinking. Instead, it is better to ask more specific questions about what happened and how they felt themselves. It is also important to realize that, although young children experience a range of emotions, they have difficulty verbally describing their feelings, except along broad dimensions, such as happy, sad, and mad.

Young children's views of right and wrong are generally based on the consequences of their actions, which Kohlberg (1976) characterized as a "preconventional" level of moral reasoning. For example, "pushing or hitting someone is wrong because you get sent to the time-out chair." That is, an action is wrong because you get punished or scolded. In social interactions, most 3- to 5-year-olds have advanced beyond parallel play and can engage in reciprocal play sequences that involve give-and-take with other children. However, they tend to stay in one activity for only short periods of time before moving on to something else.

The last column of Table 2.1 summarizes peer interactions that are typical for early childhood (based on a review by Bierman & Welsh, 1997). These developmental characteristics are important to keep in mind when interviewing children about peer relations and friendships, as discussed in Chapter 3. Three- to 5-year-old children generally enjoy shared play activities and fantasy games. Their play often mimics familiar adult activities (e.g., playing house, playing school) or involves fantasy play with toys (e.g., cars and trucks, dolls) or shared physical activities (e.g., riding bikes, playing on the beach, running and chasing). Because young children are just beginning to learn to coordinate social behavior, peer interactions are of short duration and involve frequent squabbles and friendships that come and go. Rough-and-tumble play is typical, especially for boys, which can result in squabbles. Peers who are consistently aggressive are generally disliked, whereas peers who share, exhibit positive affect, and have an agreeable disposition are generally liked.

Questioning Strategies for Early Childhood

Interviewers can accommodate young children's developmental level in various ways, as listed as "Interviewing dos" in the top section of Table 2.2. As noted earlier, sitting at the same level can help young children feel more comfortable in clinical interviews. To facilitate communication, limit the length and complexity of your questions and comments. Garbarino and Scott (1989) suggested limiting questions to only three to five words more than the length of the child's usual sentence. This is a good rule of thumb for interviewing children of all ages, but especially young children. That is, always try to reduce the amount of "interviewer talk" in favor of increasing the amount of "child talk."

> With young children, use open-ended questions and limit your questions and comments to no more than five words more than child's usual sentence.

As another general rule, try to use open-ended questions that do not require a "yes" or "no" answer. For young children, open-ended questions should focus on concrete, familiar activities and situations. For example: "What do you like best about going to [name of preschool]?"; "What don't you like about [name of preschool]?" Using props, toys, and manipulatives (especially puppets) can also provide concrete ways for children to demonstrate actions or feelings, or to act out a situation, along with giving verbal descriptions. Using children's own terms and phrases and people's names (not pronouns) can help to tailor interview questions to children's level of understanding. Examples include using children's words for body parts, children's names for friends and family members, and using children's terms for rules and punishments at home. Frequent use of extenders ("Oh," "Um," "OK," and "I understand") will let children know you understand them and thereby encourage more conversation. Avoid long questions or sentences with embedded phrases or clauses. Do not follow every response with another question, because this will make the interview seem too much like a test or interrogation. Be tolerant of silences and pauses that allow children time to think of what they want to say. Too often, adults jump in with more questions or comments whenever children stop talking, which can easily cause them to shut down.

Developmental Characteristics of Middle Childhood

As children move into middle childhood, their communicative competence, cognitive skills, and social–emotional functioning advance markedly. These advances can greatly enhance their ability to participate in child clinical interviews. In terms of cognitive functioning (Table 2.1, second column), children enter Piaget's "concrete operational" stage at about ages 6–7 and continue in that stage until about ages 11–12. In the concrete operational stage, children can apply simple logic to tangible objects and actual event sequences. Developmental psychologists have described a variety of logical skills that come "online" during this period. For example, 6- to 11-year-old children are able to focus on more than one attribute of an object at the same time, such as height and width (decentration). They understand that changing the appearance of a set of objects, such as a stack of 10 blocks, does not change the quantity (conservation). They have a concrete understanding of the reverse relationship of simple operations, such as addition (2 + 2 = 4) and subtraction (4 − 2 = 2) (reversibility). Elementary teachers often capitalize on these concrete reasoning skills by using manipulatives to teach abstract concepts. An example is using graduated colored rods to teach math concepts. Middle childhood also is a time of rapid advances in vocabulary and ability to communicate with peers and adults.

In terms of social–emotional functioning (Table 2.1, third column), middle childhood is the time when most children master "recursive thinking." This type of cognition involves the ability to imagine what another person might be thinking ("I like him, and I think he likes me"). This is an important social–cognitive skill because it allows children to consider another person's perspective in a social interaction—to put themselves in the other person's shoes, so to speak. Children in this stage not only can understand and answer questions about how they think or feel in certain situations, but also how others might think or feel.

Six- to 11-year-olds' views of right and wrong are generally based on rules and social conventions, which Kohlberg (1976) characterized as a "conventional" level of moral reasoning. For example, "Fighting on the playground is wrong because it is against school rules." Children at this level of moral reasoning often have "black-and-white" views of rules as absolute principles with no exceptions. This absolutist viewpoint can often lead to arguments with peers or authority figures about whether the rules were broken or whether certain rules apply in specific situations. In fact, some children adopt a very righteous attitude about rules at home and school and have great concerns about whether they and others are treated fairly according to those rules. Children's understanding of, and compliance with, rules are also prerequisites for their participation in structured games and sports.

Middle childhood is a time when children develop a clearer sense of self-competency in several arenas, including academic skills, athletics, and social interactions with peers. The ability to regulate affect, especially excitement and anger, improves in middle childhood and thereby enhances participation in competitive games and activities. Though some people may have political or religious beliefs that eschew competition, it is important to understand that a desire to compete and a desire to excel are normal aspects of development in middle childhood and adolescence.

Peer interactions in middle childhood (Table 2.1, fourth column) reflect growth in cognitive and social–emotional functioning. Structured board games, group games, and team sports with complex rules are common activities with peers. Games and sports can often lead to squabbles as children negotiate the rules and try to understand them. A child's failure to comply with the rules is a typical source of complaints by other children to parents and teachers. This is the time when children struggle between appealing to authority figures for help versus trying to solve problems among themselves. Friendships in middle childhood tend to be more stable than in early childhood. Best friends are usually children of the same sex, though there can always be exceptions. As in early childhood, aggressive children tend to be disliked, but socially withdrawn children can also be disliked or rejected. Peers who are friendly, helpful, and supportive are usually most liked. Acceptance into the peer group becomes much more important in middle childhood. Peer groups are often shaped by classroom groupings, neighborhood contacts, and structured social activities (e.g., Girl Scouts, Boy Scouts, team sports). Chapter 3 discusses peer relations and friendships in more detail as well as problems with bullying and victimization during middle childhood and adolescence.

Questioning Strategies for Middle Childhood

Because of their improved language skills, 6- to 11-year-olds can respond better to interview questions than they could at earlier ages (see Table 2.2). Nonetheless, it is important to take time to establish rapport early in the interview. One of the best ways to do this is to begin by asking children about their favorite activities and interests. For example, the SCICA protocol begins by asking, "What do you like to do in your spare time, like when you're not in school?" Most children can easily talk about something they like to do. This entrée into the interview will not only build confidence and help them feel comfortable, but will also give them the sense that you are interested in their views. Chapter 3 presents additional "warm-up" questions.

Another key strategy is to listen to what children say without casting judgments on their responses. For many children, the clinical interview presents a unique situation: a one-on-one discussion with an adult who is not trying to teach them something or to shape their behavior or attitudes in some way. Many children, especially those with emotional and behavioral problems, may not have had such an experience. It is therefore not surprising that they might be wary and reticent about sharing their feelings and opinions. When you listen without expressing judgment, you show children that you are truly interested in their perspectives. Listening without judgment includes trying to avoid both positive and negative judgmental statements. When children hear many positive statements or too much praise (e.g., "So you like reading, that's great," or "I really like your drawing"), they may begin to respond only in ways that they think will please the adult. In the clinical interview, your goal is not to help children feel better, as it might be in therapy, but instead to help them feel comfortable enough to share their genuine views on important issues. When children hear comments that hint of negative judgments (e.g., "I'll bet that made your mother mad"), they may feel threatened and stop responding, or they may become more defensive and argumentative. As an alternative, you can show empathy by restating and paraphrasing the thoughts and feelings children express. If appropriate, you can then ask children to elaborate on their responses with "tell me more" statements (e.g., "Sounds like your brother really makes you mad when he gets into stuff in your room—tell me more about that"). As with younger children, you can also use extenders ("Um," "OK," "Uh-huh") to show that you understand.

> **Listen to what children say without casting either positive or negative judgments. Show empathy by restating and paraphrasing children's thoughts and feelings.**

Following children's lead in the conversation is also a key strategy. This means allowing children to control the sequencing of topics and tolerating the sometimes meandering, "illogical" nature of their conversations. Using a written protocol of topics and questions, such as the SCICA protocol (McConaughy & Achenbach, 2001), can help you keep track of what has been discussed and what remains to be covered. The SCICA protocol is organized in a modular fashion that proceeds from less sensitive topics (e.g., activities and interests) to more specific and potentially more sensitive topics (e.g., school, peer relations, family relations, feelings). The Semistructured Student Interview in Chapter 3 (McConaughy, 2012; Appendix 3.1) is modeled on the modular format of the SCICA. It covers topics related to the child's activities and interests, academic performance, and social interactions. Using either protocol, you can adjust the sequence of topics in response to cues from the child.

As with younger children, you should generally phrase initial interview questions in an open-ended fashion (e.g., "What do you like best in school?", "What do like least?"), and then follow these with more specific probes that encourage children to elaborate on their thoughts and feelings (e.g., "So you don't like math? What is it about math that you don't like?"). When children have trouble elaborating on their responses, you can provide multiple-choice options that cover a variety of possible experiences (e.g., "Sometimes children don't like math because it is too hard, or they don't understand it, or it is boring. How do you feel about math?").

Despite their improved language skills, many children at this stage are still unaccustomed to in-depth conversations with adults, perhaps because they lack appropriate opportunities. Parents' work schedules and children's own programmed activities outside the home may leave little time for prolonged conversations. To facilitate communication with children at the middle childhood level, Table 2.2 lists several interviewing "dos": Talk about familiar settings and activities; provide contextual cues, such as pictures and examples; and rephrase and simplify questions when the child has misunderstood or not responded. Table 2.2 also lists several interviewing "don'ts": Avoid constant eye contact that may make children uncomfortable; avoid too many factual questions; avoid questions about abstract concepts; and avoid questions with obvious right or wrong answers.

Avoiding rhetorical questions is another key interviewing "don't." Rhetorical questions are implied requests or commands that are stated in the form of a question (e.g., "Would you like to . . . ?"). Because of their concrete level of reasoning, children under age 11 or 12 can easily misunderstand such questions as presenting true options for doing or not doing what is requested.

When children choose not to follow the request, then you are left in a quandary of trying to persuade them to change their minds, or of taking back your request. Such situations can quickly set the stage for oppositional behavior as well as undermine trust. To avoid this problem, give direct requests or polite "commands" as a way to transition to new topics or activities. For example: "Tell me about your friends—who are some of your friends?"; "Now let's talk about your family. . . ."; "Draw a picture of your family doing something together." Such requests carry a clear message of the interviewer's expectations and can still be stated in a warm and friendly manner.

It is also good to avoid or minimize the number of "why" questions. It is a common practice of language arts teachers to instruct children about the "wh" questions: *who, what, where, when,* and *why* (they also add *how* to this list). Although elementary-age children are often asked "why" questions, they may have difficulty answering them when the focus is on the reasons for their own behavior or for other people's behavior. Motivation for behavior is an abstract concept that is hard for some 6- to 11-year-olds to understand and articulate because they have difficulty taking a third-person point of view to explain human interactions. Instead, they tend to focus more on actions and event sequences than on the motives behind the actions. For example, in one of my studies of children's ability to summarize short stories, fifth-grade children tended to emphasize action sequences, or "what happened," more than characters' motives or "why it happened" (McConaughy, Fitzhenry-Coor, & Howell, 1983). This does not mean that elementary-age children are incapable of understanding motives. Nevertheless, because motivation is a difficult concept, asking "why" questions in clinical interviews often leads to "I don't know" responses or shut down.

Even adolescents, who may be more capable of focusing on motivation, will sometimes become unresponsive to "why" questions if they perceive them as accusations, threats, or tests. Such reactions are especially likely from children who have had conflicts with authority figures. An alternative to the "why" question is to use the reflective technique of repeating children's phrases and then following with a polite or soft command, such as "Tell me more about that." You can also ask, "What did you do when that happened?" and then probe for feelings and reactions, "How did that make you feel?" or "What did you think about that?"

Developmental Characteristics of Adolescence

Adolescence generally includes ages 12–18, at least in terms of physical development, regardless of intellectual ability. As all parents and teachers know well, the early years of adolescence can be rocky as children undergo hormonal changes leading to adulthood. By age 11 or 12, children normally move into Piaget's "formal operational" stage of cognitive development (Table 2.1, second column). This stage involves the ability to reason abstractly and apply logical rules for solving problems in several arenas. Normally developing adolescents become more systematic in their approach to academic tasks and social problem solving. They enjoy applying their new reasoning skills to hypothetical situations. You might characterize this time as the "what if" stage of development, because that is a frequent question adolescents pose to adults and peers. This new and growing ability for hypothetical reasoning can make many adolescents seem argumentative. At the same time, do not assume that every adolescent is capable of formal operational thought. Adolescents with below-average intelligence or mental retardation, in particular, are unlikely to master abstract logical thinking. Therefore, it behooves interviewers to have some knowledge of adolescents' cognitive ability or to screen briefly for ability. Vocabulary and general language skills are often good indicators of intellectual ability, except for individuals with verbal learning disabilities.

In terms of social–emotional functioning (Table 2.1, third column), many adolescents can take a third-person view of what they and other people are thinking (i.e., thinking about thinking). This has been described as "metacognitive thinking," because it allows individuals to simultaneously imagine both sides of a social interaction. That is, they can understand their own perspective and the perspective of another person, as well as how both perspectives may be viewed by someone else (e.g., "She thinks that I like him and that he likes me"). Although metacognitive thinking represents another advance in social reasoning, it can also lead to embarrassing complications, especially in romantic relationships. Some adolescents who are experiencing emotional and behavioral problems may not have developed the capacity for this type of thinking, which can be a major factor in the poor quality of their social relations with peers and adults.

Adolescence is the time when many individuals reach Kohlberg's (1976) level of "postconventional moral reasoning," though this ability may not develop until ages 17 or 18 in some, or not at all in others. At this level, judgments of right or wrong are based on individual principles of conscience or religious or philosophical ideals (e.g., "Violence is wrong because it goes against principles of a safe and just society"; "Stealing is wrong because it infringes on people's personal property rights"; "Lying is wrong because it violates trust"). As adolescents learn to reason according to moral principles, they may also experiment with different ideals and values, which can lead to conflicts with family and peers. Many adolescents struggle with identity issues, which can lead to self-consciousness, and they often experience intense shifts in emotions. As they become more socially aware, adolescents look to peer groups for social acceptance, which is extremely important to them.

Peer interactions among adolescents (Table 2.1, fourth column) often involve "hanging out" and communicating with friends. This can take the form of talking in groups, sending notes, making phone calls, and more recently, talking and texting on cell phones, and socializing on the Internet through social networks (e.g., Facebook), e-mail, and online chat groups. Managing their time on the Internet and cell phones can be a challenge with some adolescents, as discussed further in Chapter 4. Along with shared activities, intimate self-disclosure often characterizes friendships, especially for girls. Squabbles and arguments at this stage often erupt over relationship issues, characterized by gossiping, betraying of secrets, and shifting loyalties. Researchers have described these types of problems as "relational aggression" in contrast to physical aggression (Crick & Grotpeter, 1995; Crick, Ostrov, & Kawabata, 2007), as discussed further in Chapter 3.

Adolescence is also the time for emerging romantic relationships, which may occur as early as ages 11 and 12, or even sooner for some. Some adolescents experience distress about their sexual identity, which can be especially painful if they are ostracized by peers or family. As in earlier stages, aggressive and antisocial peers are generally disliked, though aggressive and antisocial adolescents may be accepted into deviant peer groups and gangs. Socially withdrawn individuals and those with odd or atypical behavior may also be rejected and ostracized. Peers who are cooperative, helpful, attractive, and competent tend to be liked. In adolescence, peer status is generally defined by group norms, including cliques and clubs. As one adolescent, Karl Bryant, put it in his clinical interview, "You know who all the different types are in this school. We have the druggies, the alcoholics, the preppies, the jocks, the smart kids, and the geeks." Chapter 3 uses Karl's case as an example of interviewing adolescents about problems in peer relations.

Questioning Strategies for Adolescence

When children enter adolescence, their improved reasoning and language abilities make it easier for them to participate in clinical interviews. However, as Merrell (2008a) cautioned, you should not assume that interviewing adolescents is like interviewing adults. Many of the interviewing dos and don'ts discussed for middle childhood apply to adolescence. There are also special challenges for interviewing adolescents. Their growing social awareness, coupled with self-consciousness and an insecure sense of identity, make it doubly important to establish rapport and trust early in the interview. It is especially important to show respect and openness to their unique points of view. When adolescents feel a lack of respect, they are likely to shut down or may become resistant or belligerent. At the same time, you also need to explain the limits of confidentiality clearly, as discussed in an earlier section, so that adolescents will not feel betrayed by reports to other persons later. Sometimes when adolescents hear that interview information may be shared with other people, they may be unwilling to disclose certain types of information. This is a necessary risk for all clinical interviewing. Discussing exactly what will and will not be reported can help to reduce such concerns. Chapter 4 discusses confidentiality issues with adolescents in more detail.

> **With adolescents, show respect and be prepared for shifts in emotions. Ask questions to explore their feelings, but also show respect for need for privacy.**

As when interviewing younger children, it is important to solicit adolescents' thoughts and feelings without making judgmental comments. Some adolescents may enjoy the interview process and share their perspectives freely. Others may be more resistant, particularly those who have had frequent clashes with authority figures and those who associate clinical interviews with stressful experiences, such as abuse investigations and potential removal from their home. Also be prepared for emotional lability and signs of stress. As Merrell (2008a) noted, adolescence has often been characterized as a time of "storm and stress." It is not unusual to see an adolescent begin a clinical interview in a cheerful, engaging manner and then quickly become agitated and angry as the interviewer broaches more sensitive topics. The interview with Karl Bryant, discussed in Chapters 3 and 5, is a good example. Other adolescents may seem anxious or depressed at different points during an interview. It is important to acknowledge such shifts in feelings and ask questions to explore those feelings further, while at the same time respecting adolescents' sense of privacy and their defenses against exploring or revealing painful experiences. When discussions turn to problem situations, you can query adolescents about their perspectives on causes and motives. You should also ask about possible alternative solutions to the problems. Such questions about problem-solving strategies are especially useful for evaluating adolescents' level of social and moral reasoning.

Because adolescents are at higher risk for suicide than are younger children (Reynolds & Mazza, 1994), it is important to ask screening questions about suicide risk and to pursue any indications of suicidal ideation or attempts. When interviewees raise issues that suggest suicide risk, interviewers should ask directly about suicidal thoughts and attempts, such as whether they have made any plans and have access to methods, such as pills or weapons. In Chapter 9, David Miller discusses the assessment of suicide risk in detail.

In addition to most of the interviewing don'ts listed in Table 2.2 for middle childhood, you should also avoid using psychological terms (e.g., *psychosis, inferiority complex*) with adolescents, even if they appear to understand them. Avoiding such terminology will help to alleviate adolescents' fears that they are being interviewed because someone thinks they are crazy or thinks they need a "shrink." It is better to use everyday language as much as possible to help adolescents understand normal processes of human behavior and emotions.

You should also be mindful of adolescents' developmental level when applying clinical diagnoses. A lack of normative standards for diagnoses is one of the shortcomings of the DSM-5 and its precursors. Although some adult DSM-5 diagnostic categories may be appropriate for adolescents, caution is still warranted when applying such diagnoses. For example, just because an adolescent displays emotional lability in the clinical interview, you should not assume that this lability is strong evidence of a mood disorder, such as major depression or bipolar disorder. If you use standardized self-reports and standardized parent and teacher rating scales to accompany clinical interviews, you will have a better basis for making clinical judgments about deviance than if you rely only on interview information. For example, the ASEBA (Achenbach & Rescorla, 2001) and BASC-2 (Reynolds & Kamphaus, 2004) provide norms for judging deviance in parent and teacher reports and youth self-reports of behavioral and emotional problems, as discussed in Chapters 4, 6, and 7.

ALTERNATING VERBAL AND NONVERBAL COMMUNICATION

Too much direct questioning can make clinical interviews tedious and unpleasant for children of all ages. One way to avoid this is to alternate between verbal and nonverbal means of communication—a common tactic used in test batteries assessing cognitive ability. There are several ways to interject nonverbal techniques into clinical interviews. One commonly used strategy is the Kinetic Family Drawing (KFD; Burns, 1982) technique, wherein the child is asked to "draw a picture of your family doing something together." The KFD is used routinely in the SCICA for children ages 6–11 and is optional for ages 12–18. After the child completes the drawing, you can inquire about family members and relationships. Chapter 5 discusses KFD procedures in detail, with illustrative examples and interview excerpts.

> **The KFD, "thought bubbles" with cartoons, and incomplete sentences are methods for interjecting nonverbal activities into clinical interviews.**

"Thought bubbles" provide another way to elicit thoughts and feelings from 6- to 11-year-olds who can think about different people's perspectives (Hughes & Baker, 1990). For this technique, draw a simple cartoon that depicts two or more characters in a problem situation. Then draw an empty thought bubble over the head of each character and ask the child to fill in the bubble with what the character is thinking and feeling. You can write children's responses into the bubbles if they have difficulty writing or do not like to write. Older children can complete their own thought bubbles. Then ask children to tell you more about what the characters think and feel and what might happen next. Thought bubbles are good techniques for exploring children's level of social cognition and their understanding of the causal relations between thoughts, feelings, and behaviors. However, you should not assume that what children say in the thought bubbles for cartoon characters necessarily represents their own thoughts and feelings. Instead, you can ask children directly how *they* might think or feel in a similar situation.

Incomplete sentences offer another alternative to direct questioning for children who can understand different perspectives. This technique involves presenting sentence stems that focus on a particular person or feeling situation and then asking the child to complete the sentences. Examples include "My mother thinks I am _____"; "My teacher thinks I am _____"; and "I feel upset when _____." Chapter 4 discusses these and other examples of incomplete sentences in more detail.

Play materials can be used with 3- to 5-year-olds and other children who are reluctant to engage in conversation. Effective play materials for clinical interviews include wooden blocks, doll family figures and additional adult and child figures, dollhouse furniture, and a dollhouse, if available. While children are playing, you can interject open-ended questions about the play events and play family relationships. As with thought bubbles, you should not assume that children's play necessarily reflects what they have experienced in their own lives. For example, for children who portray violent play with doll figures, you might comment, "There is a lot of fighting going on in that family. What happens in your house? Tell me what people do in your house." It is important to ask such questions in order to determine whether children's violent play represents their own real-life experiences or worrisome violent fantasies; after all, children can view violence from many sources, other than their homes lives, such as TV, movies, video games, and in their schools and neighborhoods. Other authors (e.g., Garbarino & Scott, 1989; Greenspan & Greenspan, 2003; Hughes & Baker, 1990) provide more discussion of play interviews as well as other nonverbal techniques such as using puppets and dolls, feeling thermometers, emotional flash cards, and social problem-solving vignettes.

If time allows, you can incorporate brief achievement tests or fine and gross motor tasks into child clinical interviews to provide breaks from verbal questioning. Such tasks offer opportunities to observe children's responses to structured school-like tasks and motor activities, in contrast to responses to direct questioning. For example, the SCICA protocol includes brief achievement tests of reading and math, a writing sample, and gross motor screening (e.g., hopping, playing catch) as optional tasks for children ages 6–11. If such tasks are included, they should not take more than about 15–20 minutes, so as not to turn the interview into a test situation. Some children may show more anxiety and report more school problems during achievement testing than during open-ended questioning; others may become more resistant, restless, or manipulative; and still others may act more self-assured and enthusiastic, or start joking and clowning during testing. Such contrasts in behavior can provide valuable clinical information about children's functioning under different task demands.

DEALING WITH LYING

As indicated at the beginning of this chapter, one of the main goals of child clinical interviews is to learn children's own perspectives on their functioning. However, sometimes interviewers may be concerned that children are lying or "stretching the truth" in their interview statements. Data collected with the ASEBA forms give a good indication of how often different informants reported that children lie or cheat. (On the ASEBA forms, lying and cheating are combined into one question.) Table 2.3 shows the percentage of children in the ASEBA normative nonreferred samples and clinically referred samples for whom "lying or cheating" was endorsed as "sometimes or somewhat true" or "very true or often true" (Achenbach & Rescorla, 2001). You can see in Table 2.3 that 24–29% of nonreferred 11- to 18-year-olds reported on the YSR that they had lied or cheated sometime in the past 6 months. Similarly, on the CBCL/6–18, 22–31% of parents of nonreferred children reported that their child had lied or cheated in the past 6 months. On the TRF, 2–13% of teachers reported that nonreferred children had lied or cheated in the past 2 months. These findings show that even some children who are considered to be "normal" (i.e., not having severe problems) sometimes lie or cheat.

TABLE 2.3. Percentage of Children Reported to Have Lied or Cheated

	Youth self-reports on the YSR[a]	Parent reports on the CBCL/6–18[a]	Teacher reports on the TRF[b]
Nonreferred girls	24	22	2
Nonreferred boys	29	31	13
Referred girls	43	66	32
Referred boys	52	71	43

Note. Data from Achenbach and Rescorla (2001). YSR, Youth Self-Report; CBCL/6–18, Child Behavior Checklist for Ages 6 to 18; TRF, Teacher's Report Form.
[a]Time frame = past 6 months.
[b]Time frame = past 2 months.

Table 2.3 shows much higher rates of lying or cheating for children referred for mental health or special education services than for nonreferred children. Among the referred children, 43–52% of 11- to 18-year-olds reported that they had lied or cheated, and 66–71% of parents, and 32–43% of teachers, reported that the children had lied or cheated. Statistical analyses revealed significantly higher scores for lying or cheating among referred than nonreferred children. Parents and teachers also reported significantly more lying or cheating among younger than older children and among boys than girls.

Because the ASEBA forms included lying and cheating in the same question, it is not clear which of the two problems was being reported for a particular child. However, the ASEBA data do indicate that it is not uncommon for children to lie or cheat, especially children who have been referred for emotional and behavioral problems. During clinical interviews, lying is more likely to occur than cheating because interviews seldom present opportunities for cheating, unless they include tasks such as achievement tests. Children might lie in clinical interviews for any number of reasons, as Hughes and Baker (1990) pointed out. They may feel threatened and afraid that their answers to certain questions will get them into trouble or lead to disapproval or reprimands. Or they may be attempting to deny memories and feelings of painful or embarrassing situations. Or they may want to impress the interviewer or gain a desired outcome or advantage.

Interviewers can reduce the potential for lying by being sensitive to situations that may inadvertently induce children to lie or "stretch the truth." One strategy is to avoid questions that might seem accusatory to a child, such as "did you" questions (e.g., "Did you take the money?") or "why" questions (e.g., "Why did you hit him?"). You should also avoid asking leading questions about children's misbehavior when you already know the answer from another source, such as a parent or a teacher. An example is asking a child whether he stole money from a teacher's desk, knowing that the teacher reported witnessing such a theft.

Young children may also appear to lie because they have difficulty distinguishing fantasy from reality or feelings from actual behavior, or they have difficulty expressing such distinctions in words. Interviewers can deal with these situations by verbalizing such distinctions for the child. For example, when a child exaggerates or describes something that obviously could not have happened, you might say, "It sounds like you really wished it could have happened that way." Or you can restate the child's feelings and then ask about reality versus fantasy, for example, by saying, "Sounds like that was really scary when your dog was hit by a car. And then you said you ran out in the middle of all the traffic and picked him up and rescued him. Was that what really happened or was that something you wished had happened?" Statements such as these help children to understand that their feelings are acceptable, and they encourage children to talk more freely about their feelings and how they wished things might have happened differently. Such statements also make it unnecessary for children to retract their statements or to admit that what they said was not exactly true or a "lie." Confronting children directly about suspected lies or exaggerations, on the other hand, is likely to be counterproductive, because it may lead them to tell more lies to save face or to defend themselves against accusations and punishments. Confronting them about lies can also make them shut down.

INTERVIEWING CULTURALLY AND LINGUISTICALLY DIVERSE CHILDREN AND THEIR PARENTS

In their ethical standards both the APA and the NASP stress the importance of considering cultural and linguistic backgrounds, along with other factors, when conducting psychological assessments:

> When interpreting assessment results, including automated interpretations, psychologists take into account the purpose of the assessment as well as the various test factors, test-taking abilities, and other characteristics of the person being assessed, such as situational, personal, linguistic, and cultural differences, that might affect psychologists' judgments or reduce the accuracy of the interpretations. They indicate any significant limitations of their interpretations. (Section 9.06; APA Ethical Principles of Psychologists and Code of Conduct, 2002)

> Psychologists use assessment methods that are appropriate to an individual's language preference and competence, unless use of an alternative language is relevant to the assessment issues. (Section 9.02 b; APA Ethical Principles of Psychologists and Code of Conduct, 2002)

> School psychologists conduct valid and fair assessments. They actively pursue knowledge of the student's disabilities and developmental, cultural, linguistic, and experiential background and then select, administer, and interpret assessment instruments and procedures in light of those characteristics. (Standard II.3.5; NASP Principals for Professional Ethics, 2010)

Based on its 2009–2010 population survey, the U.S. Census Bureau (2010) reported that out of the total U.S. civilian population (estimated 307,006,550), 79.6% identified themselves as White (65.1% as White–not Hispanic), 15.8% identified themselves as Hispanic or Latino, 12.9% as Black or African American, 4.6% as Asian, and 1% as American Indian or Alaska Native. The 2010 U.S. census also showed that 11.1% of the U.S. population was foreign born (i.e., not U.S. citizens at birth) and 17.9% spoke a language other than English at home. These statistics highlight the great diversity of ethnic, cultural, and linguistic backgrounds in our country. Because a person's cultural background can play an important role in communication and interpersonal relationships, interviewers need to be sensitive to cultural characteristics to conduct effective and valid clinical assessments. Ethnic and cultural considerations are especially pertinent to judgments about whether children are exhibiting emotional or behavioral *problems*. For example, some cultures may value inhibited or cautious behavior in children as a sign of respect and self-control. Other cultures may value more outgoing, expressive modes of interaction.

Table 2.4 summarizes general behavioral characteristics and communication patterns among four major U.S. groups—Hispanic, Asian, African American, and Native American children—compared to the "mainstream U.S." culture, as described by Vasquez-Nuttall, Li, Sanchez, Nuttall, and Mathisen (2003). Some of the characteristics in Table 2.4 may also apply to children's parents. As noted by Merrell (2008a), the degree of eye contact and acceptable physical distance between two persons are two cultural dimensions that can have immediate relevance in clinical interviews. For example, some multicultural experts have observed that White Americans tend to make eye contact with the speaker most of the time, but avoid eye contact

> **Interviewers need to be knowledgeable about and sensitive to the cultural and linguistic diversity of children and parents in order to conduct effective and valid assessments.**

TABLE 2.4. Behavioral Characteristics and Communication Patterns across Cultures

Behavior	Mainstream United States	Hispanics	Asians	African Americans	Native Americans
Eye contact	Direct eye contact	Direct eye contact with adults is unacceptable when reprimanded; lowering the eyes is a sign of respect	Looking down is considered a sign of respect	Direct eye contact is unacceptable when admonished	Very limited; tendency to lower eyes to show respect
Touching	Not accepted, except among intimate friends	Accepted and expected as demonstrations of love and acceptance	Discouraged, particularly with the opposite sex	Physical touching for expression is acceptable	Not shown in public
Distance	Personal, intimate, and social distance maintained according to relationship	Interaction at a close distance is accepted and expected	Maintained among strangers	Close physical distance with friends and family; initial distance with strangers	Distance with strangers is maintained; closeness is shown through sharing
Facial and emotional expressions	Controlled, not generally expressed	Very expressive; smiles; gestures; nose, eye, and hand movements when talking	Very controlled	Facial gestures to stress words and meanings and emotions	Controlled, not expressive
Tone of voice	Generally moderate	Rural children are soft spoken; urban children are verbal and vivacious	Soft speaking voice	Use of different voice tones and pitch for meaning	Soft speaking voice; valuation of silence and contemplation

Note. From Vasquez-Nuttall, Li, Sanchez, Nuttall, and Mathisen (2003). Copyright 2003 by PRO-ED. Reprinted by permission.

about half of the time when speaking to others. African Americans tend to make eye contact more often when speaking but less often when listening. Native Americans are likely to use indirect eye contact patterns when speaking or listening, and Asian Americans and Hispanics are likely to avoid eye contact when speaking to persons with higher status (Sue & Sue, 1999; Vasquez-Nuttall et al., 2003). Regarding physical distance, the same experts noted that a much closer physical distance between persons is accepted among many different cultural groups (e.g., Hispanics, African Americans, Indonesians, South Americans, Arabs, and French) than is commonly accepted by White/Anglo clinicians (Sue & Sue, 1999; Vasquez-Nuttall et al., 2003). Table 2.4 also summarizes general behavioral and communication patterns among the four major U.S. cultural groups regarding touching, facial and emotional expressions, and tone of voice. Merrell (2008a) discussed general characteristics and behavioral patterns of the same four groups in more detail.

While it may be helpful to keep different cultural patterns of behavior in mind, it is important to remember that much of our information on ethnic, cultural, and racial differences is based on *generalizations from group studies*, as Merrell (2008a) wisely pointed out. Therefore, you should not assume that the behavioral characteristics and communication patterns shown in Table 2.4 apply to everyone in a particular group. There are always individuals who do not fit "typical" group characteristics. To gain an accurate understanding of each individual, it is important to avoid stereotypes and overgeneralization of group differences.

Limited-English-Proficient and Bilingual Children

The diversity of the U.S. population is also reflected in the number of children who have limited English language skills or are bilingual. Several terms have been used to identify those who speak limited English, including *limited English proficient* (LEP) and *English learners* (ELs). The Elementary and Secondary Education Act, reauthorized as the No Child Left Behind Act (NCLB, 2001), relies on a definition of an LEP student as an individual

> who is aged 3 to 21; is enrolled or preparing to enroll in an elementary or secondary school; who was not born in the United States or whose native language is a language other than English; who is a Native American or Alaska Native, or a native resident of the outlying areas; and who comes from an environment where a language other than English has had a significant impact on the individual's level of English language proficiency; or who is migratory, whose native language is a language other than English, and who comes from an environment where a language other than English is dominant; and whose difficulties in speaking, reading, writing, or understanding the English language may be sufficient to deny the individual the ability to meet the State's proficient level of achievement on State assessments . . . ; the ability to successfully achieve in classrooms where the language of instruction is English; or the opportunity to participate fully in society. (NCLB, 2001, Public Law 107-110, Section 9101; Ramsey & O'Day, 2010)

In the 2007–2008 school year, the number of LEP students in the 50 states and the District of Columbia totaled approximately 4.7 million, or close to 10% of the K–12 enrollment in public schools nationwide (Ramsey & O'Day, 2010). Over 1.5 million students were identified as LEP in California, comprising 24% of the K–12 population. New Mexico, Texas, Florida, Illinois, New York, and South Carolina also had over 100,000 LEP students. Although the majority of LEP students speak Spanish as their dominant language, a 2002 survey identified over 400 different languages that were dominant among LEP students. Other languages spoken by approximately 1–2% of LEP students were Vietnamese, Hmong, Haitian Creole, Korean, Cantonese, Arabic, Russian, Navajo, and Tagalong (Kindler, 2002).

The *dominant* or *native* language is the language normally used by an individual in the home or learning environment. Sometimes the dominant language of a child may be different from the dominant language of the parent. Under the 1997 revisions of IDEA, "native language" was defined as "the language normally used by that individual, or in the case of a child, the language normally used by the parents of the child." However, the 1997 revisions of IDEA also expanded the definition of native language of the child as "the language normally used by the child, and not that of the parents, if there is a difference between the two." These distinctions are particularly relevant for bilingual children from families with parents or grandparents who do not speak English at home. However, even when a child from a non-English-speaking family uses English in school, practitioners should not assume that English is the child's "native" or dominant language. As Rhodes, Ochoa, and Ortiz (2005) pointed out, bilingualism usually develops along a continuum, depending on the child's age and generational status with respect to when the family entered the United States. They also cautioned that even if an LEP child can carry on a social conversation in English, it does not necessarily mean that he or she has sufficient English skills to perform academic tasks or to perform up to ability on intelligence tests administered in English. The same precautions are applicable to child clinical interviews, which by necessity cover sensitive and emotionally loaded topics that may difficult to discuss in a second nondominant language.

Use of Interpreters

For children and/or parents who are not fluent in English, use of an interpreter is often required for a valid assessment. The NASP ethical principles have a specific standard regarding the use of interpreters:

> When interpreters are used to facilitate the provision of assessment and intervention services, school psychologists take steps to ensure that the interpreters are appropriately trained and are acceptable to clients. (Standard II.3.6; NASP Principles of Professional Ethics, 2010)

Interpreters should be fluent in both English and the native language of child/parent and have expertise in translating and a basic understanding of the assessment process.

However, it is not immediately obvious who should serve as an appropriate interpreter, nor is it obvious how to work with an interpreter. In surveys of school psychologists, Ochoa and colleagues found that a majority who used interpreters had received little or no training in the process, and the interpreters themselves had little or no training (Ochoa, Gonzales, Galarza, & Guillemard, 1996). By contrast, the Standards for Educational and Psychological Testing (1999), developed jointly by the American Educational Research Association (AERA), APA, and the National Council on Measurement in Education NCME) clearly state:

> When an interpreter is used in testing, the interpreter should be fluent in both the language of the test and the examinee's native language, should have expertise in translating, and should have a

basic understanding of the assessment process. (Standard 9.11; AERA, APA, NCME Standards for Educational and Psychological Testing, 1999)

Rhodes et al. (2005) provided detailed guidelines for selecting interpreters. The following points summarize their key criteria:

- The interpreter should be equally fluent in English and the native language of the child or parent being interviewed or tested. Individuals who speak or understand "a little" of the native language may be helpful in impromptu or informal conversations, but these individuals should, *under no circumstances*, be used in any formal capacity as an interpreter.
- Friends and family members should *not* be used as interpreters. Using friends or family members would likely involve a breach of confidentiality for the child and/or parent. It might also lead to manipulation of information and inappropriate role reversals.
- Interpreters should have at least a high school diploma and communication skills adequate for the task. Communication skills include:
  - Ability to accurately convey meaning from one language to another.
  - Sensitivity to the style of the speaker.
  - Ability to adjust to linguistic variations within different communities.
  - Knowledge about the cultures of the people who speak the native language.
  - Familiarity with educational or psychological terminology.
  - Understanding of the function and role of interpreter.
  - Ability to stay emotionally uninvolved with the content of discussion and to maintain neutrality and confidentiality.

Rhodes et al. (2005) also discussed ways in which interviewers and test examiners can make the interpretation process go smoothly and professionally. Table 2.5 lists some of their suggestions that are especially applicable for clinical interviews with children and/or parents. Also draw-

---

TABLE 2.5. Interviewing Strategies for Using Interpreters in Clinical Interviews

Speak naturally and clearly in short, simple sentences. Do not expect the interpreter to accurately convey lengthy statements. Do not expect the interpreter to finish your thoughts or ideas for you.

Look at and speak to the child or parents(s), not the interpreter.

Monitor facial expressions of the interpreter, and child or parent(s), for apparent confusion or concern.

Monitor body language of the interpreter, and child or parent(s), for possible discomfort or resistance.

Feel free to ask the interpreter, child, or parent(s), if he/she has any questions or needs clarification on any point.

Allow extra time for interpretation and clarification.

Encourage breaks for the interpreter when needed.

Meet with the interpreter after the interview to debrief and discuss any issues that arose during the interview.

Note. Adapted from Rhodes, Ochoa, and Ortiz (2005). Copyright 2005 by The Guilford Press. Adapted by permission.

ing upon recommendations by Rhodes and colleagues, Appendix 2.1 provides general behavioral guidelines for interpreters, and Appendix 2.2 provides ethical guidelines for interpreters. Practitioners can copy these appendices and discuss them with interpreters prior to interviewing LEP children, parents, and/or other family members.

Acculturation and Cultural Self-Identity

Along with considering linguistic and cultural factors, it is also helpful to be aware of an individual's level of acculturation and sense of ethnic, cultural, or racial self-identity. *Acculturation* refers to the process of change that occurs when an individual from a different minority culture begins to adopt the cultural content or elements of another more dominant culture (Rhodes et al., 2005; Sattler, 1998). Acculturation and cultural self-identity can vary for different individuals in a particular group and can change over time. As Rhodes et al. (2005) pointed out, "Individuals can vary along a spectrum from absolutely not acculturated to fully or completely acculturated and everything in between. [In the United States,] this continuum of acculturation is very similar to, and shares a great deal of variance with, dimensions of bilingualism and the process of acquiring English as a second language" (p. 128). Like bilingualism, the level of acculturation is likely to vary depending on the individual's stage of development from childhood to adulthood and the individual's generational status with respect to introduction to the dominant culture (e.g., first-generation, foreign born, vs. second-, third-, or fourth-generation, U.S. born). Rhodes et al. (2005) also pointed out that, regardless of whether assimilation of the dominant culture is, or is not desirable, there are certain predictable patterns across generations. For example, second-generation individuals (e.g., U.S.-born children of immigrant parents) often find themselves caught between two cultures that compete for their identification and loyalty. Third- or fourth-generation individuals often consider themselves more aligned with the mainstream or dominant culture but still value certain parts of their minority cultural heritage. Different levels of acculturation can also occur across generations within the same family, as when second-generation children align themselves more with the dominant culture while parents and grandparents align themselves with their native culture.

Drawing on the work of Sue and Sue (1999), Merrell (2008a) described five developmental stages of acculturation and cultural self-identity formation experienced by members of minority ethnic, racial, or cultural groups. These stages are summarized in Table 2.6. Recognizing stages of cultural self-identity formation can be especially helpful for interviewing linguistically and culturally diverse children and adolescents. An individual's progression through the stages of cultural self-identity formation most likely will be linked to his or her general stage of cognitive and social–emotional development, as outlined in Table 2.1. For example, it would be unlikely for 3- to 5-year-olds or many 6- to 11-year-olds to have advanced to the fourth or fifth stage of cultural self-identity formation that requires introspection or integrative awareness. It is also important to recognize that not all individuals will progress through all of the five stages and that some individuals, even adult family members, may remain "stuck" in one of the earlier stages. Having an awareness of levels of acculturation and cultural self-identity formation can enhance the sensitivity and effectiveness of interviews with linguistically and culturally diverse children, parents, and family members. Chapter 6 discusses additional considerations for interviewing culturally and linguistically diverse parents.

Interviewers also need to be sensitive to their own cultural viewpoints and potential biases or prejudices toward particular ethnic, cultural, or racial groups. If you have strong negative attitudes

TABLE 2.6. Stages of Acculturation and Cultural Self-Identity Formation

Stage	Characteristics
Conformity	Depreciating attitude toward self and others of the same minority group; discriminatory attitude toward other minority groups; appreciating attitude toward dominant group
Dissonance	Conflict between depreciating and appreciating attitudes toward self, others of same minority groups, other minority groups, and dominant group
Resistance/immersion	Appreciating attitude toward self and others of same minority group; conflict between empathic and culturocentric feelings toward other minority groups; depreciating attitude toward dominant group
Introspection	Concern with basis of self-appreciation and unequivocal nature of appreciation toward others of same minority group; concern with culturocentric views toward members of other minority groups; concern with basis of depreciation of dominant group
Integrative awareness	Appreciating attitude toward self, others of same minority group, and other minority groups; selective appreciation for dominant group

Note. From Merrell (2008a). Copyright 2008 by Lawrence Erlbaum Associates. Reprinted by permission.

or stereotypes about particular groups, seek additional education and appropriate supervision or refrain from conducting interviews and other assessments of individuals from those groups. Several other sources provide more in-depth discussion of issues related to assessment of linguistically and culturally diverse children and adults, including Merrell (2008a), Rhodes et al. (2005), Sattler (1998), Sue and Sue (1999), and Vasquez-Nuttal et al. (2003). Achenbach and Rescorla (2007) also provide an extensive discussion of multicultural patterns of children's competencies and problem behavior, based on research with the ASEBA forms. Various ASEBA forms have been translated into over 85 different languages and are used in research and clinical practice around the world. Practitioners can use the different translations of the ASEBA CBCL/6–18 and YSR to obtain reports of children's competencies and problems from non-English-speaking parents and adolescents. The ASEBA TRF has also been translated into many different languages.

CONCLUDING THE CHILD CLINICAL INTERVIEW

Interviewers should have a standard protocol for ending child clinical interviews, just as they have for beginning the interviews. To conclude the interview, you can first thank the child for participating and sharing his/her thoughts and feelings. Then review statements regarding confidentiality and discuss how interview information will be shared with other people, such as parents and teachers. If there will be a follow-up meeting to discuss the interview, tell the child that you will be meeting with parents and/or teachers to talk about what you learned in the interview. (You should have told the child about such meetings at the beginning of the interview, as indicated earlier.) Explain briefly what information you want to share with others and how you will share it. You can also ask the child if there is anything else he/she wants you to share. If you will be writing a report, explain how interview material will be summarized in the report. Such disclosures are especially important for adolescents, who are likely to be more sensitive about privacy issues than are younger children.

Concluding remarks should be brief and tailored to the developmental level of the child in the same manner as opening remarks. A good general strategy is to summarize key aspects of what you learned about the child in the interview and then tell the child what general or specific issues you want to discuss with parents, teachers, or other important parties. Most children will be comfortable with this approach, especially if you explain that discussing important issues with other people can help everyone figure out how to solve identified problems. The following is an example of a concluding discussion with a 7-year-old girl:

I: Well, that was a pretty long talk about a lot of different things—school, your friends, your family, what makes you happy, sad, and mad, and things that are problems for you. I really appreciate how you shared your feelings with me. Do you remember what I said about this being a private talk?

C: Yeah, you said you wouldn't tell my mom.

I: That's right. Now, one important thing I learned was about all that fighting with your sister and how you feel you always get blamed. I think that would be important to talk about with your mom, so we can figure out better ways to deal with that. Is that OK with you?

C: Yeah, OK . . . but don't tell Mom I called Cindy a jerk.

I: No, I won't tell Mom about the "jerk" part. I'll just tell her about the fighting and how you feel you always get blamed.

C: OK.

I: I'm also going to talk to your mom and teachers about your problems finishing your work in school and how you would like some extra help.

C: OK. Can I go now? (McConaughy, 2000a, p. 184)

Some children, especially adolescents, may want more specific assurance of the privacy of their interviews. When children do have concerns about confidentiality, you can reassure them that you will not quote their exact words or specific statements that they made during the interview, as illustrated above, and you can paraphrase examples of what you will say. You can also avoid directly reporting children's interview statements in reports and meetings with other informants by referring to those informants' key areas of concern and saying that similar issues were discussed in the child interview.

When there is reason to suspect that the child poses a danger to self or others, or that the child is in danger of abuse, however, you do have legal obligations to report such information to others. In such cases, you should remind the child about the limits of confidentiality stated at the beginning of the interview. (As indicated earlier, your introductory remarks should clearly state that information is not confidential if there is reason to suspect that "you were going to hurt yourself, hurt someone else, or someone has hurt you.") Then you should discuss with the child the next steps in the reporting process. Chapter 5 addresses confidentiality and reporting obligations for child abuse. Chapters 9 and 10 address confidentiality and reporting issues around danger to self and danger to others. Also see Jacob, Decker, and Hartshorne (2011) for discussion of ethical and legal issues regarding confidentiality.

SUMMARY

Child clinical interviews offer rich opportunities to learn children's perspectives on their competencies and problems and to directly observe their behavior, affect, and interaction styles. To facilitate developmentally sensitive interviewing, this chapter discussed interviewing strategies for children at three developmental levels: early childhood (ages 3–5), middle childhood (ages 6–11), and adolescence (ages 12–18). Key aspects of cognitive functioning, social–emotional functioning, and peer interactions were summarized for each developmental level. The chapter also discussed issues regarding confidentiality, nonverbal interviewing techniques, dealing with lying, and special considerations for interviewing culturally and linguistically diverse children and parents.

General Guidelines for Interpreters

Provide evidence of your qualifications as an interpreter to the person(s) requesting your services.

Develop an understanding of the purpose of the assessment and the materials and procedures to be used prior to the start of the session.

Clarify any areas of concern or uncertainty about your role or the assessment process prior to start of the session.

Introduce yourself to the child and/or family members and explain your role in the assessment process.

Interpret everything that is said by the speaker.

Do not make assumptions regarding the importance or relevance of the information requiring interpretation. It is not your role to act as a filter or censor of information.

Reflect the pace, tone, and inflection of the speaker.

Maintain neutrality throughout the process.

Monitor any emotional reaction to the content or events discussed and decisions that are reached, but do not try to influence the discussion or emotional reactions.

Inquire about any words, terms, or statements that are unclear or unknown while the assessment is taking place.

Accurate interpretation is more important than seamless interpretation.

Maintain confidentiality of all aspects of the assessment process.

Ethical Guidelines for Individuals Serving as Interpreters

Interpreters shall keep all assignment-related information strictly confidential.

No information about the child or family shall be revealed, including the fact that the assessment is being conducted, unless the parent or legal guardian has given written consent for such disclosure by the interpreter.

Interpreters shall render the message faithfully, always conveying the content and spirit of the speaker, using language most readily understood by the person(s) whom they serve.

Interpreters are not editors and must transmit everything that is said in exactly the same way it was intended by the speaker. Interpreters must remember that they are not at all responsible for what is said, only for conveying it accurately. If the interpreter's own feelings interfere with rendering the message accurately, the interpreter shall withdraw from the assignment.

Interpreters shall not counsel, advise, or interject personal opinions.

Interpreters shall refrain from adding anything to the situation, even when they are asked to by other parties involved. They shall remain personally uninvolved and leave the responsibility of the outcome to those for whom they are facilitating communication.

Interpreters shall accept only those assignments for which they are qualified.

Interpreters shall be fluent in both the language of the interviewer (or examiner) and the child and/or family members being interviewed (or tested). Interpreters shall have expertise in translating and have a basic understanding of the assessment process.

Interpreters shall request compensation for services in a professional and judicious manner.

Interpreters shall have knowledge about fees that are appropriate to the profession and shall be informed about the current fee schedule of the national interpreter organization.

Interpreters shall function in a manner appropriate to the situation.

Interpreters shall conduct themselves in a manner that brings respect to themselves, the child and/or family members being interviewed or examined and the professions or institutions of all involved.

Interpreters shall strive to further their knowledge and skills through participation in workshops, professional meetings, interactions with professional colleagues, and/or reading of current literature in the field.

CHAPTER 3

Child Clinical Interviews
Activities, School, and Peer Relations

To conduct a comprehensive assessment, clinical interviews should cover a variety of areas that can impact children's functioning, including intrapersonal functioning, family relationships, peer relationships, school adjustment, and community involvement (Merrell, 2008a). Table 3.1 lists six broad content areas for child clinical interviews along with more specific topics within each area. The SCICA (McConaughy & Achenbach, 2001) provides a standardized format for covering these content areas with children ages 6–18. The SCICA protocol lists open-ended questions for each topic and provides space for interviewers to record notes of their observations of children's behavior and children's self-reports during the interview. The SCICA protocol also includes questions regarding parent- and teacher-reported problems and optional screening procedures to assess academic achievement and fine and gross motor skills of 6- to 11-year-old children.

The SCICA was designed to fit a multimethod assessment model, as shown in Table 1.2 in Chapter 1. To dovetail with other ASEBA instruments, the SCICA has structured rating forms on which interviewers rate their observations of children's behavior during the interview and rate children's own reports of their problems. Interviewers' ratings are then scored on a standardized profile of problem scales similar to profiles developed for other ASEBA instruments for school-age children, including the CBCL/6–18 (hereafter called CBCL), TRF, and YSR. The problem scales for the CBCL, TRF, YSR, and SCICA profiles were developed from data on large samples of children who were referred for mental health services and/or special services in schools. The SCICA rating forms and scoring profile provide quantitative scores for identifying patterns of children's problems and judging the severity of those problems relative to samples of other clinically referred children. Chapter 8 describes the SCICA rating forms and scoring profile in detail. You can learn more about the SCICA and other ASEBA forms by visiting the ASEBA website *(www.ASEBA.org)* or e-mailing the ASEBA research staff *(mail@ASEBA.org)*.

The SCICA was designed as a comprehensive child clinical interview for mental health assessments and research. In some cases, you may not want to cover all of the topics included in the SCICA. For example, school-based practitioners may want to limit their interviews to topics relevant to children's academic and social functioning and not delve into more personal matters related to the home situation and family or other issues related to functioning outside of school. To

TABLE 3.1. Content Areas for Child Clinical Interviews

I. Activities and interests

    Favorite activities
    Sports, hobbies, organizations
    Chores/job

II. School and homework

    Best liked things about school
    Least liked things about school
    Grades
    Homework
    Relations with school staff
    Worries about school
    School problems

III. Friendships and peer relations

    Number of friends
    Activities with friends
    Peers liked and disliked
    Social problems with peers (fights, being left out)
    Bullying and victimization
    Social coping strategies

IV. Self-awareness and feelings

    Three wishes
    Future goals
    Wishes for changes at home
    Feelings (happy, sad, mad, scared)
    Worries
    Strange thoughts or experiences
    Suicidal ideation

V. Adolescent issues (ages 12–18)

    Alcohol and drugs
    Antisocial behavior and trouble with the law
    Dating, romances, and sexual activity
    Sexual identity
    Cell phones, Internet, and social networking

VI. Home situation and family relations

    People in the family
    Rules and punishments
    Relationships with parents
    Relationships with siblings
    How parents get along
    Kinetic family drawing (ages 6–11)

facilitate such school-based assessment, Appendix 3.1 includes the Semistructured Student Interview (McConaughy, 2012), which includes questions covering the first four content areas listed in Table 3.1: activities and interests, school and homework, friendships and peer relations, and self-awareness and feelings. The Semistructured Student Interview does not include questions about the adolescent issues (Table 3.1, section V) or home situation and family relations (Table 3.1, section VI). Depending on your purpose, you can decide whether to use the reproducible protocol for the Semistructured Student Interview in Appendix 3.1 or the SCICA protocol and rating forms available from the ASEBA developers.

This chapter discusses the first three content areas for child clinical interviews listed in Table 3.1: activities and interests, school and homework, and friendships and peer relations. Chapter 4 discusses self-awareness and feelings and adolescent issues. Chapter 5 discusses home situation and family relations. All three chapters include sample interview questions for the various topic areas along with case illustrations of interviews with one or more of the five children introduced in Chapter 1. Relevant research findings are also reviewed to provide an empirical basis for judging the clinical significance of problems reported by children, parents, and teachers.

ACTIVITIES AND INTERESTS

Asking children to describe their favorite activities and interests is a good way to begin clinical interviews with them. These types of questions can be used as "warm-ups" to establish rapport before addressing potentially more sensitive issues, such as school functioning and peer relations. Discussing children's activities and interests can also provide some insight into their perceptions of their own competencies. You can then compare children's reports to similar reports from parents and teachers. Although this area of activities and interests may seem generally benign, validity studies for the CBCL have shown that clinically referred children score significantly lower on the Activities scale than do matched samples of nonreferred children (Achenbach & Rescorla, 2001).

> **Starting with open-ended questions about children's interests and activities is a good way to establish rapport at the beginning of clinical interviews.**

Table 3.2 lists sample questions for interviewing children about their activities and interests. It is not necessary to ask all the questions listed in this table. However, asking about video games, TV, and movies may reveal potential problems for children who spend a great deal of time in these activities at the expense of other physical activities and face-to-face social interactions. It is also good to ask children if they are responsible for performing chores at home and whether they receive an allowance or other forms of rewards in reeturn. Allowances can be especially useful as reward systems for behavioral interventions in the home setting. You can ask adolescents whether they have jobs outside of the home, and if so, how they feel about the job and their boss. All of these questions can provide insight into children's sense of responsibility and independence.

TABLE 3.2. Sample Questions about Activities and Interests

Activities and interests

What do you like to do for fun, like when you are not in school?

What are your favorite activities? What do like about _____?

What kind of music do you like? Who are your favorite musicians? What do you like about _____?

Do you play video games (e.g., PlayStation, Wii, DS)? Which ones are your favorites? Do you have video games at home? Are there any rules at home about when you can play video games or watch TV/movies?

What sports do you like? Are you on any teams?

What do you think you are best at? Tell me more about that.

Chores/jobs

Do you have any chores or jobs at home? Do you get them done?

Do you earn an allowance for chores at home? *If no*, would you like an allowance? What do you think would be a good plan for earning an allowance for chores at home?

For adolescents:
Do you have a job? Is it a paying job? How much do you earn per week?

How do you feel about your job? How do you feel about your boss?

Note. Adapted from McConaughy and Achenbach (2001) and McConaughy (2012). Copyright 2001 by Stephanie H. McConaughy and Thomas M. Achenbach and copyright 2012 by Stephanie H. McConaughy. Adapted by permission.

SCHOOL AND HOMEWORK

Assuming the length of the average school day is about 7 hours and at least 1 additional hour is required for homework, we can estimate that children devote about 50% of their waking hours each weekday to school. For children with academic, emotional, and behavioral problems, the large amount of time consumed by school can be particularly challenging. According to the 30th Annual Report to Congress on the Implementation of the Individuals with Disabilities Education Act (U.S. Department of Education, 2008), over 6 million students ages 6–21 experienced academic problems severe enough to warrant special education services. These represented 9.1% of the 2006 general school population, including 4.0% with a specific learning disability, 1.7% with a speech/language impairment, 0.9% with other health impairment (which can include ADHD), 0.7% with emotional disturbance, and 0.8% with intellectual disabilities. Among those students served under IDEA 2004, 44.6% had a specific learning disability, 19.1% had a speech/language impairment, 9.9% had other health impairments, 7.5% had emotional disturbance, and 8.6% had intellectual disabilities. These statistics represent only the most severe cases that required an individualized education program (IEP).

National surveys to develop the ASEBA school-age forms provide additional data on the prevalence of academic problems in 6- to 18-year-old children (Achenbach & Rescorla, 2001). For example, on the CBCL, parents reported "poor schoolwork" for 16–27% of nonreferred children in the normative sample and 59–72% in the clinically referred sample. Similarly, on the TRF, teachers reported "poor schoolwork" for 22–38% of nonreferred children and 62–81% of clinically referred children. Teachers also reported that 23–41% of nonreferred children and 63–78% of referred children were "underachieving, not working up to potential." These findings, coupled with the sheer amount of time spent on schoolwork, underscore the importance of addressing school experiences in child clinical interviews.

Table 3.3 lists sample questions that elicit children's views and attitudes toward school and homework. Table 3.4 lists sample questions about extracurricular school activities and relations with school staff, as well as children's worries about school and potential school problems. The initial, open-ended questions in Table 3.3 invite children to express both positive and negative thoughts and feelings about school. It is also good to ask children what they think they do best and what kind of schoolwork is hard for them. Follow-up questions can then probe for more detail, as needed, to understand children's perspectives on school issues.

For most children, homework is a necessary part of the school experience. Research studies have shown that homework has positive effects on students' academic performance and test scores (Keith & DeGraff, 1997). Research has also shown that the amount of homework completed, more than the amount of time spent on homework, is a key factor in promoting good academic achievement (Cooper, Lindsay, Nye, & Greathouse, 1998). As Lee and Pruit (1979) pointed out, homework can involve several different forms and purposes: practice assignments that review material presented in class; preparation assignments that introduce topics to be presented in future classes; extension assignments that facilitate generalization of concepts from familiar to unfamiliar contexts; and creative assignments that require integrating knowledge into new concepts or products. Homework can also help to develop children's study skills and work habits.

> **Homework has positive effects on academic performance and test scores. The *amount of homework completed* is most important in promoting good academic achievement.**

TABLE 3.3. Sample Questions about School and Homework

<u>School</u>

For children ages 6–11:
Let's talk about school.
What do you like best in school?
What do you like about _____?

What do you like the least in school?
What don't you like about _____?

How about the schoolwork?
What do you feel you are best at? How are you good at _____?
What do feel you are not so good at? What makes _____ harder for you?

For adolescents:
Let's talk about school.

What subjects/courses do you have this year?

Which subjects/courses do you like best?
What do you like about _____?

Which subjects/courses do like least?
What don't you like about _____?

Which subjects/courses do you feel you are best at?
How are you good at _____?

Which subjects/courses do feel you are not so good at?
What makes _____ harder for you?

What kind of grades do you get?
How about the hard subjects/courses. What grades do you get in those?
How do you feel about your grades?
How do your parents feel about your grades?

<u>Homework</u>

For all ages:
What about homework? Do you have homework every day or every week?
In what subjects/courses?

Do you usually get homework done on time?
What happens when you (or other kids) don't get homework done on time?

Do you have any trouble with homework?
If yes, What kind of trouble do you have?

Additional probes if trouble with homework:
Let's talk about how you do your homework.
When do you usually do homework? Is there a special time for it?
Where do you usually do your homework (e.g., in your room, at the kitchen table, in the living room watching TV)? Is there a place that works best for you?
How long do you usually work on homework each day?
Are there rules in your home about homework?

(continued)

TABLE 3.3. *(continued)*

A lot of teachers give assignments that are due much later (e.g., at the end of the week or 2 or 3 weeks later). How do those kind of assignments work out for you?
Do you get them done on time?
How do you do them (e.g., do you do a little bit each day or do you wait until later to start them)?

Does anyone help you with your homework or schoolwork?
How does that work out, having _____ help you?
If you had your way, what would help you the most?

How would you feel about having another kid/student help you in school?

How would you feel about having a teacher or another adult help you?

If you got help, where would be a good place to get it (e.g., in class, in study hall, in a private place where there are no other students around)?

When would be the best times for getting help with your schoolwork?

How would you feel about having extra time at school to get help with your work (e.g., staying after school or coming in early)?

Note. From McConaughy and Achenbach (2001) and McConaughy (2012). Copyright 2001 by Stephanie H. McConaughy and Thomas M. Achenbach and copyright 2012 by Stephanie H. McConaughy. Reprinted by permission.

TABLE 3.4. Sample Questions about School Activities and Relations with School Staff

School activities

Are you involved in any special activities in school (e.g., art, dance, music, clubs, teams)?
(If yes) What are they? Which ones do you like the best?
How much time do you spend at those activities?
(If no) Are there any special activities or teams that you would like to be in?
What keeps you from getting into _____?

Relations with school staff

Let's talk about your teachers.
Which teacher do you like best? What do you like about _____?

Which teacher do you like least? What don't you like about _____?

How do you feel about the principal/assistant principal?
Is there anyone at school who is special/very important to you?

Do you ever worry about school?
What do you worry about?

Do you ever get into trouble at school?
What kind of trouble?

If you could change something about school, what would it be?

Note. From McConaughy and Achenbach (2001) and McConaughy (2012). Copyright 2001 by Stephanie H. McConaughy and Thomas M. Achenbach and copyright 2012 by Stephanie H. McConaughy. Reprinted by permission.

Despite its potential academic benefits, homework creates problems for many children. Failure to complete homework is a frequent contributor to poor or failing grades at school (Cooper et al., 1998). Homework difficulties can also create conflicts between parents and children (Daniel, Power, Karustis, & Leff, 1999) and undermine collaboration between parents and teachers (Buck et al., 1996). Problems with homework can arise for various reasons: The directions for assignments may be unclear; the assignments may be too difficult; the assignments may be too tedious or too time consuming; children may lack organizational skills for completing homework assignments on their own; or it may be hard to find the right place and time to do homework assignments, given other competing activities in children's lives. Homework can be especially challenging for children who have ADHD and/or learning disabilities (Power, Karustis, & Habboushe, 2001) as well as for children who have behavioral and emotional problems.

Along with questions about positive and negative aspects of school, Table 3.3 lists specific questions that interviewers can ask about homework. These questions elicit children's perspectives on homework, their strategies for completing it, and any problems they might have with it. When children report trouble with homework, you can ask additional probe questions about when and where they do their homework, how long it usually takes, and whether the family has any rules about homework (e.g., no TV or video games until homework is done). Several additional questions explore children's attitudes about receiving help with homework and what form of help (e.g., peer tutoring) might be acceptable to them. Such information can be especially useful for designing individual interventions to improve homework completion and accuracy (Power et al., 2001). You can gather additional information about homework problems in parent and teacher interviews and by asking parents and teachers to complete rating scales about children's homework behavior, such as the Homework Performance Questionnaire (Power, Dombrowski, Watkins, Mautone, & Eagle, 2007).

> **Questions about homework can elicit children's attitudes toward it, what strategies they use, and what types of interventions might be most effective to improve completion and accuracy.**

Case Example: Andy Lockwood

Box 3.1 shows a segment from the school psychologist's discussion about school with 7-year-old Andy Lockwood, who was introduced in Chapter 1. Despite repeating first grade, Andy was still struggling with basic skills. Andy disliked everything in school, except nonacademic activities that were fun. If he had his way, Andy would avoid school altogether and just stay home. It was clear from even this short interview segment that Andy had a negative attitude about school. The interview also raised questions as to whether a learning disability or some other problem might be impeding Andy's academic progress. Even with special help, Andy still found schoolwork hard, particularly reading. When the school psychologist probed further, Andy could not explain exactly what about the work was so hard.

The school psychologist continued the interview by querying Andy about homework, as illustrated in Box 3.2. From this interview segment, it became clearer that Andy felt overwhelmed by schoolwork. He said, at one point, he even had homework in the summer that was left over from his last year in first grade. The interview also revealed that, at least from Andy's perspective, there were no consequences when he failed to complete his schoolwork. Instead, Andy said that his mother threw away last year's homework and that his current teacher forgets about homework.

BOX 3.1. Talking with Andy about School

INTERVIEWER: Let's talk about school. What do you like best in school?

ANDY: I don't know. I like the . . . ah, what are those? . . . I like the holidays.

I: Oh, the holidays? The holidays are the times you're not in school.

A: Yeah. We have parties. (*Smiles, squirms in seat a little.*)

I: Uh-huh. Oh, that's what you mean. You're in school, but you have parties.

A: Yeah.

I: Do you mean Halloween and stuff?

A: Yeah.

I: So you like holidays, you like the parties and stuff. What about the regular school stuff like math, reading, recess?

A: Recess.

I: Uh-huh. OK.

A: You get to go out and play a lot.

I: So you like going out and playing.

A: Yeah. You know those little miniature ATVs for kids my size?

I: Hmm.

A: Those things that are all plastic, and they have a battery that goes inside?

I: You mean the kind you can ride on?

A: Yeah.

I: All-terrain vehicles, is that what you mean?

A: Yeah. Like those Bigfoots, and they're old-fashioned and car-like. I want one of the ATVs a lot, or a Bigfoot.

I: Do you have one?

A: No. (*Frowns.*) All I have is a bike.

I: What made you think about that? We were talking about recess.

A: I don't know.

I: You were just thinking of something you like.

A: Yeah. (*Squirms in seat, fidgets with clothing a bit.*)

I: Those sound pretty neat. Well, what are some things you *don't* like in school?

A: Oh. There are lots of things. (*Smiles.*)

I: OK. What are they?

A: School.

I: (*Chuckles.*) School. School in general, huh? Sounds like you're not too wild about school.

A: No. I like staying home.

I: Oh. Well, what don't you like about school?

A: Mmm . . . it's just no fun! I don't like to have to do all that work and stuff. I just want to get up and play with my friends a lot and have them be home so I can be home and be with them.

(continued)

I: So you think that you have a lot of work to do?

A: A lot!

I: Did you have more work this year than last year? Or did you always have a lot of work?

A: Alllways! (*Draws out word for emphasis.*)

I: Always a lot, huh? Mmm. Is the work easy or hard?

A: Hard.

I: Mmm. Tell me what's hard.

A: (*Shrugs, pauses.*) But one of the things that is easy is 100 + 100. It's 200. (*Smiles.*)

I: So 100 + 100 is easy. How about other plusses and take-aways?

A: Easy. Math is easy.

I: All of math is easy?

A: Yeah. I said math is easy.

I: OK. I wasn't sure.

A: Most of it.

I: Uh-huh. So math is easy. So what is hard for you then?

A: Hard for me . . . ? (*Looks confused.*)

I: You said some things were hard . . . I was wondering what was hard.

A: Oh. Lots of things. (*Looks around room, swings feet.*)

I: Can you give me an example?

A: Mmm . . . I don't know. There's things that are hard.

I: How about reading? Is that easy or hard?

A: Kind of hard and kind of easy. (*Pauses.*) Half easy, half hard.

I: OK, so reading is sort of half and half. Sounds like just doing all the work is hard.

A: Yeah.

Obviously, the school psychologist will need more information from other sources to clarify the nature of Andy's academic problems. Nonetheless, these interview segments suggest that school interventions for Andy might include a restructuring of assignments and the amount of work required as well as provision of positive behavioral supports and incentives to improve his motivation and productivity.

FRIENDSHIPS AND PEER RELATIONS

Friendships and peer relations play critical roles in children's social–emotional development (Bierman, 2004; Bierman & Welsh, 1997; Parker, Rubin, Price, & DeRosier, 1995). Friendships involve mutual, dyadic relationships that are not the same as mere acceptance in the peer group. Popular children tend to have more close friends than rejected children. However, some popular children may not have any close friends, and some rejected children may have one or more close friends (Parker & Asher, 1993).

BOX 3.2. Talking with Andy about Homework

INTERVIEWER: How about homework? Do you get homework?

ANDY: Yes.

I: How much homework do you usually have?

A: A lot!

I: A lot. How much is a lot?

A: I still have homework from last year when I was in school that started that year. (*Makes face.*)

I: I don't understand. Do you mean you still have homework from last year when you were in school?

A: Yeah, for last year when we were in school with my other teacher. You know, like near the end of the year, last year, when we were in school.

I: Did you do that homework?

A: No, we threw that away.

I: Oh?

A: Because my mom didn't want me to do it. It was too far back.

I: Oh, so you threw that homework away. What about this year? Do you have homework this year that you have to finish at home?

A: Yes. (*Squirms restlessly in seat.*)

I: Do you get it done?

A: No. Not very much.

I: Uh-huh. OK. What happens when you don't get it done?

A: Nothing.

I: You don't get into trouble or anything?

A: No.

I: Oh, OK. Tell me more about that.

A: She just forgets about it. (*Squirms in seat.*)

I: The teacher forgets about it?

A: Yeah.

I: What about your mom? What does she say about the homework?

A: She says try . . . (*pause*) . . . but I don't have to do it.

I: OK. So nothing happens when you don't do your homework.

A: Yeah.

I: OK. Now, were you in first grade last year?

A: I stayed back.

I: Oh, you stayed back . . . you mean, in first grade this year. How do you feel about that?

A: She was mean, the teacher from last year. She was mean.

I: What was mean about her?

A: I don't know. She was just mean. (*Looks slightly unhappy.*)

I: So now you have a new teacher. What do you think about her? I won't tell her what you say.

(continued)

A: She's nice. (*Smiles.*)

I: Oh, OK. What makes her nice?

A: I don't know . . . she doesn't yell.

I: Anything else about her?

A: I don't know.

I: You told me you stayed back this year. I was wondering what you thought about staying back. Did you think that was a good idea or not a good idea?

A: I didn't mind. (*Looks around room.*)

I: Hmm. Was it easier for you?

A: (*Brightens.*) Yeah, *much* easier. And I have a good chance of passing this year.

I: Oh, you do? OK.

Bierman and Welsh (1997) cited three qualities that distinguish friendships from mere peer-group status: similarity, reciprocity, and commitment. Friends are often similar in age, gender, and socioeconomic status, though there can be exceptions to any of these characteristics. Reciprocity involves the give-and-take of friendships. For young children, reciprocity is concrete: Friends like the same things, play games together, share toys, take turns, and do not hit or call names. For adolescents, reciprocity becomes more abstract and psychological: Friends share their intimate thoughts and feelings as well as interests and activities, and are loyal, trustworthy, and sincere.

As children get older, peer groups become increasingly important influences on the way they behave, think, and feel in social situations. On the positive side of the picture, developmental research has shown significant associations between positive peer relations and good social adjustment (Bierman, 2004). Social interactions with peers provide an arena for development of many important social skills. For elementary-age children, peer interactions offer opportunities to learn reciprocity and perspective taking, cooperation and negotiation, and social norms, conventions, and problem solving. For adolescents, good peer relations can support the development of self-identity and autonomy.

> **Research has shown that positive peer relations are significant predictors of good social adjustment, whereas poor peer relations are significant predictors of social maladjustment.**

On the negative side of the picture, poor peer relations can be a strong predictor of concurrent and future social maladjustment (Bierman, 2004; Bierman & Welsh, 1997; Parker et al., 1995). In addition, poor peer relations can contribute to stress, feelings of loneliness, poor self-worth, anxiety, depression, and antisocial behavior. Research has also shown a strong association between social maladjustment and hostile attribution biases (Crick & Dodge, 1994). That is, socially rejected and aggressive children tend to attribute hostile intent to peers (e.g., "He bumped into me on purpose"), which often leads to fights and other negative social interactions.

Although poor peer relations are potent "markers" for maladaptive social–emotional development, Bierman and Welsh (1997) cautioned that "it has not been clear whether poor peer relations are simply the effects of other disorders or whether they play an active role in exacerbating negative developmental trajectories" (p. 329). For example, Bierman and colleagues found that aggressive children who were rejected by peers demonstrated severe attention deficits, emotional dysregulation, and internalizing problems more often than did aggressive, nonrejected children (Bierman, Smoot, & Aumiller, 1993). Other problems may thus contribute to peers' rejection of some aggressive children, but not others. Coie (1990) has also argued that being deprived of positive peer relations may inhibit the development of the prosocial skills and empathy that promote good social adjustment.

Risk Factors for Peer Rejection

The findings from clinical and developmental research underscore the importance of focusing on children's friendships and peer relations in clinical assessments. Peer rejection is particularly important to assess, as are prosocial skills that lead to peer acceptance. Research has shown a strong association between peer rejection and aggressive behavior among children of all ages (Coie, Dodge, & Kupersmidt, 1990). However, not all aggressive children are rejected by their peers. As Bierman (2004) pointed out, aggressive behavior can take on different forms, including physical aggression intended to inflict bodily harm on someone (e.g., hitting, kicking), verbal aggression intended to derogate or control another person (e.g., yelling, insulting, threatening), and social aggression (or relational aggression) intended to cause embarrassment or loss of social

> Not all children who are aggressive are socially rejected. Children who are more emotionally reactive and aggressive when threatened are more likely to be rejected.

standing to someone (e.g., spreading rumors, tattling, cheating in a game). Some children ("effective aggressors") can control their aggressive behavior and use physical force or intimidation to gain dominance, lead others, or get their own way. These children often have the necessary social skills to establish friendships and gain peer acceptance. Other children ("ineffective aggressors") are more emotionally reactive and more likely to explode into a tantrum or become physically aggressive when they are threatened or assaulted by someone else. These children are more often rejected by peers and may become victims of harassment and bullying (Bierman, 2004; Perry, Perry, & Kennedy, 1992). A later section in this chapter discusses bullying and victimization in more detail.

To evaluate whether an aggressive child is also likely to be rejected by peers, Bierman and Welsh (1997) advised focusing on the following key risk factors:

- Does the child exhibit a wide range of conduct problems, including disruptive or hyperactive behavior or attention problems, as well as physical aggression?
- Does the child have deficits in positive social skills?
- Does the child have opportunities for positive peer interactions?
- Is the child a member of a deviant peer group, such as a gang, or does the child act aggressively alone, perhaps driven by feelings of injustice and/or need for revenge?
- Is the child's aggressive behavior physical and "instrumental" (i.e., done for a purpose; e.g., demonstrating physical superiority or warding off a fight), or is the child's aggressive behavior "reactive" (i.e., arises from poor control of emotional arousal and anger)?

Other risk factors appear to be associated with peer rejection combined with social withdrawal. Furthermore, some socially withdrawn or isolated children may be neglected by their peers, but not out rightly rejected. Neglected children may simply prefer solitary play or constructive and manipulative play that does not require social interaction. Children who are neglected by peers at one age may improve their status later, as they move into new peer groups or expand their interests. However, children who are socially withdrawn *and* rejected are less likely to improve their peer status (Coie & Kupersmidt, 1983). To evaluate whether a socially withdrawn child is also likely to be rejected, Bierman and Welsh (1997) advised focusing on the following risk factors:

> **Not all children who are socially isolated are socially rejected. Children who are socially withdrawn *and* rejected are least likely to be accepted later on.**

- Does the child tend to be reticent, anxious, and/or avoidant in social interactions (e.g., "hovering" on the edge of peer groups because he/she does not know how to enter into a group)?
- Does the child have low levels of positive social skills?
- Is the child ostracized for "odd" appearance, disabilities, or "atypical" social behavior?
- Is the child lonely or depressed, or does he/she have a negative perception of his/her social competence?
- Is the child a victim of teasing, harassment, or bullying by peers?

Interviewing about Friendships and Peer Relations

Clinical interviews offer good opportunities to assess children's perspectives on their friendships and peer relations. As discussed in Chapter 2, the nature of children's reports about social interactions will vary depending on their developmental level. Children's perspectives on their social relations may also be quite different from what their parents and teachers report. Differences in perspectives may indicate a lack of awareness of social problems by one or the other informant, which should be considered when planning interventions. Even when different informants agree that children have social problems, child clinical interviews can provide important insights into possibilities for addressing the problems.

Table 3.5 lists sample questions about friendships and peer relations for child clinical interviews. Initial questions elicit children's reports about activities with friends and their perceptions of liked and disliked peers. Later questions address possible social problems, including social isolation and fighting. The open-ended format of most questions encourages children to freely express their feelings and opinions about potentially sensitive issues. You can then follow up with probe questions to explore risk factors for poor peer relations or rejection, including physical aggression, limited social problem-solving skills, social anxiety, depression, or poor anger control.

> **Questions about peer relations should explore risk factors for poor relations, including aggression, social withdrawal, poor social problem solving, anger control, and anxiety or depression.**

Case Example: Bruce Garcia

Box 3.3 illustrates how 9-year-old Bruce Garcia responded to some of the interviewer's questions about his social interactions. Although Bruce was cooperative throughout the interview, he had difficulty expressing his ideas, and his conversation was sometimes loose and tangential. In response to initial questions about peer relations, Bruce expressed considerable distress about

TABLE 3.5. Sample Questions about Friendships and Peer Relations

Friends

How many friends do you have?
Do you think that is enough friends?
Are your friends boys or girls?
How old are your friends?

What do you do with your friends?
Do they come to your house?
Do you go to their house?
How often?

Tell me about someone you like.
What do you like about _____?

Tell me about someone you don't like.
What don't you like about _____?

Social problems

Do you have problems getting along with other kids?
What kinds of problems do you have?
What do you try to do about _____?

Do you ever feel lonely or left out of things?
What do you do when that happens?

Do you ever get into fights or arguments with other kids?
(*If yes*) Tell me more about that.
Are they yelling fights or hitting fights?
Does that happen with only one other kid or with a group of kids?
What usually starts the fights?
How do they usually end?
What are some ways you could solve that problem, besides fighting?

Do you have trouble controlling your temper?

Note. From McConaughy and Achenbach (2001) and McConaughy (2012). Copyright 2001 by Stephanie H. McConaughy and Thomas M. Achenbach and copyright 2012 by Stephanie H. McConaughy. Reprinted by permission.

other children's refusal to follow the rules of a game—a typical response for his age. However, it soon became apparent that Bruce's arguments during play situations sometimes deteriorated into physical fighting. His responses to follow-up questions about fighting painted a vivid picture of a child who was a victim of teasing and physical harassment by peers.

Unfortunately, Bruce also appeared to have limited social skills for coping with peer-related problems. The only solution he could imagine for the teasing he received at the bus stop was to ask an adult to intervene by giving the offenders a detention. However, Bruce did not think that would work very well. Bruce also appeared to have few, if any, positive friends in school. The one child he liked may have been a bad influence (Jamie, who "sneaks around like a robber"). Bruce could not name any other children who were friends. Coupled with poor social problem-solving skills, Bruce's confusion and odd mannerisms exhibited during the interview (indicated in italics) would put him at further risk for peer rejection and victimization.

BOX 3.3. Talking with Bruce about Peer Relations

INTERVIEWER: Tell me what you like to do for fun.

BRUCE: Play games. (*Makes odd movements, twitches, fidgets with clothes.*)

I: What kind of games do you like to play?

B: Marbles.

I: Tell me a little more about marbles.

B: I was playing . . . playing with Jason. He went first. He played a big marble. It has little designs on it. And I played my little one. It had blue on it. I played him, and I won. On the last game, I said "Keeps" . . . because there's no take-outs. Do you know what *take-outs* means? (*Gets up and wanders about the room while talking.*)

I: I'm not sure. What does it mean?

B: You can't take out the marble. If somebody wins, you can't take out the marble. You just can't keep your marble, because they've won it. That's what Jason did. (*Still standing, facing interviewer.*)

I: He took out his marble?

B: Yeah, and he wouldn't even give it. Because I won. (*Looks away.*)

I: Then what happened?

B: He got mad at me. He said, "It was funs," and I said, "It was keeps." We both said it was "keeps," and then at the end of the game, he said it was "funs." (*Sits down in chair.*)

I: What did you think about that?

B: I thought he was out of his mind, because I won, and he just didn't want to lose that game. (*Looks intensely at interviewer, then looks away.*)

I: What did you do about it when Jason took his marble and said it was "funs" instead?

B: I got mad at him, and he was irked. (*Gets up and paces around the room.*)

I: You got mad at him? What happens when you're mad?

B: Well, he got mad at me first, because he thought it was "funs," and I thought it was "keeps," and he got so mad at me. It happened before when I let him have some of my marbles. I had to because I gave him the last marble, and he tried to steal my marbles. (*Still pacing while talking.*)

I: Did he get them?

B: Nope.

I: What did you do to keep him from getting them?

B: I told him you shouldn't. After that, I tried to get away from him. Get him away from me. (*Long pause.*) Sort of like a little fight . . . so I could get away from him.

I: What kind of little fight?

B: I mean, trying to get the kid away from me. I just had to fight him so he wouldn't get my marbles. I stuffed them away like this. (*Shows interviewer how he stuffed marbles into his pocket.*) And then after the fight was done, I yelled that he's a stealer, because he tried to steal my marbles. If I'd let him, he would've stolen my marbles. (*Comes back to chair and sits down; does not look at interviewer.*)

I: Sounds like you didn't let him. What kind of a fight was it? A yelling fight? A hitting fight?

B: A punch fight and a yelling fight. Both. (*Grimaces and makes odd face.*)

(continued)

I: Did anybody get hurt?

B: No. Definitely not. He's more than I am in pounds. (*Fidgets with string on pants.*)

I: But you fought anyway.

B: (*Long pause before answering.*) Yeah.

I: Do you get into fights with other kids?

B: Sometimes.

I: How much do you get into fights?

B: Not very often.

I: Like would you say every day?

B: No way! (*Looks around the room.*)

I: What do you mean "No way?" Do you mean, more than that or not as much as that?

B: Not as much as that.

I: Do you get into fights with kids other than Jason?

B: Yeah, sometimes. In the winter, I got into one. This one I think was a couple of days ago. I didn't start the fight. He just wanted to . . . (*pauses a long time to think*)—there were all kinds of kids *ganging up* on me because they didn't like me a lot. So Chuck thought I was real wimpy and then he jumped . . . *everyone* jumped on me and threw me to the ground. I was like this. (*Lies on floor, covers head, goes limp, then sits up.*)

I: So you were down like that? Then what happened?

B: And then Sam tried to kick me (*pauses, grimaces*) . . . tried to kick me in the stomach. And the second time, he did. And then they thought I would cry, and I didn't.

I: Does that happen? Do kids pick on you or gang up on you?

B: Not very often. Well, yeah, they pick on me. (*Looks sad.*)

I: Do you get teased?

B: No . . . yes. They pick on me . . . tease me . . . for no reason.

I: How do you feel when they gang up on you or tease you?

B: I felt that it wasn't very fair, because I didn't do anything to them to deserve it. (*Looks mad.*)

I: What do you do about it if somebody is picking on you?

B: I just stand there. (*Looks away, stares off into space.*)

I: What could you do if you didn't want them to pick on you? (*Bruce continues to stare off into space.*) Did you hear my question? What could you do the next time?

B: Get on the bus . . . get on the bus. (*Looks confused, stares blankly.*)

I: Does this happen when you're waiting for the bus?

B: Yeah. Waiting on the bus . . . 3 or 4 o'clock, or something. And riding on the bus . . . all I have to do is tell all of them to get detentions. For detentions they have to stay after school probably until 4 o'clock, and their mother has to pick them up.

I: Do you mean you could say to them, "You're gonna get a detention?" Or do you mean you'd tell a teacher?

B: No. I would just try to be last in line, so everybody would be on their seats. And all I'd have to do is tell the bus driver and ask him if he thinks they deserve a detention. I'd say, "Can you give them a detention? I want them to have it."

(continued)

I: Do you think that would work?

B: Probably . . . I don't think so, because some of the kids don't even *care* if they get detentions.

I: What else could you do?

B: (*Long pause*) I don't know.

I: So that's the only thing you've thought of so far? Asking the bus driver to give them a detention?

B: Yeah.

I: OK. Well let's talk more about the kids. Tell me about a kid that you like a lot. (*Long pause; Bruce does not respond.*) Is there somebody that you like a lot?

B: Uh . . . Jamie.

I: What do you like about Jamie?

B: Sometimes he does something daring. Like he tried to sneak so nobody would see him . . . what's it called—somebody who sneaks around? (*Shows facial tic, plays with hair, rocks back and forth in seat.*)

I: I'm not sure what you mean.

B: Robber. (*Rubs his arm back and forth in circles on the table.*)

I: Like a robber? Jamie sneaks around like a robber?

B: (*Continues to rub the table in circles.*) Yeah. I'm his partner and I do what he says. And he's really nice. And there's other fourth and fifth graders . . . they're both my friends too.

I: Is Jamie the one who's in fourth grade?

B: The kid that has a red jacket on I think is in fourth grade, and the one that has a blue jacket on is in fifth grade. (*Looks confused.*)

I: Do you know those kids' names?

B: No, I don't . . . (*pause*) I can't remember.

Case Example: Karl Bryant

The clinical interview with 12-year-old Karl Bryant, shown in Box 3.4, illustrates a very different pattern of poor peer relations compared to Bruce. Karl was more often the perpetrator than the victim of physical aggression. Karl engaged easily in conversation during the interview and was eager to talk about his problems. When he discussed his interests, he was happy and even charming, to the point of seeming overly confident about his abilities. Although Karl sometimes fidgeted with objects or his clothing, he was only slightly restless or distracted and showed little anxiety.

In the interview segment, Karl described physical fights at school with a sort of relish. He freely admitted that he initiated some of these battles to seek revenge for insults or to right some perceived injustice. As Karl described his fights, he became more and more agitated. He reported having a very bad temper and said that anger built up inside him until he blew up and lost control. Karl also seemed to have concerns about fairness at school that bordered on obsessional, but he did not accept any personal responsibility for his actions. An example was his story about attempting to "restrain" another child and feeling indignant when the teachers did nothing to stop other children from pushing him around. Karl showed no remorse or guilt for fighting or being cruel toward other children. In Karl's mind, everyone deserved exactly what they got from him.

BOX 3.4. Talking with Karl about Peer Relations

INTERVIEWER: Tell me a little more about how things go at school. Like, have you ever gotten into trouble at school?

KARL: Not lately.

I: In the past 6 months, have you gotten any detentions, or anything like that?

K: Just two. Maybe more, I don't remember.

I: Is it hard to remember?

K: Yeah. I don't keep track.

I: Well, what did you get two for?

K: See, that's another thing I want to talk to you about.

I: OK.

K: Mr. Smith, our principal, he says just because I get in a fight with somebody or a kid punches me in the head and gives me a bloody nose . . .

I: Uh-huh.

K: And I'm supposed to go and tell a teacher, and the teacher doesn't do a thing. (*Squirms in seat, looks angry.*) Well, I went back to that kid and I floored him. I threw him up against the wall. I was really furious. I was out of it. Everybody was trying to stop me, and I just wouldn't let up. And I pounded him, thinking because the teacher wouldn't do anything. So I just pounded the kid—I mean, I just lost it completely.

I: So then what happened?

K: I went into the office. They tried to sit me down, and I wouldn't—I just wanted to get him so bad. (*Voice gets louder and louder.*) The principal gave *me* a detention because he had to get one. (*Looks angry.*)

I: What do you mean "because *he* had to get one"?

K: His parents said that he needs a detention every morning, if he gets into a fight. Because he started it and everything, he got a detention, so I had to. That's baloney! (*Looks angry, loud voice.*)

I: What's baloney?

K: I mean, I get into a fight and I pound somebody, and the other person isn't so badly into it. When he just comes out and pushes me, I'll push him back. I get the worst rap. They get off easier. He says there are different punishments for different things that are done. Well, that's baloney! (*Loud voice*)

I: What do *you* think about that?

K: It's worthless. His *ways*. Everybody hates him. (*Looks intensely at interviewer; angry expression.*)

I: How do you feel about him—the principal?

K: I hate him! (*Loud voice, still angry*) Nobody likes him in the school, except the teachers.

I: Do you think . . . ?

K: (*Interrupts.*) Truthfully, I hate him. I don't like him at all.

I: Do you think he's fair or unfair?

K: He's not fair about anything! (*Looks angry.*)

I: So about this detention—was that fair or unfair?

(continued)

K: Definitely unfair! And then he gave me another detention for a kid by the name of Mike. He started a fight with me in school, and he thought he was Mr. Macho because he thought he was the strongest kid. Well, I proved him wrong. (*Looks smug, gestures with hands.*)

I: What did you do?

K: Just for restraining the kid . . . just for *restraining* him . . . because he tried to ram into me. You know, he put his shoulder on me and tried to hit me in the stomach. I picked him up right off the ground and put him on the ground until the teacher got there. I didn't even touch him for it. (*Squirms in seat, changes positions several times, gestures to stress his point.*)

I: Did you hit him?

K: No. I just restrained him. I just brought him to the ground and I held him there until a teacher came. (*Calmer voice*)

I: Uh-huh. And you didn't hit him or kick him or anything?

K: I didn't *touch* him. I just picked him up. All I did is, he came running, and I moved. (*Gets up to show move.*) I picked him up right by his shirt, and I set him on the ground, and I held him there. (*Shows how he set kid down.*)

I: So how hard did you set him on the ground? Did you knock him down?

K: No. I just grabbed him. He pushed *himself*, really, he pushed himself onto the ground. (*Calmer, quieter voice*)

I: Hmm . . . so that time, it sounds like you feel you didn't lose it like you did that first time.

K: Right.

I: So what was the difference? Why didn't you lose your temper that time like you did with the first time?

K: All I did was *restrain* him. (*Voice gets louder.*) He was trying to *hit* me, and he didn't. But the kid before had *hit* me. He'd been pushing me, throwing stuff at me—rocks, sticks. And the teacher wouldn't do *anything*. (*Loud voice*) Finally, he hit me in the head, right in the nose. (*Gestures to show punch in nose.*)

I: Oh, that's when you got that bloody nose, huh?

K: Yeah. And that's when I let loose on him.

I: What did you do then?

K: I really pounded the crap out of him.

I: So it sounds like when somebody does something to you, then you get really mad and it's hard to. . . .

K: (*Interrupts. Looks agitated.*) Not necessarily—it's just when a *teacher* won't do anything.

I: Oh. So *that's* the big thing? Is it when a teacher won't do anything?

K: Yeah—when the teacher won't do anything about it when they're pushing me. It's like, *why*? (*Gestures dramatically.*)

I: Uh-huh.

K: You know, it's like if somebody complains to them about me, or something (*Imitates teacher's sing-song squeaky voice*), "Oh, Karl, go sit up against the wall." You know. But if it's them doing something, "Oh, they won't do that again. Just leave them alone." (*Imitates teacher's voice again.*)

I: Oh, I think I get it now. So, what you think is that when you're doing stuff to other kids, the teacher will do something about it, but when they're doing it to you, the teachers don't do anything about it.

(continued)

K: Exactly! Exactly! (*Sighs and looks calmer.*)

I: And you don't think that's fair?

K: Yeah. And I will prevent that!

I: You'll prevent it?

K: Right. Like I have certain friends who get into a lot of trouble. They don't care if they get in trouble. I just tell them to go at it, because I don't need them to fight my battles.

I: So how is it that you'll prevent it?

K: I don't take it. The next time that person touches me, I *flog* 'em.

I: So you flog them.

K: Yeah. For instance . . . (*Pauses, looks suspicious*) . . . wait a minute, who are you going to tell all this to?

I: Tell what to?

K: What we're talking about. Are you going to tell the principal or my teachers?

I: This is a private talk. Remember what I told you in the beginning? I won't tell your parents or teachers what we talked about, unless you say it's OK . . . unless I think you're going to hurt someone else or someone has hurt you.

K: Well, you're not going to probably believe *this*, but I pinned a kid up in a tree. (*Grins, chuckles.*)

I: You pinned a kid up in a tree.

K: Me and another kid picked him right up, and we put him in a tree—a big pine tree. We stood up on the roof and we stuck him in the tree, on a branch. (*Looks pleased, smiles.*)

I: Uh-huh.

K: He kept ramming, ramming. He kept throwing a ball and hitting us with a whiffle ball bat. So I just said, "*Get up* there," and pushed him up in the tree. (*Gestures to show how he put the boy up in the tree.*) Because he was pushing us, you know.

I: And did he get hurt?

K: No. But he looked really scared and started crying.

I: What did you do when he started crying?

K: Nothing. We just made him stay up there.

I: Did anybody see that?

K: No. Thank goodness.

I: Thank goodness?

K: Because we really would have gotten into trouble.

I: And how did you feel afterward? Like, did you feel bad for making the kid cry?

K: No way! He deserved it—I won't take it!

I: Did you feel bad that you might get in trouble, like, if the teachers saw you?

K: No. Like I said, he deserved it. He pissed me off! (*Pauses, looks for reaction from interviewer.*) Well, I mean he got me mad. (*Pauses.*) He had it coming.

I: So it sounds like *fairness* is really important to you.

K: Yeah. I mean, because I don't care if I get in trouble. But when I get mad, I won't put up with . . . when somebody's bugging me. (*Pauses, looks worried.*) And I've got all kinds of worries about other things, other things. (*Pauses, uses sing-song voice.*) Like worrying about divorces, worrying about my future life, or something. (*Pauses, moves around in seat, grabs at shirt collar and shirt tails.*)

(continued)

I: Tell me about those worries.

K: Like I have problems with schoolwork and everything, and it's all built up in me, and when some-body hits me, I just lose it. All that anger comes out, and I just lose it. (*Looks agitated.*)

I: So are you trying to tell me that you're going around school worrying about divorce and your future life and stuff like that?

K: No. No! Just the *work*.

I: So it sounds like you have problems with schoolwork.

K: Right. My teacher *loads* it on, and I can't take it, and she *hollers* at me. She *screams* at me. (*Voice gets louder.*) She says *I* always do stuff, and nobody else does anything.

I: Like what kind of stuff?

K: Like she makes me stay after school for not doing my work, but not the other kids. So I get so much anger built up, I mean, it's like when somebody does something to me, that's it, I just lay 'em out. (*Looks agitated, angry, grabs at shirt.*)

I: So you just blow up when you get all this anger built up.

K: Yeah.

I: Well, how often do you feel that way, with all that anger?

K: Pretty often.

I: Would you say it's every day or every week?

K: I don't know.

I: Can you give me an idea?

K: It's just that it gets built up in me. I guess every week. Well *usually* every day. I mean, I think about things, and I can't take it. I've got to *shut my mouth* or else I get in trouble. (*Pauses, looks directly at interviewer.*) You know, by just firing right back. It's like my teacher is the bullet and I've got the trigger. (*Gestures with hand, as if holding a gun at interviewer; looks angry.*)

The two interview segments in Boxes 3.3 and 3.4 suggest that social skills interventions might help both Bruce and Karl improve their peer relations. However, the form of such interventions would have to be different for each boy. For Bruce, the focus should be more on developing social skills and coping strategies to reduce his vulnerability to teasing and bullying. For Karl, the focus should be more on anger control, aggression replacement training, and advancing his level of moral reasoning. Karl's statements at the end of the interview segment also suggested a need for further assessment of his risk for violence beyond the physical fighting he described in the interview. In Chapter 10, William Halikias discusses procedures for assessing violence threats and children's risk for violence.

BULLYING AND VICTIMIZATION

Over the past three decades, an extensive research literature has emerged on bullying and victimization among school-age children and adolescents. This literature offers some important lessons for evaluating children's behavior in the context of their social interactions. Most experts view bullying as a subset of aggressive behavior, though there is no clear consensus on an exact definition of bullying. Norwegian scholar Daniel Olweus, who was a pioneer in studying bullying, defined bullying as aggressive behavior that includes an imbalance of power between the perpetrator and the victim, is intentionally harmful, and occurs repetitively (Olweus, Limber, & Milhalic, 1999). The *imbalance of power* means that the bully is usually stronger than the victim in some way (e.g., physically bigger or stronger) or has higher status among peers (e.g., more popular, smarter) (Swearer, Espelage, & Napolitano, 2009).

Researchers have identified different forms of aggression, some of which are considered to be bullying, whereas others are not. Dodge (1991) made the distinction between *proactive* aggression versus *reactive* aggression. Proactive aggression (or instrumental aggression) is a form of bullying because it includes behavior directed at a victim to obtain a desired outcome, such as gaining property, power, or affiliation. By contrast, reactive aggression is not a form of bullying because it arises from anger or frustration on the part of the perpetrator as a result of an aversive event or action of someone else. Others have made distinctions between *direct* (overt) aggression versus *indirect* (covert)

> **Bullying includes an imbalance of power, is intentionally harmful, occurs repetitively, can be overt or covert aggression and physical or nonphysical relational aggression.**

aggression (Olweus, 1993; Crick, 1995), both of which can be forms of bullying. Direct (overt) aggression includes physical fighting (e.g., pushing, shoving, kicking) and verbal threatening behavior (e.g., name-calling, teasing) that involves a face-to-face confrontation. Indirect (covert) aggression includes verbal aggression that is not face-to-face and involves a third party (e.g., rumor spreading).

Finally, Crick and colleagues coined the term *relational aggression* to describe nonphysical aggression in which the perpetrator manipulates or harms the victim's social standing or reputation within the peer group (Crick & Grotpeter, 1995; Crick et al., 2007). Relational aggression can be direct, such as when peers indicate they will no longer be a person's friend if that person does not do what they say, or indirect, such as when peers spread rumors behind a person's back so that others will not like that person. Relational aggression (e.g., social isolation, rumor spreading) is a subtler form of bullying than physical aggression. The increased use of cell phones, text messaging, e-mail, and social network sites on the Internet has opened new venues for relational aggression, now referred to as *cyberaggression* (Williams & Guerra, 2007)

Prevalence of Bullying and Victimization

As Swearer, Espelage, and Napolitano (2009) pointed out, bullying and victimization do not fall into simple "either–or" roles for children. Although some individuals might act primarily as bullies and others are usually victims, many children move in and out of different roles, sometimes acting as the bully, sometimes being the victim, and other times acting as a bystander. With this role fluidity in mind, Swearer and colleagues view bullying and victimization as involving dynamic

> **Bullying is not a "normal" part of growing up. Bullying peaks in middle school grades, but also occurs among elementary and high school students.**

social relationship problems that depend on the social–ecological circumstances or contexts surrounding the behavior (e.g., aggression at home, peer groups that bully, lack of supervision in school settings). Research has also shown that bullying is not a "normal" part of growing up. Although bullying seems to peak in the middle school years, forms of bullying also occur among elementary and high school students.

The exact prevalence of bullying and victimization is hard to estimate because research studies have used different measures and different definitions of bullying. Nonetheless, there is good evidence that bullying is relatively common in American schools. A 1998 survey of 15,686 American students in grades 6–10 found that 30% reported frequent involvement in bullying or victimization, with 13% reporting bullying others, 11% reporting frequently being a victim of bullying, and 6% reporting being both a bully and a victim (Nansel et al., 2001). A 2006 web-based survey of 15,185 students in grades 4–12 found that 41% of students reported frequent involvement in bullying or victimization (two or more times in the past month), with 8% reporting bullying others, 23% reporting being a victim of bullying, and 9% reporting being both a bully and a victim (Bradshaw, Sawyer, & O'Brennan, 2007).

The Bradshaw et al. (2007) study was especially interesting because they surveyed both students and school staff ($N = 1,547$) and reported separate findings for elementary school (grades 4 and 5), middle school (grades 6–8), and high school (grades 9–12). Their results revealed significant discrepancies between student and staff perceptions of the prevalence of bullying and victimization. When school staff members were asked, "What percentage of students do you think have been bullied two or more times during the past month?", over 70% estimated that 15% or fewer students had been bullied. Over 70% of elementary staff, 40% of middle school staff, and 57% of high school staff estimated that 10% or fewer of students had been bullied. By contrast, prevalence rates of frequent victimization reported by students were 34% for elementary school, 33% for middle school, and 23% for high school.

Bradshaw et al. (2007) also reported findings on specific aspects of bullying and victimization, including the location of bullying, perceived reasons for bullying, and responses to bullying. Students at all three levels reported that the most common reason for being bullied was for the way they "look, talk, or dress." Table 3.6 shows the percent of students in elementary, middle, and high school reporting different forms of victimization. The most common form of victimization reported by students was

> **Students report higher rates of student victimization from bullying than reported by teachers in all grades.**

TABLE 3.6. Forms of Victimization Reported by Students

Form of victimization	Percent Reporting Victimization		
	Elementary school	Middle school	High school
Direct verbal			
Name-calling	41	44	31
Threats	21	27	24
Teasing	43	43	36
Sexual comments or gestures	Not asked	24	24
Direct physical			
Push or shove	28	32	24
Hit, slap, or kick	21	29	22
Steal belongings	20	27	22
Indirect or relational			
E-mail or blogging	3	10	11
Spreading rumors or lies	37	36	24
Leaving out	30	29	24

Note. From Bradshaw, Sawyer, and O'Brennan (2007). Copyright 2007 by the National Association of School Psychologists. Bethesda, MD. Reprinted with permission of the publisher. *www.nasponline.org.*

direct verbal bullying (e.g., name-calling, teasing), followed by relational aggression (e.g., spreading rumors or lies and leaving out), and then direct physical aggression (e.g., pushing and shoving).

Approximately 70% of students and school staff in the Bradshaw et al. (2007) survey reported having witnessed bullying within the past month. Middle school students and staff were more likely to have witnessed bullying than elementary and high school students and staff. Students and staff were also asked what they did when they witnessed bullying. As shown in Table 3.7, 35–40% of middle and high school students said that they ignored it or did nothing, and 25% said that they tried to stop it. Only 6–11% reported the incident to an adult. Surprisingly, 12–13% said that they would join in the bullying. When asked about retaliation, 73–76% of middle and high school students felt it was OK to hit someone who had hit them first, compared to only 35% of elementary school students.

Bradshaw et al. (2007) found large discrepancies between students versus school staff in their perceptions of how school staff intervened in bullying and whether the interventions were effective. Table 3.8 shows how school staff said that they responded to bullying. Very few staff reported ignoring bullying or doing nothing. Large percentages said that they intervened with the bully or the victim. Over 86% of school staff believed that they had effective strategies for handling a bullying situation. By contrast, upon reporting bullying to an adult at school, 34% of middle school students and 26% of high school students felt that school staff did nothing to follow up, and over 50% of students reported that they had "seen adults in school watching bullying and doing nothing." Moreover, 62% of middle school students and 57% of high school students believed that school staff made the situation worse when they intervened.

Predictors of Bullying and Victimization

Bradshaw et al. (2007) reported that over 50% of middle school students and staff and over 30% of high school students and staff thought bullying was a moderate or serious problem in their school. The seriousness of bullying and victimization was also underscored by findings in a report of the U.S. Secret Service from an interview-based investigation of friends, families, and neighbors of 41 school shooters between 1974 and 2000 (Vossekuil, Fein, Reddy, Borum, & Modzeleski, 2002). Although the Secret Service did not establish a clear profile of school shooters, one commonality that did emerge was that 71% of shooters had been victims of a bully. This finding does not mean that students who are victims of bullying are likely to become perpetrators of such extreme vio-

TABLE 3.7. Middle and High School Student Responses to Witnessing Bullying

Student response	Percent middle school	Percent high school
Ignore it or do nothing	35	40
Try to stop	25	25
Join in	12	13
Report it to an adult in school	11	7
Report it to a parent	11	7
Tell another student	16	10

Note. From Bradshaw, Sawyer, and O'Brennan (2007). Copyright 2007 by the National Association of School Psychologists, Baltimore, MD. Reprinted with permission of the publisher. *www. nasponline.org.*

TABLE 3.8. School Staff Responses to Witnessing Bullying

	Percent Reporting Response		
Staff response	Elementary school	Middle school	High school
Ignored it or did nothing	1	4	4
Intervened with bully	74	86	61
Intervened with victim	68	79	52
Talked to other staff	51	60	29
Talked to an administrator	37	63	27
Referred to guidance counselor or school psychologist	42	53	18
Talked to bully's parents	24	18	9
Talked to victim's parents	19	17	8

Note. From Bradshaw, Sawyer, and O'Brennan (2007). Copyright 2007 by the National Association of School Psychologists, Baltimore, MD. Reprinted with permission of the publisher. *www.nasponline.org.*

lence, but it does raise concerns about assessing children's experiences with bullying and victimization and making schools safer places where all students feel protected and valued (Espelage & Swearer, 2003).

Although no simple conclusions can be drawn to predict who will become a bully or a victim or both, and under what circumstances, some trends have emerged from research that can be helpful to mental health practitioners and school psychologists as they evaluate children with such problems. Of particular interest is a meta-analytic study by Cook, Williams, Guerra, Kim, and Sadek (2010) who examined the relative strength (effect sizes) of individual characteristics and contextual variables for predicting bullying and victimization among nondisabled children in kindergarten through 12th grade. From 1,622 studies published between 1970 and 2006, they selected 153 English language studies that focused on predictors of bullies, victims, and bully/victims and that included quantitative information that could be computed into effect size estimates (Pearson correlation coefficients). The individual predictors included externalizing behavior, internalizing behavior, social competence, self-related cognitions, other-related cognitions, and academic performance. Contextual predictors included family/home environment, school climate, community factors, and peer status.

Cook et al. (2010) identified several individual and contextual predictors of the three groups (bully, victim, bully/victim) that are relevant for prevention and intervention programs. Of most interest are those predictors that showed at least medium effect sizes (correlations above .29). The strongest individual predictors of *being a bully* were high externalizing behavior and negative other-related cognitions, and the strongest contextual predictor was negative peer influence. The strongest individual predictor of *being a victim* was low social competence, and the strongest contextual predictor was negative peer status. High internalizing problems were the next strongest predictor of being a victim (correlation = .25). The strongest predictors of *being both a bully and victim* were negative self-related cognitions, low social competence, high externalizing behavior, and poor academic performance. The strongest contextual predictors of bully/victim status were negative peer influence, negative peer status, and negative school climate.

Cook et al. (2010) also reported some general trends and moderators of predictive associations. Boys tended to be more involved than girls as a bully, victim, or both bully/victim. Family/home environment, negative school climate, and community factors were influences on being a bully, victim, or bully/victim, though not always to the same degree. Another common predictor across the three groups was poor social problem-solving skills, but the effect sizes for social problem solving were small compared to other predictors. Age influenced the effects of the individual predictors on being a bully, but in different ways. Externalizing behavior was more strongly associated with being a bully in the childhood years than in adolescence, whereas internalizing behavior was more strongly associated with being a bully in adolescence than in childhood.

Considering all of the significant predictors, Cook et al. (2001) provided the following summaries of the characteristics of bullies, victims, and bully/victims:

- The typical *bully* is one who exhibits significant externalizing behavior, has internalizing symptoms, has both social competence and academic challenges, possesses negative attitudes and beliefs about others, has negative self-related cognitions, has trouble resolving problems with others, comes from a family environment characterized by conflict and poor parental monitoring, is more likely to perceive his or her school as having a negative atmosphere, is influenced by negative community factors, and tends to be negatively influenced by his or her peers.
- The typical *victim* is one who is likely to demonstrate internalizing symptoms, engage in externalizing behavior, lack adequate social skills, possess negative self-related cognitions, experience difficulties solving social problems, come from negative community, family and school environments, and be noticeably rejected and isolated by peers.
- The typical bully/victim is one who has comorbid externalizing and internalizing problems, holds significantly negative attitudes and beliefs about himself or herself and others, is low in social competence, does not have adequate social problem-solving skills, performs poorly academically, and is not only rejected and isolated by peers, but is also negatively influenced by the peers with whom he or she interacts. (pp. 75–76)

The above descriptions show the complexity of influences on bullying and victimization with several characteristics shared by all three groups. They also underscore the role that social context plays in the development and maintenance of bullying. Both individual and contextual variables need to be considered in evaluating children's involvement in bullying and victimization and in developing effective prevention and intervention strategies (Swearer et al., 2009).

Interviewing about Bullying and Victimization

As in the case examples of Bruce and Karl, children may spontaneously report experiences with bullying and/or being a victim of bullying when they are responding to open-ended questions about friends and peer relations. You can then ask more specific questions about these experiences, using some of the sample questions listed in Table 3.9 from the Semistructured Student Interview (Appendix 3.1). If experiences with bullying and victimization have not been discussed, you can use these same questions to broach the topic. As with other parts of the child clinical interview, you still need to follow the child's lead in the conversation and take care not to make this part of the interview seem like a drill or a series of accusations. Talking with perpetrators of bullying is likely to elicit strong emotions (anger, hatred) and perhaps some feelings of guilt or at least apprehension about possible punishments. Talking with victims of bullying is also likely to bring out strong emotions (sadness, anger) and feelings of helplessness. Some children may also feel that they are somehow at fault for causing others to bully them.

TABLE 3.9. Sample Questions about Bullying and Victimization

I would like know about bullying at your school. What do you think bullying is?

(Follow the child's lead to say:)
That's a good description. Bullying is when a kid who is stronger or more important tries to hurt or threaten another kid or puts that kid down. Bullying includes things like fighting, hitting, or shoving, or calling names, threatening, or teasing, or leaving someone out on purpose, or saying that you won't be another person's friend. It is not bullying when two kids who are both strong argue or fight with each other.

Is bullying a problem at your school?
(*If yes*) Tell me more about that.

Victimization

Has bullying been a problem for you?
(*If yes*) How is it a problem? What happens? Who bullies you?

What does _____ do to bully you?
What does _____ say/tease you about?
(*Probe*: What you wear? What you look like? The way you talk or act? Maybe he/she says "You're stupid" or "You're gay"?)
How does that make you feel?

What do you do when that happens?
(*Probe*: Tell a teacher/principal? Ignore/walk away? Call names back? Hit him/her? Make a plan to get back at him or her.)
Does that solve the problem for the next time?

What do the other kids do when _____ is bullying you?

If someone bullies you, do think it is OK to hit that person?

What else do you think you could do to solve that problem?

Bullying

How about you? Do you sometimes bully other kids?
(*If no*) Do you tease or pick on other kids?

(*If yes*)) Tell me more about that.
Who do you bully/pick on?
What do you do?
How you feel when you do that?

What do the other kids do when that happens?

What happens next? Does anyone get into trouble?

Are there any rules in your school or classroom about how kids are supposed to act toward each other?

What do you think would be good ways to solve the problem of bullying at your school?

Note. From McConaughy (2012). Copyright 2012 by Stephanie H. McConaughy. Reprinted by permission.

To begin, you can ask the child "What do you think bullying is?" This will start the discussion with the child's own view. After reflecting back the child's statements, you can state the general definition of bullying shown in Table 3.9 to ensure that both of you are thinking of the same types of behaviors. It is also important to clarify that bullying involves an imbalance of power between the bully and the victim, by stating, "It is not bullying when two kids who are both strong argue or fight with each other." You can then proceed to open-ended questions about victimization to learn details of what happened, what the child was bullied about, and what the child did or might do next time. Table 3.9 also lists open-ended questions about bullying behavior. These questions are likely to be more threatening to some children because of fears of punishment or disapproval from the interviewer. You also need to think about the limits of confidentiality and, when appropriate, inform the child about reporting obligations when there is an indication of danger to others.

> Interview questions about bullying and victimization can address the frequency, types of bullying experienced or witnessed, and strategies children use for coping with bullying.

Finally, a good way to close interviewing about bullying and victimization is to ask children, "What do you think would be good ways to solve the problem of bullying at school?" As shown in the Bradshaw et al. (2007) survey, children may have very negative perceptions of the effectiveness of certain school interventions. They may also have creative ideas about other possible solutions. In an interesting qualitative study, Cunningham, Cunningham, Ratcliffe, and Vaillancourt (2010) asked 62 Canadian students in grades 5–8 what they thought their schools were doing about bullying and what would be other ways to help stop bullying. The researchers used open-ended questions with small focus groups to encourage an exchange of ideas. The students offered a variety of suggestions for bullying prevention strategies, as shown in Table 3.10. Some strategies were endorsed by a majority of groups (e.g., organizing antibullying campaigns, posting antibullying reminders, and increasing monitoring and supervision), whereas others were endorsed by fewer groups (e.g., mandating school uniforms and informing parents).

The students' suggestions were grounded in their own perceptions and experiences and were quite practical. Many of their suggestions were also consistent with research findings on effective prevention. For example, for antibullying campaigns, students advised that presentations should never be too long so that kids don't space out and fail to listen; videos would be more engaging than just letting the principal or a teacher do the talking; police officers, in particular, might be especially effective because kids look up to them as people in charge; students might listen more to other students than to adults; antibullying posters should be placed where students will see them frequently (e.g., near the water fountain); and posters should focus on solutions and consequences, rather than just saying *"Don't bully!"* Students also had suggestions for improving peer relationships (e.g., making an effort to include new students or isolated students into a group) and promoting prosocial behaviors (e.g., teaching social skills and appropriate assertive responses to bullying).

SUMMARY

Child clinical interviews are essential components of most assessments of children's behavioral and emotional functioning. The flexibility of semistructured clinical interviews makes them well suited for obtaining children's views of their activities, feelings, and life circumstances. Both the SCICA

TABLE 3.10. Bullying Prevention Strategies Suggested by Student Focus Groups

Prevention strategies	Number of groups endorsing strategy
Organizational and structural approaches	
Increase monitoring and supervision	8
Organize recess activities	8
Mandate school uniforms	3
Restructure high-risk settings	8
Relational approaches	
Include isolated students	6
Restructure peer groups	6
Mobilize older student influences	7
Teach social skills	7
Improve parenting	5
Antibullying campaign	
Provide inclusive definitions	5
Organize antibullying presentations	11
Post antibullying reminders	9
Responding to bullying	
Encourage assertive responses	
Engage bystanders	5
Encourage reporting	7
Organize discussion groups	7
Give meaningful consequences	10
Inform parents	4

Note. Adapted from Cunningham, Cunningham, Ratcliffe, and Vaillancourt (2010). Copyright 2010 by Taylor & Francis Group, LLC. Reprinted by permission. *www.taylorandfrancis.com.*

(McConaughy & Achenbach, 2001) and the Semistructured Student Interview (McConaughy, 2012) in Appendix 3.1 provide standardized formats for child clinical interviews. This chapter discussed questions and strategies for interviewing children about their activities and interests, school and homework, friendships and peer relations, and experiences with bullying and victimization. Relevant research findings were discussed to guide interviewers in addressing these topics. Segments of clinical interviews with Andy Lockwood, Bruce Garcia, and Karl Bryant (all pseudonyms) illustrated the give-and-take of semistructured clinical interviews with children. Chapters 4 and 5 discuss additional questions and strategies for addressing other content areas shown in Table 3.1.

Semistructured Student Interview

Child's name _____ Age _____ Gender _____
First   Middle   Last

Interviewer's name _____ Date ____/____/____
First   Middle   Last   Month Day Year

CONFIDENTIALITY AND PURPOSE OF THE INTERVIEW

We are going to spend some time talking together, so that I can get to know you and learn about what you like and don't like. This is a private talk. I won't tell your parents or your teachers what you say unless you tell me it is OK. However, I would have to tell other people if you said you were going to hurt yourself, hurt someone else, or that someone has hurt you. Do you understand?

If the interview will be discussed at a meeting with parents and teachers and/or in a written evaluation report: Later I will be meeting with your parents and/or teachers to talk about what I learned about you. At the end of our talk today, we can discuss what I will say and how to say it. Do you understand?

I. ACTIVITIES AND INTERESTS	RESPONSES/OBSERVATIONS
What do you like to do for fun, like when you are not in school? What are your favorite activities? What do like about _____?	
What kind of music do you like? Who are your favorite musicians? What do you like about _____?	
Do you play video games (e.g., PlayStation, Wii, DS)? Which ones are your favorites? Do you have video games at home? Are there any rules at home about when you can play video games or watch TV/movies?	
What sports do you like? Are you on any teams? What do you think you are best at? Tell me more about that.	
Jobs/Chores Do you have any chores or jobs at home? Do you get them done? Do you earn an allowance for chores at home? (*If no*) Would you like an allowance? What do you think would be a good plan for earning an allowance for chores at home?	

(continued)

	RESPONSES/OBSERVATIONS

Jobs/Chores *(cont.)*

For adolescents:
Do you have a job? Is it a paying job? How much do you earn per week?
How do you feel about your job? How do you feel about your boss?

II. SCHOOL

For children ages 6–11:
Let's talk about school.
What do you like best in school?
What do you like about _____?

What do you like the least in school?
What don't you like about _____?

How about the schoolwork?
What do you feel you are best at? How are you good at _____?
What do feel you are not so good at? What makes _____ harder for you?

For adolescents:
Let's talk about school.
What subjects/courses do you have this year?

Which subjects/courses do you like best?
What do you like about _____?

Which subjects/courses do you like least?
What don't you like about _____?

Which subjects/courses do you feel you are best at? How are you good at _____?

Which subjects/courses do feel you are not so good at? What makes _____ harder for you?

What kind of grades do you get?
How about the hard subjects/courses: What grades do you get in those?
How do you feel about your grades?
How do your parents feel about your grades?

Homework

For all ages:
What about homework; Do you have homework every day or every week?
In what subjects/courses?

(continued)

Homework *(cont.)*	**RESPONSES/OBSERVATIONS**

Homework *(cont.)*

Do you usually get homework done on time?
What happens when you (or other kids) don't get homework done on time?

Do you have any trouble with homework?
(*If yes*) What kind of trouble do you have?

Additional probes if trouble with homework:
Let's talk about how you do your homework.
When do you usually do homework? Is there a special time for it?
Where do you usually do your homework (e.g., in your room, at the kitchen table, in living room watching TV)? Is there a place that works best for you?
How long do you usually work on homework each day?
Are there rules in your home about homework?

A lot of teachers give assignments that are due much later (e.g., at the end of the week or 2 or 3 weeks later). How do those kind of assignments work out for you?
Do you get them done on time?
How do you do them (e.g., do you do a little bit each day or do you wait until later to start them)?

Does anyone help you with your homework or schoolwork? How does that work out, having
_____ help you?
If you had your way, what would help you the most?

How would you feel about having another kid/ student help you in school?
How would you feel about having a teacher or another adult help you?

If you got help, where would be a good place to get it (e.g., in class, in study hall, in a private place where there are no other students around)?

When would be the best times for getting help with your schoolwork?

How would you feel about having extra time at school to get help with your work (e.g., staying after school or coming in early)?

(continued)

School Activities

Are you involved in any special activities in school (e.g., art, dance, music, clubs, teams)?
(If yes) What are they? Which ones do you like the best?
How much time do you spend at those activities?
(If no) Are there any special activities or teams that you would like to be in?
What keeps you from getting into _____?

Relations with School Staff

Let's talk about your teachers.
Which teacher do you like best? What do you like about _____?

Which teacher do you like least? What don't you like about _____?

How do you feel about the principal/assistant principal?
Is there anyone at school who is special/very important to you?

Do you ever worry about school?
What do you worry about?

Do you ever get into trouble at school?
What kind of trouble?

If you could change something about school, what would it be?

III. FRIENDSHIPS AND PEER RELATIONS
Friends

How many friends do you have?
Do you think that is enough friends?
Are your friends boys or girls?
How old are your friends?

What do you do with your friends?
Do they come to your house?
Do you go to their house?
How often?

Tell me about someone you like.
What do you like about _____?

Tell me about someone you don't like.
What don't you like about _____?

RESPONSES/OBSERVATIONS

(continued)

73

	RESPONSES/OBSERVATIONS

Social Problems

Do you have problems getting along with other kids?

What kinds of problems do you have?

What do you try to do about _____?

Do you ever feel lonely or left out of things?

What do you do when that happens?

Do you ever get into fights or arguments with other kids?

(*If yes*) Tell me more about that.

Are they yelling fights or hitting fights?

Does that happen with only one other kid or with a group of kids?

What usually starts the fights?

How do they usually end?

What are some ways you could solve that problem, besides fighting?

Do you have trouble controlling your temper?

Bullying and Victimization

I would like know about bullying at your school.

What do you think bullying is?

Follow the child's lead to say:

"That's a good description. Bullying is when a kid who is stronger or more important tries to hurt or threaten another kid or puts that kid down. Bullying includes things like fighting, hitting, or shoving, or calling names, threatening, or teasing, or leaving someone out on purpose or saying that you won't be another person's friend. It is not bullying when two kids who are both strong argue or fight with each other."

Is bullying a problem at your school?

(*If yes*) Tell me more about that.

Victimization

Has bullying been a problem for you?

(*If yes*) How is it a problem? What happens? Who bullies you?

What does _____ do to bully you?

What does _____ say/tease you about?

(*Probe*: What you wear? What you look like? The way you talk or act? Maybe he/she says "you're stupid" or "you're gay"?)

How does that make you feel?

(continued)

	RESPONSES/OBSERVATIONS

Victimization *(cont.)*

What do you do when that happens?
(*Probe*: Tell a teacher/principal? Ignore/walk away?
Call names back? Hit him/her? Make a plan to get
back at him/her?)

Does that solve the problem for the next time?

What do the other kids do when _____ is
bullying you?

If someone bullies you, do think it is OK to hit that
person?

What else do you think you could do to solve that
problem?

Bullying

How about you. Do you sometimes bully other
kids?
(*If no*) Do you tease or pick on other kids?

(*If yes*) Tell me more about that.
Who do you bully/pick on?
What do you do?
How do you feel when you do that?

What do the other kids do when that happens?
What happens next? Does anyone get into trouble?

Are there any rules in your school or classroom
about how kids are supposed to act toward each
other?
What do you think would be good ways to solve
the problem of bullying at your school?

IV. SELF-AWARENESS AND FEELINGS
Feelings

Tell me more about yourself.
What makes you happy?
What makes you sad? What do you do when you
are sad?
What makes you mad? What do you do when you
are mad?
What makes you scared? What do you do when
you are scared?

(continued)

75

Screening Questions for Anxiety, Depression, Suicidal Risk	**RESPONSES/OBSERVATIONS**
Do you feel unusually anxious or worried about things?	
(If yes) Tell me more about your worries.	
Have you ever felt very sad or depressed for a long period of time?	
(If yes) Tell me more about that.	
Have you ever been so sad that you wished you were dead?	
Have you been thinking about hurting yourself or killing yourself?	
Have you ever tried to harm or kill yourself?	
(If yes, probe for suicide plans, preparations, and available methods).	
How do you feel most of the time?	
What do you need the most?	
Wishes	
If you had three wishes, what would you wish for? Reasons for each?	
If you could change one thing about yourself, what would it be?	

Notes/Summary

CHAPTER 4

Child Clinical Interviews

Self-Awareness, Feelings, and Adolescent Issues

Chapter 3 discussed interviewing children about their activities and interests, school, and friends. These are familiar topics for most children and thus may be relatively easy to talk about, even when children have problems in these areas. This chapter moves into topics that are more sensitive and may be harder for some children to talk about: self-awareness and feelings and issues more specific to adolescents, including alcohol and drug use, antisocial behavior and trouble with the law, dating and romances, sexual activity, and sexual identity. It also discusses adolescents' use of digital communication (cell phones, Internet, and social networking sites) and problems that may create. Although these topics are presented in a certain sequence, you should feel free to change the sequence, as needed, to follow a child's lead in a conversation. If a child seems reluctant to discuss certain topics, you can switch to other topics and then return to the sensitive topics when the child seems more comfortable or more willing to discuss them. You can also save topics that are likely to be most sensitive for the end of your interview, so as not to jeopardize rapport for less sensitive topics.

SELF-AWARENESS AND FEELINGS

Clinical interviews provide good opportunities to assess children's degree of self-awareness and feelings. Goleman's (1995) theory of emotional intelligence provides a useful framework for interpreting children's responses to questions about self-awareness and feelings. Goleman described five main domains of emotional intelligence, each of which builds upon the other. The first domain is *knowing your own emotions*, or *self-awareness*, which is the ability to recognize a feeling in yourself as it happens. Goleman considered self-awareness to be the keystone to emotional intelligence. The next domain is *managing emotions*, which means handling or controlling your feelings so that they are

> Emotional intelligence develops in stages, each of which builds upon the other. Knowing your own emotions (self-awareness) is the beginning stage of emotional intelligence.

appropriate to the situation and do not become overwhelming. The third domain is *motivating yourself*, which involves marshaling your emotions to serve a specific goal. Sometimes this can take the form of "pumping yourself up" to achieve a goal, or it can mean controlling your emotions by delaying gratification or stifling impulsiveness in order to achieve a later goal. The fourth domain, *recognizing emotions in others*, involves thinking about what another person is thinking or feeling. This is often termed *empathy* and requires the ability to engage in recursive thinking, as discussed in Chapter 2. The fifth domain, *handling relationships*, involves managing your response to other people's emotions and usually requires the metacognitive ability to take a third-party perspective on social interactions (also discussed in Chapter 2).

In clinical interviews, you can routinely ask children about their feelings when discussing topics such as school, peer relations, and family relations. Interspersing questions about feelings is a good way to assess the first two domains of emotional intelligence: recognizing and managing feelings. You can also ask children direct questions that tap into their self-awareness and feelings, as shown in Table 4.1.

TABLE 4.1. Sample Questions about Self-Awareness and Feelings

Wishes

If you had three wishes, what would you wish for? Reasons for each?

What would you like to be when you're older/grown up?

If you could change one thing about yourself, what would it be?

Feelings

Tell me about yourself.
What makes you happy?
What makes you sad? What do you do when you are sad?
What makes you mad? What do you do when you are mad?
What makes you scared? What do you do when you are scared?
What do you worry about?

How do you feel most of the time?

What do you need the most?

Have you ever had any strange experiences or things happen that you don't understand?

Screening questions for anxiety, depression, suicidal risk

Do you feel unusually anxious or worried about things?
(*If yes*) Tell me more about your worries.

Have you ever felt very sad or depressed for a long period of time?
(*If yes*) Tell me more about that.

Have you ever been so sad that you wished you were dead?
Have you been thinking about hurting yourself or killing yourself?
Have you ever tried to harm or kill yourself?
(*If yes, probe for suicide plans, preparations, and available methods.*)

Note. From McConaughy and Achenbach (2001) and McConaughy (2012). Copyright 2001 by Stephanie H. McConaughy and Thomas M. Achenbach and copyright 2012 by Stephanie H. McConaughy. Reprinted by permission.

Three Wishes

Asking children to state "three wishes" is a technique that is commonly used with young children, but it can also be very effective with adolescents. Children's wishes can provide some insight into their level of imagination and their desires. Asking what they want to be when they grow up and what they would change about themselves are additional questions that tap into children's goals and sense of ideal self.

In my research to develop the SCICA (McConaughy & Achenbach, 2001), 6- to 11-year-olds often expressed wishes for concrete things (e.g., toys, money, pets) or fun activities (e.g., to go to Disney World). Another common response was more wishes (e.g., a lot of wishes; a million wishes). These typical wishes reflect children's desires for fun and happiness, despite problems they might have reported earlier in the interview. Other SCICA participants expressed specific wishes for improvements in their home situations or relationships (e.g., for Dad to be home; to have a better, nicer sister; a mother to take care of the children). Others expressed wishes to be better at an activity, sport, or academic skill (e.g., to be good at soccer; to be a better reader). These types of wishes, coupled with other interview content, can provide insights into which issues are especially poignant for children.

Bruce Garcia's three wishes were "to be on the Dolphins' team—the last best player"; "to go to Florida" (where the Dolphins play); and "to be the tallest person in the whole world." Bruce's wishes were consistent with other interview statements reflecting his desire to be stronger and taller. They also reflected a somewhat obsessional preoccupation with his favorite football team. Karl Bryant's wishes were "to live in a mansion with a pool, Jaguars, and Porsches" and "everlasting life for the whole family—that no one would ever die." He did not give a third wish. Karl's first wish reflected his desire for a grandiose lifestyle, which was consistent with earlier statements suggesting that he wanted to be important and respected. His second wish reflected concerns about the safety of family members. In Chapter 8, you will learn that Karl had witnessed episodes of violence in the home as a young child.

Questions about Basic Feelings

Direct questions about basic feelings (happy, sad, mad, scared, and worried) can assess how well children recognize their own feelings and whether they can differentiate among feelings. You can then probe for the behaviors that feelings elicit by asking, "What do you do when you are sad/mad/ scared?" After asking questions about basic feelings, you can query children about their most predominant mood ("How do you feel most of the time?") and what they perceive as their basic needs ("What do you need the most?").

Elementary school children can usually identify something that makes them happy. Often their responses reflect their concrete operational level of reasoning. Examples from the SCICA research participants were "getting presents for my birthday," "money," "getting toys," and "Mom giving me treats." Some responses also revealed children's concerns about family problems and peer relations: "having Dad back home," "getting my own way," and "kids letting me in the game." Elementary school children seemed to have more difficulty talking about sad than happy feelings, and some had trouble differentiating sad from mad. For example, the SCICA question "What makes you sad?" elicited more "don't know"

> **Young children find it easier to talk about positive than negative feelings like sad and mad. Some may also have trouble differentiating mad from sad.**

responses than questions about other feelings. Other responses to the question about sadness were "when a pet dies," "when someone dies," "when I get punished," and "when my sister slaps me."

Children seemed to find it easier to say what makes them mad than what makes them sad. The most typical SCICA responses involved sibling conflicts: "My brother punches me"; "My brother breaks my toys"; "My brother/sister gets into fights with me"; and "My sister gets more attention." Other typical responses to the mad question were "getting punished," "not getting my own way," and "people picking on me." Responses to the SCICA question "What makes you scared?" included "scary movies," "dragons," "Dracula," "the dark," "monsters in my room," "chicken pox," and "bad dreams." Sample answers to "What do you worry about?" were "not passing a grade" and "parents not taking care of me."

Sample responses from SCICA participants give some idea of what clinically referred 6- to 11-year-olds might say about their feelings. Three additional research studies provided further insights into the types of worries reported by "normal" children who had not been referred for clinical services. Not surprisingly, Vasey and Daleiden (1994) found that children expressed different types of worries as they grew older: 5- to 6-year-olds worried most often about threats to their physical well-being, whereas 8- to 12-year-olds worried about their behavioral competence, social evaluation, and psychological well-being.

Muris, Meesters, Merckelbach, Sermon, and Zwakhalen (1998) reported the following top 10 most intense worries among normal 8- to 13-year-olds: school performance, dying or illness of others, getting sick themselves, being teased, making mistakes, appearance, specific future events (e.g., a party), parents divorcing, whether other children like them, and the well-being of their pets. Henker, Whalen, and O'Neill (1995) reported the following 10 most frequent worries in children in grades 4–8 (approximate ages 10–14): academic or school-related problems, health and safety issues, environmental degradation, social relations, death and dying, social ills, positive disposition (e.g., "Am I doing the right thing?"), family relations, environmental disasters, and drugs. Knowing what worries are most typical for children of different ages can help you determine whether worries expressed by particular children are unusual compared to their peers.

Strange Thoughts and Suicidal Ideation

Though few children report strange or psychotic thoughts, it is still good practice to screen for such critical problems (e.g., "Have you ever had any strange experiences or things happen that you don't understand?"). When interviewing adolescents, you can also ask more direct questions to screen for anxiety, depression, and suicidal ideation, if you have not covered these in other sections of the interview. Table 4.1 lists the following examples of screening questions: "Do you feel unusually anxious or worried about things? (*If yes*) Tell me more about your worries. Have you ever felt very sad or depressed for a long period of time? (*If yes*) Tell me more about that."

Whenever children express very sad feelings and/or concerns about death, you need to probe further for suicidal ideation by asking questions such as "Have you ever been so sad that you wished you were dead? Have you been thinking about hurting yourself or killing yourself? Have

> **When children express very sad feelings and/or concerns about death, it is important to probe further for suicidal ideation or behavior.**

you ever tried to harm or kill yourself?" If children answer such questions affirmatively, you should probe for potential suicide plans, preparations to carry out plans, available methods (e.g., pills, guns), plans regarding place or setting, and whether there are any deterrents to suicide. When you suspect that a child is seriously considering suicide, you need to explain that his/her suicidal intents cannot be kept confidential and then discuss what will happen next. After the interview is completed, you must take immediate protective action, such as notifying parents, a child protection team, or a local crisis center, depending on the circumstances and legal requirements. Chapter 8 discusses the assessment of suicide risk in detail and provides guidelines for taking protective actions.

Incomplete Sentences

Another way to explore children's self-awareness and feelings is to use the incomplete sentences technique. This involves presenting children with sentence stems that focus on particular content areas and then asking them to complete each sentence as they wish. Examples are "What I like best is _____. What I like least is _____." There are numerous versions of incomplete sentences. Appendix 4.1 is a reproducible worksheet of incomplete sentences drawn from Hughes and Baker (1990) and my own clinical work. You can pick and choose from this list, as well as add your own sentences to tap specific issues or concerns.

To introduce the incomplete sentences, you can say:

"Here are some sentences I'd like you to finish for me. It will help me to get to know you and learn how you think and feel about things. You can say whatever you think, and I will write what you say right here [point to the blank in the sentence]. There aren't any right or wrong answers—it is just what you think and feel. Here is the first one [read sentence]."

Read each sentence and record responses for young children who have limited writing skills. You can give older children the option of writing their own answers or having you write their responses for them. Try to avoid making the task seem like a test. After children finish the sentences, you can select certain ones and ask children to tell you more about that thought or feeling.

Appendix 4.2 is a reproducible worksheet of additional incomplete sentences, taken from Merrell (2008b), that focuses specifically on feelings. Merrell recommended using incomplete sentences about feelings in cognitive-behavioral therapy for children with anxiety or depression. He also described several other techniques for addressing feelings in therapy: a worksheet listing comfortable and uncomfortable feelings, a self-rating form for evaluating how hard it is to express certain feelings, and a self-rating inventory of hypothetical situations that evoke different feelings. You can incorporate some of these techniques into clinical interviews as well as using them in therapy. Such indirect techniques may be especially effective with children who are resistant or unresponsive to direct questioning about feelings. Incomplete sentences and other similar techniques may not be very effective with children under age 8 who cannot engage in recursive thinking about their own thoughts and feelings.

Case Example: Catherine Holcomb

The interview with 11-year-old Catherine Holcomb, shown in Box 4.1, provides a good example of asking direct questions about feelings. Catherine, who was introduced in Chapter 1, lived with her mother and one older brother. In an early part of the interview, Catherine had reported that she still felt very sad about her father's death, which had occurred when she was 7 years old. At first, Catherine was reluctant to discuss her sad feelings. However, after she became more comfortable, the interviewer reopened the topic of her father's death as an entrée to explore her experience of basic feelings.

BOX 4.1. Talking with Catherine about Feelings

INTERVIEWER: Tell me a little bit about your father. You said earlier that your father died? When did that happen?

CATHERINE: Just about 4 years ago. (*Looks sad, avoids eye contact.*)

I: When you were about 6 years old?

C: No, I was about 7, and Billy was about 10.

I: What kind of a person was your father?

C: He was nice. (*Fleeting eye contact, then looks away.*)

I: Tell me a little bit about him . . . you know, what you remember.

C: Well, I remember going on a lot of camping trips with Dad. He loved going on camping trips. And we'd go canoeing a lot. We have a big canoe. He called it Thunder, because it sounds like thunder. It's a really big canoe.

I: So you remember going on camping trips and things. How do you feel about all that now?

C: Sad. (*Fidgets with pant leg, looking down.*)

I: You're still sad about it. Do you talk about that with your mother?

C: No. (*Sounds sad, looks away.*)

I: Do you talk about it with anybody?

C: No. (*Pause, looks sad, sniffs, wipes a tear.*)

I: It sounds like it's hard to talk about, and you still feel sad about it.

C: (*Long pause*) I just wish my father was still alive. (*Fidgets with clothes, looks down.*)

I: Sounds like you miss him.

C: I do. (*Chokes up, looks about to cry.*)

I: Did you cry when he died?

C: Uh-huh. (*Rocks in chair, looks down.*)

I: Does it still make you cry sometimes?

C: Uh-huh.

I: How often do you think about that?

C: I think about it a lot.

I: Do you think about it when you're in school?

C: Yeah. (*Speaks softly.*)

I: What do you think about in school?

C: (*Long pause, no reply*)

I: Is it kind of hard to talk about that?

C: (*Nods "yes"; no verbal reply.*)

I: I can see it's hard to talk about it. Let's talk about some of your other feelings. What kind of things make you happy?

C: If I got a puppy for my birthday. (*Pauses.*) Christmas is fun. I get presents.

I: So you want a puppy for your birthday. Like that puppy you told me about earlier?

C: (*Brightens, nods "yes."*)

(continued)

I: And it makes you happy to get presents at Christmas. How about what makes you sad. You told me about one thing that makes you sad. Are there some other things that make you sad?

C: (*Pauses.*) I can't think of any.

I: When you're feeling sad, do you ever feel so sad that you wish *you* weren't alive?

C: No. (*Looks down.*)

I: You don't feel that sad?

C: No.

I: Have you *ever* felt so sad that you wished *you* weren't alive?

C: No.

I: What do you think about when you're sad?

C: I really don't think about anything.

I: You don't think about anything? Just kind of being sad, huh? (*Nods "yes."*) What about *mad*? What kind of things make you mad?

C: If somebody hits me.

I: Does that ever happen to you, people hitting you?

C: Sometimes people hit me.

I: Where does that happen? At home . . . or at school?

C: At home . . . my brother hits me sometimes.

I: Sometimes?

C: Uh-huh.

I: What do you do when he hits you?

C: I get mad . . . and go to my room.

I: Do you ever hit him back?

C: Sometimes I hit him back. He can get very irritating. (*Voice gets louder and sounds annoyed.*)

I: Your brother can get very irritating, huh? How is he irritating?

C: Like he might do something . . . like he might start pounding his fist on my toes. And then when I told him to stop, he wouldn't listen to me. He'd keep on doing it. I'd say it louder, and then I'd start screaming at him. (*Squirms in seat.*)

I: So first you tell him to stop, and he keeps on doing it. Then you scream at him and get mad. Then what would happen?

C: I would leave and go to my room.

I: What kind of things make you *scared*?

C: Sometimes my brother hides, and when I walk into my room, he scares me.

I: So he hides on you and scares you. Does that *really* make you scared?

C: Yes . . . he jumps out and scares me.

I: What other kinds of things are you afraid of?

C: Sometimes I'm afraid of having bad dreams. I don't like having bad dreams. (*Looks agitated, squirms in seat, rubs clothing.*)

I: What kind of bad dreams do you have?

C: I had one where I was in my closet, and there were green hands on my shoulders. (*Pulls at shirt.*)

(*continued*)

I: What would the green hands do?

C: They were just sitting on my shoulder and talking.

I: Talking green hands? What was bad about that dream?

C: It was just scary.

I: What did the green hands say?

C: I don't remember. I woke up.

I: Do you ever have any good dreams?

C: Uh-huh. (*Laughs a little, giggles, smiles at interviewer.*)

I: What is a good dream you've had?

C: (*Looks happier.*) I had a big black horse.

I: A big black horse. Tell me about that one.

C: Well, I got this horse, and I kept working it and showing everybody, and I woke up before I could even get on the horse. (*Giggles.*)

I: (*Interviewer laughs too.*) So you were walking around showing him and everything, and you didn't get to get on him? The big black horse. Do you like horses?

C: Uh-huh.

I: Do you ever get to ride horses?

C: Not very much. Only when I'm down at Moose Lake.

I: Moose Lake. What is that?

C: It's a camp in the summer. They have horseback riding . . . archery. Now I don't have to be led anymore.

I: You don't have to be led?

C: I used to have to be led, and now I don't have to.

I: Does that mean you can ride by yourself?

C: Uh-huh. It's fun. (*Looks at interviewer smiles, pauses*.) One time I was riding on a horse, and he started to run.

I: How did you feel then?

C: I was scared. He was fast.

I: I remember riding a horse, and it was kind of scary when he ran.

C: (*Brightens up and looks at interviewer.*) It's fun riding horses.

I: You really like to do it. Is Moose Lake a place that you stay overnight?

C: Not when I was a kid. I'm old enough now, if I want to go. But I don't now.

I: You don't want to stay overnight?

C: (*Nods "no."*) Billy does, though.

I: Why don't you want to stay overnight?

C: It's scary. I don't want to stay by myself.

I: OK. Let me ask a different question. What would you say you *need* the most?

C: (*Pauses.*) Uh . . . food.

I: Food? What do you mean, you need food?

C: You need food to keep living. (*Looks sad again, quiet voice.*)

I: Oh. So if you're going to keep living, you need food. OK.

The interviewer began by asking what Catherine remembered about her father. She then moved into assessing the frequency and pervasiveness of her sad feelings. Catherine reported that she was often sad, even during school hours, which may help to explain the inattentiveness and apathy reported by her teachers. During this conversation, the interviewer learned that Catherine had never talked with anyone, including her mother, about her sad feelings. The fact that she was willing to discuss such painful feelings in the clinical interview suggested that, at this stage of her development, Catherine might be amenable to psychotherapy. Her negative responses to probe questions about thoughts of dying also indicated that she did not appear to be currently at risk for suicide.

The interview segment with Catherine also illustrates how she responded to questions about other basic feelings. Her reports of getting mad when her brother hit her or irritated her were typical of children her age. However, the intensity of her negative feelings still suggested that her poor relationship with her brother was an important issue for Catherine. She also reported being scared of bad dreams and being afraid to go to summer camp. These fears seemed somewhat immature for an 11-year-old. In another part of the interview, Catherine reported that she sometimes would crawl into her mother's bed at night when she has a bad dream or stomachache. In this interview segment, Catherine's expression of her fears and recurrent feelings of sadness raised the possibility of a mood disorder, though more information would be needed from other sources to make such a diagnosis.

ADOLESCENT ISSUES

Alcohol and Drugs

Each year since 1975, the National Institute on Drug Abuse has sponsored a nationwide survey, Monitoring the Future, to measure national trends in the use of alcohol, nicotine, and other illicit substances by adolescents. The data from this annual survey are especially useful to keep in mind when interviewing adolescents about their substance use. The 2009 sample for the survey included over 46,000 students in 8th, 10th, and 12th grades in 389 schools across the nation (Johnston, O'Malley, Bachman, & Schulenberg, 2010). (The national survey also included college students and adults through ages 50.) The 2009 results showed that in grades 8, 10, and 12 combined, 33% of students reported use of any illicit drug in their lifetime and 26% reported use of any illicit drug in the past year. Illicit drugs included marijuana, hallucinogens, crack, cocaine, heroin and other narcotics and tranquillizers not under a doctor's orders.

> According to Monitoring the Future (2010), 26% of students in grades 8, 10, and 12 reported having used an illicit drug in the past year.

The bad news was that after a decade of gradual decline from 1997 and leveling off between 2007 to 2008, marijuana use showed a slight but significant increase in 2009. Across grades 8, 10, and 12 combined, in 2009, 29% of students reported having tried marijuana in their lifetime. In the past year, 33% of 12th graders, 27% of 10th graders, and 12% of 8th graders reported having used marijuana. The slight increase in use was accompanied by a decline in adolescents' beliefs about how much risk marijuana poses. For example, the percent of students seeing great risk in regular marijuana use in 2005 versus 2009 fell from 74 to 70% among 8th graders and 58 to 52% among 12th graders.

Across the three grades combined, the annual use of other illicit drugs was 6–7% for inhalants, Vicodin (a prescription painkiller), and amphetamines (including nonprescription use of the stimulants Ritalin, Adderall, and methamphetamine). Annual use was 4% for Oxycontin (another prescription painkiller) and hallucinogens (including LSD and ecstasy/MDMA). Annual use of other illicit drugs across the three grades combined ranged from less than 1 to 3%.

> **Monitoring the Future (2010) reported alcohol use by 55% of American students in their lifetime and 48% in past year.**

Another disturbing trend was the continued widespread alcohol use among American adolescents. In 2009, across grades 8, 10, and 12 combined 55% reported having consumed alcohol (more than a few sips), and 36% reported having been drunk in their lifetime. In 2009, 48% reported having consumed alcohol in the past year, and 29% reported having been drunk in the past year.

The good news was a decline in cigarette use over the past 12–13 years, following a dramatic increase in adolescent smoking earlier in the 1990s. In 2009, cigarette use reached the lowest level among 12th graders, with 20% reporting being current smokers. However, cigarette smoking was still high among American students, with 20% having tried cigarettes by 8th grade and 44% having tried cigarettes by 12th grade. And the 20% current use by 12th graders is still cause for concern.

The general trends from the Monitoring the Future survey underscore the need for continuing concerns about use of alcohol, cigarettes, and illicit drugs among U.S. youth. To give a more differentiated picture of current use, Table 4.2 lists the percentages of 8th-, 10th-, and 12th-grade

TABLE 4.2. Percentage of Adolescents Reporting Substance Use in the Past 30 Days in 2009

Type of substance	8th grade	10th grade	12th grade
Alcohol	15	30	44
Cigarettes	7	13	20
Marijuana/hashish	7	16	21
Smokeless tobacco	4	7	8
Amphetamine (without prescription)	2	3	3
Tranquilizers (without prescription)	1	2	3
Inhalants	4	2	1
Hallucinogens other than LSD	1	1	1
Methamphetamine (crystal meth, "ice")	—	—	< 1
Cocaine	1	1	1
Crack cocaine	1	0	1
LSD	1	1	1
Ecstasy (MDMA)	1	1	2
Steroids	< 1	< 1	1
Heroin	< 1	< 1	< 1
Any illicit drug, including marijuana	8	18	23
Any illicit drug, excluding marijuana	4	6	9

Note. Based on Johnston, O'Malley, Bachman, and Schulenberg (2010).

students reporting use of various substances over the 30 days preceding the 2009 survey. Consistent with the lifetime and annual data, alcohol, cigarettes, and marijuana top the list, with 20–44% of 12th graders reporting their use. Three to 8% of 12th graders reported use of smokeless tobacco, amphetamines without a doctor's prescription, and tranquilizers without a prescription. Other drugs were used by 1–2%, and heroin, steroids, and methamphetamine (crystal meth, "ice") were used by less than 1% of 12th graders.

The data in Table 4.2 were drawn from self-reports by a large national sample of students without distinguishing between normal "nonreferred" students versus those who had been referred for clinical services. To add to this picture, Table 4.3 shows the percentage of nonreferred versus referred 11- to 18-year-olds who reported using alcohol, tobacco, or drugs for nonmedical purposes over the past 6 months on the YSR (Achenbach & Rescorla, 2001). Significantly more referred than nonreferred adolescents reported substance use on the YSR. The percentage of adolescents reporting substance use was somewhat lower on the YSR than on the Monitoring the Future survey, probably because of the broader age range and differences in sampling and questionnaire methods.

Adolescence is certainly a time of experimentation. As you can see from the data in Tables 4.2 and 4.3, for many youth, experimentation includes using alcohol and drugs. When considering such data, it is important to distinguish between substance use as experimentation versus substance abuse and dependency. Accordingly, Sattler (1998) delineated five stages of substance use: experimentation arising from curiosity, risk taking, or peer pressure; social use to gain acceptance in a peer group; instrumental use to manipulate emotions and behavior; habitual use that can lead to abuse; and finally, compulsive use or addiction that leads to dependency. These progressive stages are good to keep in mind when evaluating the severity of adolescents' substance use.

The widespread substance use among U.S. youth certainly puts them at risk for developing substance abuse or dependence. For this reason, it is important to screen for alcohol and drug use in clinical interviews. Table 4.4 lists some open-ended questions that cover tobacco and alcohol use, plus general drug use. When adolescents do report use of substances, you should probe further

TABLE 4.3. Percentage of Adolescents Reporting Alcohol or Drug Use on the Youth Self-Report

YSR problem item[a]	Nonreferred girls	Nonreferred boys	Referred girls	Referred boys
I drink alcohol without my parents' approval	14	10	17	17
I smoke, chew, or sniff tobacco	10	6	28	25
I use drugs for nonmedical purposes (do not include alcohol or tobacco)	4	16	16	13

Note. Items are from the Youth Self-Report (YSR; Achenbach, 2001). Copyright 2001 by T.M. Achenbach. Reprinted by permission.

[a]YSR problem items endorsed as "somewhat or sometimes true" or "very true or often true" over the past 6 months by children ages 11–18.

to determine the frequency of use and whether such use has created problems for them. When adolescents report frequent use that suggests possible substance abuse or dependence, you should try to assess their desire for change and readiness for help or treatment. For example, you can ask adolescents if they have ever received help or treatment and whether they want help or treatment now. If you suspect that an adolescent has a severe alcohol or drug problem, then you may want to do more in-depth interviewing regarding his/her substance use. Sattler (1998) provided several interview protocols for such purposes.

Antisocial Behavior and Trouble with the Law

In addition to asking adolescents about substance use, it is important to screen for antisocial behavior that may lead to trouble with the law. Other sections of the clinical interview may naturally present opportunities to ask about such problems, for example, when discussing activities with friends or family. You can then follow up such discussions with probes about activities that may have led to trouble with the law. If you do not have opportunities to ask such questions earlier in the interview, you can ask directly about trouble with the law and gang activities, as shown in Table 4.5.

Researchers on conduct disorders have described two different developmental paths for antisocial behavior. One pattern involves early onset (e.g., age 6 or younger) of aggressive and antisocial behavior that seems to be strongly associated with children's temperaments and poor parent–child relationships. Another pattern involves later onset of antisocial behavior among adolescents who associate with troubled or delinquent peers (Moffitt, 1993, 2003; McMahon & Frick, 2007). Children who show early onset of aggressive, antisocial behavior tend to have severe problems that continue into adulthood. Very early interventions are crucial for changing such patterns of behavior. However, adolescents who begin antisocial behavior later in life may or may not continue

---

TABLE 4.4. Sample Questions about Alcohol and Drug Use

Do you smoke or chew tobacco?
(*If yes*) How often?

Have you ever drunk beer, wine, or liquor?
(*If yes*) When and how often?

Have you ever been drunk from alcohol?
(*If yes*) When and how often?
Do you think you have a problem with alcohol?
Have you ever received any help/treatment for alcohol problems?
Do you want help/treatment for alcohol problems now?

Have you used drugs/been high on drugs?
(*If yes*) When and how often?
What kind of drugs?
Do you think you have a problem with drugs?
Have you ever received any help/treatment for drug problems?
Do you want help/treatment for drug problems now?

Note. From McConaughy and Achenbach (2001). Copyright 2001 by Stephanie H. McConaughy and Thomas M. Achenbach. Reprinted by permission.

TABLE 4.5. Sample Questions about Trouble with the Law

Have you ever been in trouble with the law or police?
(*If yes*) What kind of trouble?
What happened when you got in trouble with the law/police?

Have you ever been in any traffic accidents/had any traffic tickets?
(*If yes*) What kind of accidents?

Do you belong to a gang?
(*If yes*) Tell me about the gang.
Has your gang ever gotten into trouble with the law or police?

Note. Reprinted from McConaughy and Achenbach (2001). Copyright 2001 by Stephanie H. McConaughy and Thomas M. Achenbach. Reprinted by permission.

such patterns into adulthood. A lot depends on the consequences adolescents experience in response to their antisocial behavior. If they are arrested and put into the criminal justice system, their expected outcomes are bleak. If, instead, they enter into treatment programs or court diversion programs, they may change their course of behavior. For example, problem-solving training and multisystemic treatment programs have shown promising results with antisocial adolescents (Henggeler & Schaeffer, 2010; Kazdin, 2010).

> **Antisocial behavior develops along two pathways: early onset, associated with children's temperaments and poor parent–child relationships or later onset via association with delinquent peers.**

To provide some background on the prevalence of adolescents' antisocial behaviors, Table 4.6 shows the percentages of 11- to 18-year-olds who reported antisocial behavior on the YSR (Achenbach & Rescorla, 2001). You can see that rates of all such problems were higher in clinically referred than nonreferred children. Still, over one-third of nonreferred children reported that they break rules and associate with kids who get into trouble. These data underscore the importance of asking adolescents about such behaviors in clinical interviews. When adolescents do report such problems, you can explore options for changing antisocial behaviors before they lead to serious social or legal consequences.

Dating, Romances, and Sexual Activity

According to the 2009 Youth Risk Behavior Surveillance System (YRBSS), conducted by the U.S. Centers for Disease Control and Prevention, 46% of students in grades 9–12 nationwide reported having had sexual intercourse sometime in their life and 34% reported being currently sexually active (Eaton et al., 2010). Overall, the prevalence rates of ever having had sexual intercourse were comparable among males (46%) and females (46%), but prevalence varied across race/ethnicity, with Black (65%) and Hispanic (49%) students showing higher rates than White students (42%). The highest prevalence rate was among black male students (72%). Six percent of students nationwide reported having had sexual intercourse before age 13, and 14% reported having had four or more sexual partners.

> **Forty-six percent of students in grades 9–12 reported having had sexual intercourse sometime in their life, and 34% reported being currently sexually active.**

TABLE 4.6. Percentage of Adolescents Reporting Antisocial Behavior on the Youth Self-Report

YSR problem item[a]	Nonreferred girls	Nonreferred boys	Referred girls	Referred boys
I break rules at home, school, or elsewhere	34	43	77	81
I hang around with kids who get into trouble	35	44	49	55
I cut classes or skip school	12	10	26	26
I run away from home	3	4	22	18
I set fires	2	6	7	14
I steal at home	3	4	10	18
I steal from places other than home	3	4	15	20

Note. Items are from the Youth Self-Report (YSR; Achenbach, 2001). Copyright 2001 by Thomas M. Achenbach. Reprinted by permission.
[a]YSR problem items endorsed as "somewhat or sometimes true" or "very true or often true" over the past 6 months by children ages 11–18.

Increased sexual feelings can certainly add a vital and exciting dimension to the lives of adolescents. Being attracted to someone and developing intimate relationships are opportunities for growth. However, early onset of sexual activity and high frequency of sexual partners put adolescents at significant risk for HIV infection and other sexually transmitted diseases (STDs), and, for girls, teenage pregnancy. It was somewhat encouraging to learn that among the 34% of students who were currently sexually active, 61% reported that either they or their partner had used a condom. However, only 20% reported that they or their partner used birth control pills. Teenage pregnancy and single motherhood, in particular, raise additional risks for dropping out of high school, receiving fewer employment opportunities, and ending up dependent on welfare.

Asking about sexual activity in clinical interviews may create discomfort for many adolescents. Discussion of sexual practices with adolescents may also be a sensitive, or even taboo, topic in the minds of some parents and school staff. For example, some Christian fundamentalist parents in my clinical practice explicitly asked whether my child clinical interview would include questions about sex. Some school districts may also have specific policies about sex-education and discussing sexual practices with students. For school-based assessments, it is important to know about such policies. When adolescents, or adults, do have concerns about sexual practices it is important to explain your purpose for discussing such topics. For example, you can explain that you may want to ask about dating and romantic relationships to learn more about an adolescent's social interactions and whether he/she is at risk for unsafe sexual behavior.

Table 4.7 lists sample questions interviewers can ask about dating, romances, and sexual activity. These are only intended as screening questions. Use your own judgment about their appropriateness for each interviewee. In some cases, you should also consider matching the gender of the interviewer and interviewee. For example, it may not be appropriate or wise for a male interviewer to ask girls questions about their sexual activity, especially when there is reason to suspect that they have experienced sexual abuse. When you do ask such sensitive questions, do so

TABLE 4.7. Sample Questions about Dating, Romances, and Sexual Activity

Do you date/go to dances or parties?
Tell me about dating. Do you usually go out with a group or just yourself and a boy/girl?

Do you have a boyfriend/girlfriend?
Tell me a little bit about your boyfriend/girlfriend.
What do you like about him/her?
What do you usually do together?

Have you had sex with your girlfriend/boyfriend?
(*If yes*) How often?
Have you had sex with other people, say last month or last year?
Do you do anything to have "safe sex"? (Explain *safe sex* if interviewee looks confused.)
Do you/your boyfriend use a condom? Do you/your girlfriend use birth control pills?
How would you feel if you/your girlfriend got pregnant? What would you do?

in a neutral, professional manner, and be prepared to handle any embarrassment that may arise. Ask only enough questions to evaluate risk without violating the adolescent's sense of privacy. Also be cautious that your questions are not misinterpreted as showing personal interest. If an adolescent's reports lead you to suspect ongoing abuse or imminent risk for abuse, you must break confidentiality and follow legal reporting requirements, as discussed in an earlier section. Inform the adolescent of these requirements and remind him/her of the limits of confidentiality that you stated at the beginning of the interview.

Sexual Identity

Developing a secure sense of self-identity and the capacity for intimate relationships are key challenges during the adolescent years. Establishing one's sexual identity is a fundamental aspect of these developmental challenges. Most adolescents clearly identify themselves as heterosexual, though some may question this at times. A minority, however, will discover that they are attracted more to their same sex than the opposite sex. Research studies have shown that about 5–8% of adolescents identify themselves as gay, lesbian, or bisexual, and another 6–7% report that they are unsure of their sexual identity. Data collected from 2001 to 2009 by the YRBSS produced the following median prevalence rates of sexual identity reported by students in grades 9–12: 93% heterosexual, 1.3% gay or lesbian, 3.7% bisexual, and 2.5% unsure (Kann et al., 2011). Another survey of over 13,921 American high school students found that 86% identified themselves as heterosexual; 7.7% as gay, lesbian, or bisexual; and 6.7% as sexually questioning (Espelage, Aragon, Birkett, & Koening, 2008). The YRBSS also asked respondents about sexual contacts. Median rates were 53.5% who reported sexual contact with the opposite sex, 2.5% who reported sexual contacts with the same sex, 3.3% who reported sexual contact with both sexes, and 40.5% who reported no sexual contacts.

Many gay, lesbian, and bisexual youth report being bullied in some form, some of which is targeted directly at perceived or actual sexual orientation (homophobic bullying). For example, D'Augelli (2002) found that 81% of gay, lesbian, and bisexual youth reported that they had been

> **Approximately 5–8% of students identify as gay, lesbian, or bisexual, and 3–7% are not sure of their sexual identity. All are at risk of homophobic bullying.**

verbally abused; 38% had been threatened with physical assault; 6% had been assaulted with a weapon; and 16% had been sexually assaulted. Rivers (2001) found that 58–82% of gay, lesbian, and bisexual youth experienced name-calling, assault, and teasing; 59% had had rumors spread about them; and 27% felt socially isolated.

Research studies have documented a variety of negative educational and psychological outcomes among victims of homophobic bullying. In a large online survey of California students in grades 7–11, 7.5% of respondents reported having been bullied because of perceived or actual sexual orientation (California Safe Schools Coalition & 4-H Center for Youth Development, University of California, Davis, 2004). Compared to nonbullied students, victims of homophobic bullying were more likely to have lower grades, to have missed school because they felt unsafe, and to have engaged in health risk behaviors (e.g., substance use, driving under the influence of alcohol). Risk for suicide was a particular concern. Forty-five percent of victims of homophobic bullying reported seriously contemplating suicide, and 35% reported making a suicide plan. Compared to heterosexual youth, gay, lesbian, and bisexual youth in the YRBSS study also showed significantly higher rates of most risk behaviors measured, including behaviors that contributed to violence, attempted suicide, tobacco use, alcohol use, other drug use, sexual behaviors, and weight management problems (Kann et al., 2011).

Rivers and Noret (2008) reported more encouraging results from a study of 106 students in grades 7–9 in the United Kingdom. They found no significant differences between matched samples of heterosexual students versus students who reported attraction to the same sex, on measures of general alcohol consumption, cigarette smoking, marijuana and drug use, depression or anxiety, and other health risk behaviors. However, same-sex-attracted youth were more likely to have concerns about their sexual orientation, were lonely, and occasionally drank alcohol alone. It is important to note that the same-sex-attracted youth in the U.K. study had not "come out" at school except to report their sexual orientation on the survey instrument. Therefore, they may not have been exposed to the homophobic bullying experienced by participants in other studies.

For the majority of adolescents who consider themselves heterosexual, issues of sexual orientation or sexual identity may seldom arise in clinical interviews, and there is no need to mention the topic. Others who are gay, lesbian, or bisexual, or questioning their sexual orientation may welcome the opportunity to discuss their concerns with a caring and nonjudgmental adult. Still other gay, lesbian, bisexual, or questioning youth may find questions about sexual identity embarrassing or offensive. Therefore, you need to approach issues about sexual identity with sensitivity and respect. To broach the topic, you might say, "Some boys/girls your age wonder if they are gay/lesbian. How about you? Do you ever wonder about this?" If the adolescent acknowledges concerns about sexual identity, you can follow up by saying, "Tell me more about that. Have you shared these thoughts and feelings with anyone else? Do other people tease or bully you because they think you are gay/lesbian? How does that make you feel? What do you do about that?"

When interviewees report being teased or bullied in general, this disclosure can provide a good entrée to questions about the type of bullying and whether it has anything to do with sexual orientation. Reports of depression, anxiety, and loneliness can also be followed up with inquiries about sexual orientation when appropriate. When interviewees do report being gay, lesbian, or bisexual, or are questioning their sexual orientation, it is important to screen for suicidal thoughts or behavior, given the research evidence about suicide risk. You should be clear in your assurances of confidentiality in discussing sexual orientation and clear about the limits of confidentiality when you suspect risk for suicide or abuse. You should also be well apprised of support services for gay, lesbian, or bisexual youth within the school and local community.

Cell Phones, Internet, and Social Networking

Digital communication by cell phones and computers is now commonplace in the lives of children and adolescents in the developed world. A Pew Internet study of 800 American 12- to 17-year-olds showed that 93% used the Internet and 75% owned a cell phone (Lenhart, Ling, Campbell, & Purcell, 2010; Purcell, 2010). Internet use was highest among Whites with college-educated parents and household incomes above $50,000. Cell phone ownership increased with age (58% of 12-year-olds vs. 83% of 17-year-olds), but there were only small ethnic differences in cell phone ownership (Whites, 78%, Blacks, 75%, and Hispanics, 68%). Seventy-five percent of adolescent phone owners had unlimited texting, with 54% reporting texting daily and about half sending 50 or more messages a day. Boys typically sent and received about 30 texts per day, whereas girls typically sent or received 80 texts per day. As might be expected, texting activity increased with age, with 12- to 13-year-olds sending and receiving about 20 texts per day and 14- to 17-year-olds sending and receiving 80 texts per day. The vast majority of texts were sent to friends, but texts were also sent to boyfriends or girlfriends, parents and siblings, or other family members. Another Pew Internet study of 799 12- to 17-year-olds showed that among those that used the Internet, 80% accessed social networking sites, such as Facebook, and/or used Twitter (Lenhart et al., 2011).

Although digital communication and the Internet have certainly changed human interactions in many positive ways, they also present some hazards. Internet aggression, or "cyberbullying," is a growing concern among parents, educators, and mental health professionals, as well as children. As discussed by Swearer et al. (2009), cyberbullying can take forms similar to face-to-face relational aggression, including gossiping, spreading rumors, making threats, or sending rude, embarrassing, or harassing messages or photos. Cyberbullying can be especially injurious when messages and images are rapidly disseminated to broad audiences. In a 2011 Pew Internet study, although 69% of adolescents who used social networking sites felt that their peers were mostly kind to one another, 20% felt that their peers were mostly unkind, and 11% reported that "it depends" (Lenhart et al., 2011). Eighty-eight percent reported that they had seen someone being mean or cruel to another person on a social networking site, ranging from 12% who had witnessed such behavior "frequently" to 47% who had witnessed it "only once in a while." Fifteen percent reported that they had experienced cruel or mean behavior on a social networking site in the past 12 months. Respondents also reported a variety of negative outcomes resulting from cruel or mean social networking comments, including face-to-face arguments or confrontations with someone, physical fights, ending of a friendship, problems with parents, feeling nervous about going to school the next day, and getting in trouble in school (Lenhart et al., 2011).

> **Cyberbullying via cell phones and Internet can be especially injurious when messages and images are rapidly disseminated to broad audiences.**

Another concern is adolescents' use of cell phones and the Internet to send and receive sexually explicit messages, pictures, and videos, now referred to as *sexting*. Cell phones are the most common media for sexting, but such messages can also be sent by e-mail, instant messaging, or social networking sites. Segool and Crespi (2011) explained that sexting involves producing and disseminating a sexually explicit message or image with full consent or volition of the person depicted. This is in contrast to sending a sexually explicit message or image without the person's consent, which could be a form of cyberbullying. According to an Associated Press/MTV poll, 18% of teenagers reported that another person had sent them naked pictures or videos of themselves via a cell phone or the Internet, and 10% reported having sent a naked picture or video of themselves to others (Knowledge Networks, 2009).

Sexting—sending/receiving sexually explicit messages/ pictures/videos—raises concerns for underage adolescents, including possible criminal charges of child pornography.

Segool and Crespi (2011) warned that the legal implications of sexting can dramatically change a young person's life course. When involving underage children and adolescents, the transmittal of an image of oneself or another person in a seminude or nude state can result in criminal charges of child pornography. Segool and Crespi reported that under federal law, and most state laws, child pornography is defined as any visual depiction produced by electronic, mechanical, or other means, where the production involves a person under age 18 engaging in sexually explicit conduct. They described court cases in four states where adolescents were charged with child pornography for sending nude, seminude, or sexually explicit pictures of themselves to friends or classmates. In a Pennsylvania case, three 13-year-old girls used cell phones to send topless images of themselves to male classmates. In a Florida case, a 16-year-old girl and 17-year-old boy exchanged digital photos of themselves engaged in sexual activity. In a New Jersey case, a 14-year-old girl posted nude photos of herself on MySpace. In a Washington State case, three middle school students were charged for distributing a nude cell phone image of one student to numerous classmates. If convicted, the charges could have led to sentences in jail or juvenile detention centers and registration as sex offenders. In the four cases reviewed, the legal charges were eventually reduced, but they still resulted in convictions requiring probation, therapy, or court diversion programs.

Segool and Crespi (2011) reported that several states have considered or enacted legislation to decrease penalties for minors engaging in consensual sexting. Nonetheless, the legal consequences are important to consider, as are the harmful social–emotional repercussions that may occur from bullying, taunting, and loss of privacy after such images are disseminated. As examples, Segool and Crespi (2011) cited two cases of adolescent girls who committed suicide after nude images of themselves had been transmitted to hundreds of students in area schools. Online sexual solicitation and exploitation are additional major concerns, with 15% of adolescents having been targeted in unwanted sexual solicitation in a year on the Internet (Ybarra & Mitchell, 2004).

The clinical interview offers opportunities to explore possible problems stemming from inappropriate use of cell phones and the Internet. Because their reasoning and judgment are still developing, adolescents may not fully understand or consider the risks and potential harm of some of their cell phone and Internet activities, particularly sexting. Some may be overly trusting of close friends and not consider how easily private images and messages can be forwarded to large audiences. Others may transmit embarrassing or sexually explicit images of themselves or others as a joke without considering the potentially harmful effects. Still others may transmit such images or messages intentionally as a form of cyberbullying. Table 4.8 lists sample questions that you can use to screen for potential problems involving use of cell phones and the Internet. You should use your own judgment on the appropriateness of such questions for each individual. It is important to ask the questions in an open and nonjudgmental manner and to be sensitive to the embarrassment that questions of this nature may arouse.

TABLE 4.8. Sample Questions about Cell Phone and Internet Use

Do you have a computer at home?
(*If yes*) How much time do you spend on the computer each day?
What do you do on the computer (e.g., homework, play games, contact friends)?

Do you use Facebook or MySpace or something like that?
(*If yes*) How do you feel about Facebook/MySpace?
How often do you post on Facebook/MySpace?
Have you ever had any unpleasant experiences on Facebook/MySpace?
(*If yes*) Tell me about that.

Do you have a cell phone?
(*If yes*) How often do you talk on your cell phone each day?
Who do you call most of the time?
What else can you do on your cell phone besides talking to people (e.g., send text messages,
    take pictures, send pictures, use the Internet)?
Has anyone ever sent you mean or cruel messages on your cell phone or on the Internet?
(*If yes*) Tell me about that.

Have you ever sent mean or cruel messages to another on your cell phone or on the Internet?
(*If yes*) Who did you send them to? What were the messages?

What about sexual messages or photos? Has anyone ever sent you a naked picture or video
    on your cell phone or on the Internet?
(*If yes*) How did that make you feel? Did you tell anyone about it?
Have you ever sent naked pictures of yourself to anyone else?
(*If yes*) What happened when you did that? How did that make you feel?

Standardized Self-Report Scales

In addition to direct interviewing, adolescents can be asked to complete standardized self-report scales to assess potential problems and competencies. Table 4.9 lists examples of standardized self-report scales that assess a broad spectrum of internalizing and externalizing problems, attention problems, social skills, and adaptive functioning. Chapter 9 discusses additional self-report scales for assessing anxiety and depression. Completing standardized self-report scales requires the ability to reflect on one's own behavior and feelings. For this reason, most self-report scales are intended for children ages 8 or older. A good practice is to ask interviewees to complete a self-report scale prior to the appointment for the clinical interview. You can then review responses ahead of time and ask questions about key problems identified on the self-report. This can be a good strategy for introducing sensitive topics such as alcohol and drug use, antisocial activities, thought problems, sexual issues, and suicidal thoughts or behavior. As an example, the ASEBA Youth Self-Report includes the following items:

I drink alcohol without my parents' approval.
I use drugs for nonmedical purposes
I set fires
I steal from home.
I steal from places other than home.

I hear sounds or voices that other people think are not there.
I see things that other people think aren't there.
I think about sex too much.
I wish I were of the opposite sex.
I think about killing myself.
I deliberately try to hurt or kill myself.

Any one of these items scored present warrants follow-up in the clinical interview.

Confidentiality Issues with Adolescents

Confidentiality and trust are often delicate issues with adolescents. For example, adolescents who use alcohol or drugs or have committed illegal acts may be reluctant to report such problems for fear of getting into trouble. Others may not want to discuss certain interactions with friends or sexual activity out of embarrassment or fear that someone else will find out about them. You should carefully consider your ethical and professional responsibilities for dealing with confidentiality before beginning clinical interviews with adolescents. And you should clearly state the limits on confidentiality at the beginning of the interview, as discussed in Chapter 2. As indicated earlier, ethical and legal standards require you to break confidentiality when there is reason to suspect harm or danger to self, harm or danger to others, or child abuse. APA and NASP ethical standards do not explicitly require breaking confidentiality to report illegal substance use or criminal behavior that does not present a danger to others. (See Jacob et al., 2011, for more detailed discussion of legal and ethical issues regarding confidentiality.)

> **Interviewers should be knowledgeable about their ethical responsibilities concerning confidentiality and inform adolescents of the limits of confidentiality at the beginning of their clinical interviews.**

One approach is to inform adolescents ahead of time that you will report concerns about substance use or illegal activities to their parents or guardians. You may also want to report unsafe sexual practices that increase health risks or risks for exploitation or abuse. Such reports are necessary when these issues are the main reasons for referral or are the focus of assessment for specific treatment programs. For example, some clinics and treatment programs require adolescents to sign a release allowing clinicians to share information about substance abuse or illegal activities with parents. When you take this route, you run the risk that interviewees will deny such problems. It is, therefore, important to establish rapport early on and to explain clearly the purpose of your interview and assessment.

In other cases, you may choose to keep reports of substance use or illegal activities confidential in order to help an adolescent move toward acknowledging the severity of the problems and accepting appropriate treatment. The federal Public Health Services Act (1987) includes comprehensive privacy rules that protect the confidentiality of patient records for persons, including minor adolescents, who enter into substance abuse treatment programs (Confidentiality of Alcohol and Drug Abuse Patient Records, 1987). In addition, at least 20 states give minors the right to seek drug treatment without their parents' consent (Gudeman, 2003). In any case, you should have a clear strategy for dealing with the limits of confidentiality prior to interviewing adolescents about their substance use or illegal activities, as well as their sexual activity.

TABLE 4.9. Examples of Published Standardized Self-Report Scales

Instrument	Items and scales	Normative samples	Publisher
Academic Competence Evaluation Scales—Student Form (ACES; DiPerna & Elliott, 2000)	68 items *Competence/Adaptive Scales* Academic Enablers Total Score, Interpersonal Skills, Engagement, Motivation, Study Skills, Academic Skills Total Score, Reading/Language Arts, Mathematics, Critical Thinking	Combined norms for boys and girls, grades 6–8 and 9–12	Pearson 19500 Bulverde Road San Antonio, TX 78259 800-627-7271 *www.psychcorp.com*
ASEBA Youth Self-Report (YSR; Achenbach & Rescorla, 2001)	105 problem items and 14 competence *Problem Scales* Total Problems, Internalizing, Externalizing, Withdrawn/Depressed, Somatic Complaints, Anxious/Depressed, Social Problems, Thought Problems, Attention Problems, Rule-Breaking Behavior, Aggressive Behavior, Obsessive–Compulsive Problems, Posttraumatic Stress Problems, Affective Problems, Anxiety Problems, Attention-Deficit/Hyperactivity Problems, Oppositional Defiant Problems, Conduct Problems *Competence/Adaptive Scales* Total Competence, Activities, Social Positive Qualities	Separate norms for boys and girls, ages 11–18 Multicultural norms	Research Center for Children, Youth, & Families, Inc. One South Prospect Street Burlington, VT 05401-3456 802-656-5130 *www.aseba.org*

(continued)

TABLE 4.9. *(continued)*

Instrument and scales	Items and scales	Normative samples	Publisher
Behavior Assessment System for Children–2 Self-Report of Personality (BASC-2 SRP; Reynolds & Kamphaus, 2004)	139–185 items *Problem Scales* Emotional Symptoms Index, Inattention/Hyperactivity, Internalizing Problems, School Problems, Attitude to School, Attitude to Teachers, Sensation Seeking, Atypicality, Locus of Control, Social Stress, Anxiety, Depression, Sense of Inadequacy, Somatization, Attention Problems, Hyperactivity, Alcohol Abuse (18–25), School Maladjustment (18–25) *Content Scales* Anger Control, Ego Strength, Mania, Test Anxiety *Competence/Adaptive Scales* Personal Adjustment, Relations with Parents, Interpersonal Relations, Self-Esteem, Self-Reliance	Separate norms for boys and girls, ages 8–11, 12–21, and 18–25	Pearson 19500 Bulverde Road San Antonio, TX 78259 800-627-7271 *www.psychcorp.com*
Behavioral and Emotional Rating Scale (2nd edition)—Youth Rating Scale (BERS-2-Y; Epstein, 2004)	57 items *Competence/Adaptive Scales* Total Strengths Score, Interpersonal Strengths, School Functioning, Intrapersonal Strengths, Family Strengths, Affective Strengths, Career Strengths	Separate norms for boys and girls, ages 11–18	PRO-ED 8700 Shoal Creek Boulevard Austin, TX 78757-6897 800-879-3202 *www.proedinc.com*
Conners Comprehensive Behavior Rating Scales—Self-Report (CBRS-SR; Conners, 2008)	179 items *Problem Scales* Emotional Distress, Defiant/Aggressive Behaviors, Academic Difficulties, Hyperactivity/Impulsivity, Violence Potential Indicator, Physical Symptoms, 12 DSM-IV-TR Disorders *Validity Scales* Positive Impression, Negative Impression, Inconsistency index	Separate norms for boys and girls, ages 8–12 and 13–18	MHS P.O. Box 950 North Tonawanda, NY 14120-0950 800-456-3003 *www.mhs.com*

Instrument	Items and Scales	Norms	Source
Millon Adolescent Clinical Inventory (Millon, 1993)	160 items *Problem Scales* 30 scales with 5 dimensions	Separate norms for boys and girls, ages 13–19	Pearson 19500 Bulverde Road San Antonio, TX 78259 800-627-7271 *www.psychcorp.com*
Minnesota Multiphasic Personality Inventory—Adolescent Version (MMPI-A; Butcher et al., 1992)	478 items *Problem Scales* 7 validity scales, 10 clinical scales, 31 clinical subscales, 15 content scales, 31 content component subscales, 11 supplementary scales	Separate norms for boys and girls, ages 14–18	Pearson 19500 Bulverde Road San Antonio, TX 78259 800-627-7271 *www.psychcorp.com*
Personality Inventory for Youth (PIY; Lachar & Gruber, 1995)	270 items *Problem Scales* Cognitive Impairment, Impulsivity/Distractibility, Delinquency, Family Dysfunction, Reality Distortion, Somatic Concern, Psychological Discomfort, Social Withdrawal, Social Skills Deficits	Separate norms for boys and girls, ages 9–19	Western Psychological Services 12031 Wilshire Boulevard Los Angeles, CA 90025-1251 800-648-8857 *www.wpspublish.com*
Social Skills Improvement System—Student Form (SSIS-S; Gresham & Elliott, 2008)	75 items *Problem Scales* Total Problems, Internalizing, Externalizing, Bullying, Hyperactivity/Inattention, Autism Spectrum *Competence/Adaptive Scales* Total Social Skills, Communication, Cooperation, Assertion, Responsibility, Empathy, Engagement, Self-Control	Separate norms for boys and girls, ages 8–12 and 13–18	Pearson 19500 Bulverde Road San Antonio, TX 78259 800-627-7271 *www.psychcorp.com*
Youth's Inventory–4R (YI-4R; Gadow & Sprafkin, 2008)	125 items *Problem Scales* 13 DSM-IV-TR Disorders *Screening Items* 6 DSM-IV-TR Disorders *Inconsistency Scale*	Separate norms for boys and girls, ages 12–18	Checkmate Plus P.O. Box 696 Stony Brook, NY 11790-0696 800-779-4292 *www.checkmateplus.com*

Note. ASEBA = Achenbach System of Empirically Based Assessment; DSM-IV-TR = *Diagnostic and statistical manual of mental disorders–fourth edition, text revision* (American Psychiatric Association, 2000).

Case Example: Kelsey Watson

Fourteen-year-old Kelsey Watson's case illustrates the special issues that can arise with adolescents. Kelsey grew up in a semirural community, where she had experienced a great deal of instability in her home life. Her biological father was an alcoholic who had left the family when Kelsey was a young child. Her mother suffered from bipolar disorder and had been hospitalized several times for psychiatric treatment. When her mother was sick, Kelsey was cared for by various relatives. At age 12 Kelsey moved to a large city to live with a maternal aunt for a year. There she attended an alternative school for children with learning and behavioral problems. She ran away from her aunt's home several times and became involved with a street gang. At age 13 Kelsey was hospitalized in a psychiatric unit because of suicide attempts. She was diagnosed with major depressive disorder and placed on antidepressant medication (Prozac). After her release from the hospital, Kelsey returned to live with her mother for 6 months. Then, at age 14, Kelsey was placed in the custody of the state social service agency because of unmanageable behavior and runaway episodes. She moved into a residential group home but continued to have home visits with her mother.

After Kelsey entered the group home, she began attending eighth grade in the local school district. There she was referred for a psychological evaluation of her behavioral and emotional functioning. The psychologist's clinical interview with Kelsey was a critical component of the evaluation. The psychologist took special care to establish rapport with her, while at the same time explaining the purpose of the interview. Kelsey arrived dressed in a black tank top and short black skirt. She had spiked hair with purple streaks and wore rings in her nose, left eyebrow, and both ears. She had a tattoo on her right arm. The psychologist greeted her without commenting on her appearance. She explained that the interview was part of Kelsey's evaluation and that she would be writing a report summarizing what she learned. She told Kelsey that they could talk about what would go into the report at the end of the interview. Because Kelsey had a history of suicide attempts, the psychologist made sure that Kelsey understood the limits of confidentiality. She clearly explained the legal requirements for reporting any concerns that Kelsey might hurt herself or hurt others or that she might be in danger of being hurt by someone else. Kelsey said she understood these limits and agreed to participate in the interview.

Although Kelsey was nervous and tense at first, she was cooperative and seemed eager to discuss her feelings and personal issues. In fact, she seemed to thrive on the individual attention. The interview covered many of the topics discussed in this chapter and Chapter 3 (see Table 3.1), along with adolescent issues regarding alcohol and drugs (Table 4.4), trouble with the law (Table 4.5), and dating and romances (Table 4.7).

Kelsey's interview raised particular concerns about several key adolescent issues. First and foremost was Kelsey's accounts of past suicide attempts and self-injury. Kelsey said, "I cut my wrists with glass and razor blades and tried to OD on caffeine pills. That's how I ended up in the mental hospital." She said that slashing her wrists made her feel "good, sort of like a high." When questioned further, Kelsey said she was no longer cutting herself and currently did not have any thoughts of killing herself. She thought that if she died, "she would probably go somewhere—heaven or hell—probably to hell." Sometimes, she said, she still felt like she wanted to die—"it was confusing"—but she reported no current plans to commit suicide. Kelsey noted that she was currently seeing a "shrink" at the group home, but that she and her therapist had not developed a contract regarding suicide.

A second concern was Kelsey's prior association with deviant or fringe peer groups when she lived in the city. Kelsey reported that at least one of her wrist-slashing episodes was part of a "cult thing" that she did with her city friends. Kelsey described herself as a "Satanist." She said that she and her friend Jillian had slashed their wrists together and then had tried to drink their own blood "to give themselves more power." Kelsey's reports of past cult activities were certainly worrisome, but she did not mention any past or current antisocial activities that had led to trouble with police. Kelsey said that she continued to write letters to Jillian, but had had no other contact with her or other city friends since she had returned home.

A third concern was Kelsey's reported use of alcohol and drugs. She freely admitted to getting drunk on beer and wine several times in the past, as well as using marijuana, LSD, pills (Valium), and heroin. She said she liked the "nice" feeling she had the two times she had shot up with heroin. She had not tried cocaine. Most of her substance use occurred during the year she spent in the city. In the clinical interview, Kelsey said she continued to use marijuana about once a month when she could get it, and she smoked "about a pack of cigarettes a day, when I can afford them." She had not drunk any alcohol in the past month, and really didn't like it as much as marijuana. Although drugs were harder to come by now, Kelsey said she still had urges to get high.

Kelsey's active sexual behavior was a fourth concern. She reported that she started having sex at age 12 with a 14-year-old boy, José, whom she had met in the city. She "was crazy about José" and "slept with him" about six times. When the psychologist asked what she meant by "sleeping with José," Kelsey looked embarrassed but then clearly described having had sexual intercourse. Sometimes, she said, José used a condom, but not always. Kelsey wanted to "get a shot for birth control," but had never seen a gynecologist and had never visited Planned Parenthood. However, she said she would like to learn more about safe sex. Kelsey also stated that she had never been sexually or physically abused by any of her cult members in the city. After she returned home, Kelsey found a new boyfriend, Eric. She reported that they engaged in oral sex and anal sex and sometimes intercourse. She said that she "would do anything for Eric" and thought about him all the time. Kelsey also reported having had several gay friends in the city. She had once tried oral sex with a girl, but thought it was embarrassing.

The summary of Kelsey's history and her clinical interview revealed serious emotional and behavioral problems at the time of the school-based evaluation. Although she was in state custody and under treatment for depression, Kelsey remained at risk for suicide, substance abuse, and sexually related problems, including teenage pregnancy, HIV and other STDs, and sexual exploitation. Kelsey's pattern of problems called for intense interventions on several fronts, involving both school and community agencies. We will return to Kelsey's case in Chapter 8 to learn more about other people's perspectives on her functioning and potential intervention strategies.

SUMMARY

This chapter discussed the process of interviewing children about self-awareness, feelings, and special issues pertinent to adolescents—alcohol and drugs; antisocial behavior and trouble with the law; dating, romances, and sexual activity; sexual identity; and potential problems arising from use of cell phones and the Internet. Research findings were included for each topic to provide a framework for talking about these issues and interpreting children's and adolescents' interview reports. Segments of the clinical interview with Catherine Holcomb illustrated interview strategies for discussing feelings. Kelsey Watson's case illustrated special concerns that can arise with adolescents, including alcohol and drug use, risky behavior, and unsafe sexual activity.

What I Think and Feel

Directions: Here are some sentences I'd like you to finish for me. It will help me to get to know you and learn how you think and feel about things. You can say whatever you think, and I will write what you say right here [point to the blank in the sentence]. There aren't any right or wrong answers—it is just what you think and feel. Here is the first one [read sentence].

What I like best is _____.

What I like least is _____.

Most grown people are _____.

My mother thinks I am _____.

My father thinks I am _____.

My teacher thinks I am _____.

Other kids in my class think I am _____.

My friends think I am _____.

My mother makes me feel _____.

My father makes me feel _____.

My sister/brother makes me feel _____.

I am _____.

When my mother gives me jobs, I _____.

When there is no one to help me, I _____.

When my teacher tells me to do something, I _____.

When my teacher corrects me, I _____.

When I don't know what the book says, I _____.

When I have hard homework, I _____.

About My Feelings

Directions: Complete each of these sentences about feelings in your own words, using examples of how you feel.

I felt afraid when _____

_____ .

I am really good at _____

_____ .

I get excited when _____

_____ .

Most of the time I feel _____

_____ .

I am happy when _____

_____ .

I feel upset when _____

_____ .

I am sad when _____

_____ .

I am calm when _____

_____ .

I was really mad when _____

_____ .

I am thankful for _____

_____ .

I am lonely when _____

_____ .

CHAPTER 5

Child Clinical Interviews
Home Situation and Family Relations

Relations between parents and children lay the foundations for children's social and emotional development. Before children enter school, the home provides the main arena for learning how to communicate and interact with other people. Learning about the home and family functioning is especially important when evaluating children who are experiencing emotional and behavioral problems or when evaluating children who may be suffering from neglect or abuse. At the same time, interviewers need to respect the privacy of family affairs. Some parents may be reluctant to disclose details about their family affairs, including their living situation, finances, and family conflicts. Asking about family issues may also make some children uncomfortable if they think that they will get into trouble if parents or other family members learn what they talked about during the interview. Therefore, it is important to inform parents ahead of time that you want to talk with their child about home and family. It is also important to assure parents and children that you will respect the privacy of what they say, within the bounds of confidentiality discussed at the beginning of the interview.

When concerns are mostly about school functioning, it may not be necessary, or even appropriate, to delve into issues regarding home and family. In such cases, the Semistructured Student Interview (McConaughy, 2012; Appendix 3.1) may be sufficient for interviewing the child. When you want a more comprehensive clinical interview, the SCICA protocol (McConaughy & Achenbach, 2001) provides a good format for asking questions about the home situation and family relations. Drawing from the SCICA, this chapter discusses strategies for interviewing children and adolescents about home and family. Chapter 6 discusses strategies for interviewing parents.

FAMILY CONFLICTS

Conflicts between parents and children naturally occur throughout all stages of development. Some parent–child conflicts are normal features of children's gradual movement into independence as adults. However, some families experience what Foster and Robin (1997) defined as "clinically significant conflict," especially as children transition into adolescence. This more severe form of parent–child conflict has the following features: (1) repeated, predominantly verbal disputes about a variety of issues; (2) failure to produce satisfactory solutions to disagreements; (3) unpleasant or angry interactions about problem issues; and (4) pervasive negative feelings (e.g., anger, hopelessness, distrust) in the child and/or parent. Conflicts of this sort can also occur between children and other adult family members, such as stepparents, a single parent's partner, or other adults, such as grandparents, who live in the child's home.

Ample research has shown strong associations between family conflict and emotional and behavioral disorders in children, especially psychiatric diagnoses of oppositional defiant disorder (ODD) and conduct disorder (CD) (Foster & Robin, 1997). In fact, several DSM-IV-TR symptoms for ODD include negative adult–child interactions in which the child/adolescent "often argues with adults" and "often actively defies or refuses to comply with adults' requests or rules" (American Psychiatric Association, 2000, p. 102). In particular, research has linked inconsistent, harsh, and punitive parental discipline to escalating cycles of negative parent–child interactions and aggressive behavior in children (McMahon & Forehand, 2003; McMahon & Frick, 2007; Patterson, 1986). Low levels of parental monitoring have also been linked to aggressive and antisocial behavior. Furthermore, clinically significant conflicts can occur between family members and children with ADHD and children who have internalizing disorders characterized by depression or anxiety. Conflicts between parents and children with ADHD often concern issues around schoolwork (e.g., grades, homework), social interactions, and following rules at home (Barkley, 2006). Conflicts between parents and children with internalizing problems may stem from overprotectiveness and/or overcontrolling disciplinary practices, which can lead to anxiety and/or social withdrawal (Rubin & Stewart, 1996).

Children's reports of their interactions with parents and others in the home can provide one window on family relations, and their perceptions of rules and punishments may shed further light on disciplinary patterns. Interviewers can use this information, along with additional information obtained from parents, to decide whether there is clinically significant conflict in the home. In some cases, a more comprehensive family assessment may be warranted. Family assessments are usually performed by mental health practitioners outside of school, but some family assessments might be done by a school social worker, school psychologist, or consulting psychologist. School-based practitioners may also decide to recommend family therapy or parent training in cases involving high family conflict.

> **Children's reports about family interactions, along with parents' reports, can provide a basis for determining whether there is clinically significant conflict in the home.**

Table 5.1 lists sample questions, adapted from the SCICA, which you can ask children about their home situation and family relations. A good way to introduce this topic is simply to ask, "Who are the people in your family?" This open-ended question allows the child to name all people who might be considered "family," including biological or adoptive parents, a single parent's boyfriend/girlfriend or same-sex partner, stepparents, siblings, stepsiblings, foster children, and members of the extended family. If the family constellation becomes too complicated or hard to follow, then you can ask "Who lives in your home?" This question helps to clarify living situations for children who have experienced divorce or other changes in their home situation.

Additional questions can explore children's perceptions of, and feelings about, rules and punishments in the home, particularly whether they feel that the rules and punishments are fair or unfair. Asking children about chores and reward systems can also assess their perceptions of responsibilities assigned in the home and their perceptions of how family members encourage desired behavior. After learning whom the child considers to be the primary family members, you can ask more questions about how well the child gets along with various people in the family, including parents, other adults in the home, and siblings. A good way to start this conversation is to ask, "Who do you get along with best?" and "Who do you get along with least?"

TABLE 5.1. Sample Questions about Home Situation and Family Relations

Home situation

Let's talk about your family.
Who are the people in your family? Who lives in your home?
In your home, do kids have separate bedrooms? How do you like having separate bedrooms/sharing a room with _____?

Rules, punishments

What are the rules in your home?
Who makes the rules?
What happens when kids break the rules?
How do you feel about the rules? Are they fair or unfair?
What are the punishments in your home?
Do kids ever get spanked/physically punished for bad behavior?
Who usually gives the punishments?
How do you feel about the punishments? Are they fair or unfair?

Chores, rewards

Do you have any special chores/jobs at home?
Do you get an allowance? (*If yes*) What do you have to do for it?
Do you have other ways to earn money?
What happens when a kid does something really good or special?
Do kids get any special rewards or treats for doing something good?
Does this ever happen for you?

Family relations

How do you get along with the people in your family/home?
Who do you get along with best?
Who do you get along with least?

*Ask about the child's relationship with each member of the family,
as appropriate: father, mother, stepparents, other adults in
home, other caregivers, siblings, stepsiblings.*

How do your parents get along?
Do they have arguments? (*If yes*) What kind of arguments?
How does that make you feel when they argue?

Note. Reprinted from McConaughy and Achenbach (2001). Copyright 2001 by Stephanie H. McConaughy and Thomas M. Achenbach. Reprinted by permission.

KINETIC FAMILY DRAWING

As a supplement to verbal queries about the family, you can ask children to do a kinetic family drawing (KFD). Hand the child a piece of blank paper and a pencil and ask him/her to "draw a picture of your family doing something together." The KFD is a standard part of the SCICA for 6- to 11-year-olds, and is optional for 12- to 18-year-olds. Because the KFD provides a break from direct questions, it can be especially effective with younger children. The KFD can also be surprisingly effective with many ado-

> **The kinetic family drawing (KFD) is one technique that interviewers can use to provide a break from direct verbal questioning about the family.**

lescents, as long as they do not view it as a childish task. Children's descriptions of their drawings and the way they depict family interactions ("doing something together") can provide valuable insights into their perceptions of family relations. Burns (1982) provided examples of KFDs from children in many different situations, along with his own research on the KFD and clinical interpretations. However, quantitative scoring and projective interpretations of the KFD are not encouraged, because there is little research evidence supporting the validity of such approaches. After the child has completed the KFD, you can ask him/her to describe the drawing and then tell something about each family member. As an example, the SCICA protocol includes the following questions about the KFD:

Who are the people in your picture?

Ask the child if it is OK for you to write the name above each person in the picture.

What are they doing?

Tell me about the people in your picture. What kind of person is _____? Tell me three words to describe _____.

How does _____ feel in that picture?

What is _____ thinking?

Who do you get along with best/least?

What is going to happen next in your picture?

Case Example: Bruce Garcia

Figure 5.1 shows the KFD produced by 9-year-old Bruce Garcia, whose case was first presented in Chapter 3. Bruce was the middle child in a blended family of three children. Bruce drew a picture of the family having a barbecue ("barboquie") in the backyard. First he drew the house at the top of the page, rotating the paper several times as he drew. The two small rectangles attached to the house are the front and back doors. The small rectangles inside the house are bathrooms. He labeled the position of each room: den (Dn), living room (LR), kitchen (Ki), and stairs (St) to his room. He described the three wiggly ovals next to the house as "the things that prevent ants from coming in . . . [with] . . . little red stuff that looks like throw-up . . . it prevents ants from coming in." These probably depicted ant poison baits. Then he drew the barbecue pit at the bottom of the page, with the cover, the "thing to clean it . . . two pieces of big wood, a newspaper, some kindling wood, some charcoal . . . and . . . the fire." Lastly he drew the family members: his mother, his stepsister Barbie, older stepbrother Sam, and himself between Barbie and Sam (all pseudonyms).

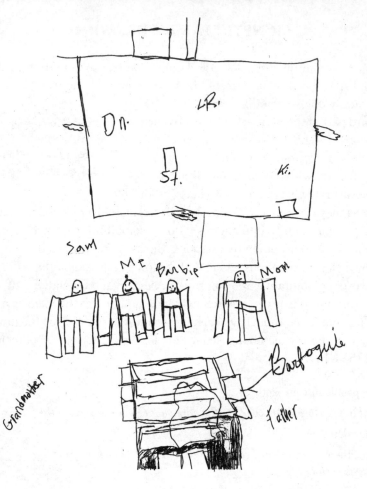

FIGURE 5.1. Kinetic Family Drawing from Bruce Garcia, age 9.

Bruce was very focused during his drawing, which took about 10 minutes to complete. He erased and redrew several parts of the picture, including changing the position of the three children in the drawing. First he drew Sam on the left side, Barbie in the middle, and himself to the right of Barbie. He drew Mom to the right of the three children. Then, as he began to describe his drawing, Bruce switched positions and erased and rewrote names to put himself in the middle of the children next to Sam. Bruce described each part of the picture as he drew. Sometimes his comments involved explanations of his drawing to the interviewer, but at other times, he seemed to be talking more to himself.

Bruce's drawing had two immediately notable features. First, his drawing of the house and the boxy shapes of the human figure drawings seemed immature for a 9-year-old, suggesting that Bruce may have some visual–motor delays. Second, his initial drawing included only the three children and his mother, which raised questions about what roles Bruce's stepfather and biological father played in his life. After Bruce completed his KFD, the interviewer asked him to talk about each family member. Box 5.1 contains a segment from this part of the interview. When the interviewer asked about his stepfather, who was missing from the drawing, Bruce added the word *Father* to the right of the barbecue. He also added the word *Grandmother* to the left of the barbecue.

BOX 5.1. Talking with Bruce about Family Relations

INTERVIEWER: So it's all done. Tell me about the people in your picture. Who do you want to talk about first?

BRUCE: My brother, Sam. (*Writes "Sam" above figure.*)

I: What kind of a guy is Sam?

B: He's a strong and tall guy.

I: What do you think about Sam?

B: (*Taps pencil on table, scratches self, looks away.*) I think . . . I think he's pretty . . . creative . . . 'cause when I barely came to my last house, he was really nice to me. He let me use his video . . . his games . . . and he's (*long pause*) . . . I can't remember.

I: Is Sam your real brother?

B: No, step . . . and about Barbie . . . she thinks she's fat. (*Writes "Barbie" above figure next to Sam.*) Change names. (*Erases "Barbie" and writes it above third figure; writes "Me" above figure next to Sam.*) Barbie's over here. OK . . . Um . . . I'm here.

I: I was wondering, why are they changing?

B: Because . . . When I think about it . . . I'm more detailed.

I: Now you're next to Sam. And then Barbie.

B: OK. Now about me is . . . (*Pauses, rubs pencil on table.*) What's the question now?

I: You were telling me about the people in the picture.

B: About me . . . I'm not a very good drawer, but I'm really good in math. I'm a really good fan of the Dolphins. Barbie is . . . she thinks she's really fat, but she's not. . . . She's pretty tall for her age, but I'm going to outgrow her. (*Rubs pencil, looks away.*)

I: So Barbie thinks she's fat, but you think she isn't. What kind of a person is she?

B: She's not sure. . . . she's pretty tall, but I'm going to outgrow her.

I: What makes you think you'll outgrow her?

B: Because she's up to here. (*Gestures with hand to demonstrate height.*) If we measured her and me head to head, I'm almost to here. (*Gestures to show his height.*)

I: Do you want to outgrow her?

B: Yes. (*Picks at ear, face.*) I'm almost the shortest kid in my class. I don't think it's fair that the girls outgrow the boys.

I: Sounds like you really want to be taller.

B: I do.

I: OK. Now let's talk about Mom. What kind of a person is Mom?

B: (*Long pause*) She's nice . . . sometimes nice . . . sometimes mean.

I: How is she nice?

B: She buys us stuff . . . she buys candy . . . sometimes she buys toys.

I: So Mom's nice when she buys candy and toys. How is she sometimes mean?

B: This morning she wasn't . . . she's sort of mean . . . sort of mean.

I: How is she mean?

(continued)

B: Says do this, do that. (*Long pause*) I get sick of it . . . don't want to. (*Looks away, avoids eye contact, squirms around in seat.*)

I: Like, do what?

B: Chores. I know I'm supposed to do chores. I don't want her to remind me.

I: So she reminds you to do your chores.

B: She says, "Do it now!" (*Imitates loud, mean voice of Mom.*)

I: What do you do then?

B: Get mad.

I: What happens when you get mad?

B: I turn into a grump . . . turn into a grump.

I: How do you turn into a grump?

B: I blow my top . . . blow my top.

I: Do you have temper tantrums?

B: Yeah . . . I blow my top . . . I get so mad . . . (*Squirms in seat, looks away.*)

I: So you blow your top?

B: Yeah, I blow my top . . . I get so mad . . . I just don't have meekness in myself. Do you know what meekness means?

I: What does it mean?

B: It means you have full control. (*Rolls pencil on the table over and over.*) You feel you just don't get mad . . . like killing and stuff that.

I: You don't have meekness.

B: I have so much anger . . . I can't get it out of myself and be really calm. (*Looks away, fidgets with drawing pad.*) I feel really mad at somebody.

I: What sort of things make you mad?

B: Saying "do this" and "do that."

I: Sounds like your mom makes you really mad.

B: She bosses me around. (*Looks glum, sad; rolls pencil on the table.*)

I: Anybody else get you mad?

B: My brother is a lot nicer than Barbie. (*Continues to roll pencil on table.*) He protects me. He's stronger than me. He grabs Barbie and says "don't do that to him." (*Shows how Sam grabs Barbie by the throat.*) My brother could easily kill my sister, but he doesn't.

I: How do you get along with Barbie?

B: I don't know . . . we don't get along.

I: How do you not get along?

B: She's mean . . . says what I do is queer. (*Rolls pencil on table.*)

I: So Barbie says what you do is queer. How does that make you feel?

B: I get mad . . . she says I'm queer . . . makes fun of me. (*Looks down, grimaces.*)

I: I can see that Barbie makes you mad. I noticed that your stepdad isn't in this picture. I was wondering about him. What kind of a person is he?

(continued)

B: He's a strong guy. . . . Is this alright? One time my sister was slapped by four 18-year-olds . . . 18-year-olds. He took all of them and throwed them against the thing. He's really strong.

I: So your stepdad seems pretty strong. What else about him?

B: He works a lot, too.

I: What does he do?

B: He does a lot of work around the house. Probably two times as much as I do in the house. He's in the army. He does a lot of work in the army.

I: How do you get along with your stepdad?

B: OK . . . (*pauses to think*) . . . and he's concerned about my life, because just before a car was coming . . . it was crossing the road . . . he saved me from getting run over by a car.

I: So you know he is concerned about your life.

B: My mom, too. They both love me very much. I can't think of anything more.

I: How do you know they love you?

B: Because they show it.

I: How do they show it?

B: They show it by . . . my stepdad pushed me back so the car wouldn't run over me . . . and Mom . . . I don't know.

I: You don't know how Mom loves you.

B: She just says she loves me very truly.

I: I also noticed that your real dad is not in your picture. Tell me about your real dad.

B: How do you know I have a real dad? (*Looks surprised.*)

I: Well, I was guessing you have a real dad because you said you have a stepdad. Do you visit your real dad?

B: Um . . . once I saw him . . . Mom took me. It takes a lot of money to get there. We went to a restaurant . . . my favorite is spaghetti. We ordered that. I asked him if he had enough money, and he said yeah, and after he said he barely had enough money to pay everything.

I: Were you worried?

B: I didn't want him to run out of money.

I: What is he like? I mean what kind of a person is your real dad?

B: He's nice. He is a real giver.

I: How is he a real giver?

B: He gave me football cards and the Dolphins' record and a poster of the Super Bowl. (*Looks away, rolls pencil on table.*)

I: Where does he live?

B: Florida.

I: How often do you get to see him?

B: Not often. Maybe I'll see him this summer. (*Looks away, taps pencil in hand.*)

I: How do you feel about that?

B: I'm excited. I might see the Dolphins. They might even live there.

Bruce's halting speech, frequent pauses, and repetitive phrases suggested difficulty with expressive language, similar to the interview segment with Bruce about peer relations in Chapter 3. His descriptions of family members tended to focus on physical features (e.g., Sam is strong and tall; Barbie thinks she's fat) and people's actions toward him (e.g., Sam lets him use his video games; Mom buys them stuff; his real dad takes them to restaurants and gives presents). Such literal descriptions of other persons are typical for children in the concrete operational stage of development.

Bruce's comments also revealed different perceptions and feelings about various family members. He appeared to have a positive perception of his stepbrother Sam and his stepfather, both of whom he viewed as his protectors. He had a more negative perception of his stepsister Barbie, and both positive and negative perceptions of his mother. From this interview segment, we learn that although Mom is "sometimes nice," she is also "sometimes mean." Bruce clearly felt bossed around by Mom, which aroused angry feelings in him. He reported having difficulty controlling his temper in such situations and contended that he wanted to have more "meekness" (an odd word choice for a child). Bruce seemed to have a positive perception of his biological father, whom he had not seen often—which did not seem to bother him much. He was concerned about how much money it cost for the trip to visit his father and have dinner with him, which suggested there may have been financial difficulties in the family. Cost may also have been the reason his mother gave for the infrequent visits with his father in Florida.

A strikingly recurrent theme was Bruce's focus on being strong and tall and his desire to be protected. This self-perception was consistent with his earlier reports about being a victim of bullying in the form of teasing and physical assaults by peers. Such reports suggested that Bruce viewed himself as powerless and in need of other people to defend him or to help him cope with social problems. Although Bruce described arguments between family members (Sam and Barbie, himself and Barbie, himself and Mom), more information would be needed to determine whether such arguments represented clinically significant conflict. Nonetheless, Bruce's intensely angry reactions to his mother's demands about chores were worrisome, because negative parent–child interactions such as these can easily lead to oppositional behavior in children.

Case Example: Karl Bryant

The KFD was also a good entrée for discussing family relations with 12-year-old Karl Bryant, whose case was also presented in Chapter 3. Karl drew a picture of his stepfather, mother, younger sister, and himself all going out to buy ice cream cones, as shown in Figure 5.2. Karl considered himself to be a very good drawer and was very meticulous in his approach. For example, he used the edge of the paper as a ruler to make straight lines, and he added shading and details to his drawing. Karl commented on his good drawing skills several times, which he considered to be one of his special talents. Even his derogatory comments about his drawing ("It's the worst drawing I have ever done") seemed boastful. In my experience, the KFD typically takes about 5–10 minutes for most children. Karl drew for at least 20 minutes, and would have continued even longer had the interviewer not intervened to ask questions.

Limiting the time for the KFD can be challenging with children such as Karl. The goal is to use the KFD to obtain children's perceptions and feelings about their family. However, you should not allow the KFD to consume too much time or take the place of talking about the family. If a child needs extra time to do the KFD, you can begin asking questions about the family before

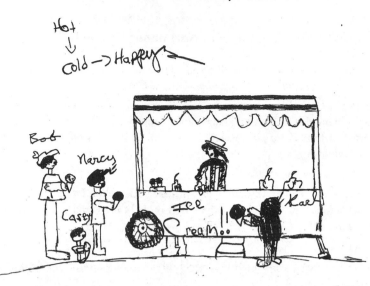

FIGURE 5.2. Kinetic Family Drawing from Karl Bryant, age 12.

the KFD is completed, as the interviewer did in Karl's case. Or you can set a time limit when you introduce the KFD by saying, "Now I would like you to draw a picture of your family doing something together. It should take about 5 minutes." Sometimes children are reluctant to do the KFD because they think they cannot draw well or they do not like to draw. In such cases, you can say, "I still want to see a picture of your family doing something together. You can draw it any way you want to. This is not a test." Most children will then go ahead with the drawing.

Box 5.2 presents excerpts of the interview with Karl about his perceptions of family members, using the KFD as a focal point. Karl was the older of two children in a blended family that included his biological mother (Nancy Ladd), stepfather (Robert Ladd), and 7-year-old sister (Casey; all pseudonyms). Karl started out painting a generally positive picture of his stepfather, whom he viewed not only his "father" but also a "friend" who treated him "fairly." Fairness was a strong and recurrent theme throughout the interview with Karl. In an earlier segment of the interview shown in Chapter 3 (Box 3.4), Karl talked a lot about how unfair he thought things were at school. In the segment shown in Box 5.2, we learn that Karl's notion of fairness was typical of a conventional stage of moral reasoning. Fairness to him meant that both children, Karl and Casey, got the same things at home (e.g., a candy bar, going somewhere with Mr. Ladd), and got the same consequences for misbehavior. Later, we learn that Bob, Karl's stepfather, was "the boss of the house" and the one who gave out the punishments. It is important to note that Karl felt that he had no say in deciding the punishments ("the decision is the decision"), and apparently that lack of input was not upsetting to him.

At the end of the discussion of the KFD, the interviewer asked Karl "Is home different from school?" Karl's perception of fairness at home contrasted sharply with his perception of extreme unfairness at school, where he felt singled out for undeserved punishments—usually detentions (see Chapter 3). The interviewer then asked Karl what advice he might give to teachers to make things fairer at school. At first, Karl seemed to think there was nothing he could do to change things ("You can't give them advice—they won't take it"). The interviewer then encouraged him

BOX 5.2. Talking with Karl about Family Relations

INTERVIEWER: Let's do something a little different. Draw a picture of your family doing something together. (*Interviewer hands drawing pad and pencil to Karl.*)

KARL: OK. I am heavily into drawing. It's one of my better subjects. I'm an artist (*Smiles.*) That's what Miss Tangier told me. I've got a good knack for drawing. My stepdad was amazed when I drew the house in perfect detail . . . simply amazed . . . he could not believe it. (*Starts drawing a structure and continues talking.*)

I: How long has he been your stepdad?

K: About 6 or 7 years. He's been through a lot with me. Like when I was burned by hot water. You should go back and ask my mom about that. He's brought me through everything. He was there and comforted me.

I: You remember that.

K: I sure do. I can't emphasize enough for every child not to play around hot water.

I: What happened?

K: (*Continues drawing while telling about event, looking up periodically.*) I was jumping around in the kitchen. My grandfather liked hot water and had just started it on the stove. We were goofing around, like on a skateboard. I brought the whole thing over. The pot landed on my head, and I got a big dent in my head. I can still feel it. (*Looks at interviewer, rubs head dramatically.*) And it burned my skin.

I: When did that happen?

K: About a year ago.

I: And your stepdad was there?

K: Yeah, he helped me. (*Starts drawing again.*)

I: Was that Bob?

K: Yes. I like him a lot.

I: What do you like about him?

K: He's funny. He treats me fairly. He's not only my father, he's a friend. If he does something, he says, "do you want to come?" He takes me everywhere.

I: How does he treat you fairly?

K: Say he gives Casey a candy bar, he'll go back and get one for me. That's just an example. If he takes Casey somewhere, then the next time he takes me.

I: Oh, so if Casey gets to go one time, you get to go the next time?

K: Yeah, he's really fair.

I: Who is Casey?

K: She's my sister. I have two families. I have relatives I haven't even met. I've got my mom's side, my stepdad's side, my real dad's side, and my stepmom's side. I have four sets of family.

I: So who all lives in your home with you right now?

K: Mom, Casey, and Bob. That's about it. (*Still carefully drawing, using the edge of the paper as a ruler for straight lines.*) This is not the most accurate drawing I've ever done. (*Erases.*) You can ask my mom how much time I spend on drawing. I have some drawings I have never even finished yet. (*More than 5 minutes have passed.*) How about the people? Who do you want in it?

(continued)

I: Anyone you want.

K: OK, I'll put in them all. (*Continues drawing structure.*) What do you think this drawing is?

I: I'm waiting to see.

K: Trust me, you will not know what this drawing means. I like drawing things that are exaggerated sometimes, and sometimes I like drawing things that are truthful. (*Continues silently for several minutes, then asks if interviewer can guess what it is.*) If anybody bumps me in the class while I'm drawing, look out.

I: What happens?

K: I scream. If anyone gets me when I'm drawing, I kill.

I: (*Karl starts drawing Mom.*) While you are drawing, tell me about your mom.

K: She's a nice person. She hollers at me sometimes and usually has a pretty good reason why she does.

I: Like what?

K: Like if I go somewhere I'm not supposed to go, if I didn't hear her correctly, she's patient with me. Like last night, I wanted to see the basketball game on TV. At first she said no, but then she said OK, you can watch the game, but you have to wake right up for me tomorrow morning. And I did. She's very patient with me.

I: Does she ever get angry with you?

K: Yeah. I mean every parent gets angry with a child every now and then.

I: Yeah, so what is she like when she is angry?

K: You don't want to know (*pause*) . . . she punches me sometimes when I do something wrong (*head down, drawing*), but it's not like she truthfully kills me.

I: So tell me more about the punching.

K: (*Ignores the question.*) Bob is a tall guy. (*Draws Bob, then Casey, then himself.*) I draw much better than this, I'm just drawing cartoons, looney tunes. I just rushed this thing so quickly, it's unreal. It's the worst drawing I have ever done.

I: You think so?

K: I know it is. If I had used my compass and a ruler, it would have been a lot better. (*Tells interviewer about another drawing he did that was much better.*)

I: Tell me about this drawing.

K: Alright. Should have put our car in, but that would have taken too long. This is my dad, Bob. This is Casey. Do you know what it is?

I: Looks like an ice cream stand.

K: You're right. We went to get ice cream because it is a hot day. This is Casey down here. This is me, and this is Mom.

I: How are the people feeling in this picture?

K: (*Pause*) Cold (*laughs*) and happy. They were hot before and now they cooled down. (*Writes* Hot → Cold → Happy.)

I: What are the people thinking?

K: I wouldn't know.

I: Well, if you imagined a story about the picture.

(continued)

K: They are thinking about what the bill will be. (*Laughs.*)

I: What does this family think about bills?

K: I don't know.

I: Does this family worry about bills?

K: No.

I: Tell me more about Mom.

K: She is a smart person. Whenever I have homework . . . I hardly ever have it, because I get it all done. She helped me with geometry, the 90-degree angles.

I: Do you ever get into arguments about homework?

K: No. I used to before with my dad, but we don't anymore. I liked working with Gail.

I: Who is Gail?

K: Stepmom.

I: So it was easier doing homework with Gail?

K: Yeah.

I: How was it easier?

K: Well, when I said an answer, she would check and say it was right and I knew it was right. My dad would say it was wrong.

I: Which dad are we talking about?

K: My real dad.

I: So you used to argue with your real dad about homework? What would happen?

K: We would just argue about it, and finally I would say "forget it" and go out in the other room.

I: What about your real mom? Do you get into arguments with her?

K: Not much anymore.

I: Does she give punishments?

K: Yeah, every kid gets punishments sometimes.

I: What are the punishments in your house?

K: No baseball—well, they can't take that away because there isn't anymore—no biking, no leaving the yard.

I: How about hitting punishments, like belts or spankings?

K: Not anymore. My mother doesn't believe in hitting anymore.

I: Did she used to?

K: Some . . . but not really. I don't really remember.

I: It's probably not fun to remember. How about Bob? Does he give punishments?

K: He's the boss of the house. He makes my mother talk to him. When she finds out what I did wrong, she talks to him and he makes the decision about the punishments. Then I get it.

I: So what are some of his punishments?

K: No TV, no going out.

I: If they say "no going out," do you stick with that?

K: Yeah, I listen to him.

(continued)

I: What if you think it's not fair?

K: I really don't have any say in that.

I: No say?

K: He says, "the decision is the decision." I don't have any say.

I: So the decision is the decision at home. What do you think about the punishments? Are they fair or unfair?

K: I have to go along with it. I have no say in whether it is fair or unfair.

I: So you have no choice in whether it is fair at home. I was wondering because earlier we were talking about school, and you said a lot of things were unfair at school, and that made you mad. (*Karl looks down and starts drawing again.*) Is home different from school?

K: Much different.

I: What makes it different?

K: The way my parents treat me compared to the school.

I: How is that?

K: (*Pause . . . drawing . . . looks down.*) They treat me more fairly. I believe it truthfully.

I: I was wondering what counts as fair to you.

K: I can't really say.

I: Well, if we wanted to give some advice to the teacher about fairness, what advice would you give?

K: You can't give them advice. They won't take it.

I: Well, let's pretend you could, what would you say?

K: Tell them to quit and get a new job. (*Laughs.*)

I: What if you were the principal of the school, what would you do to be fair?

K: For one, I would be more open. I would let kids come into my office, and I would listen to them. I would give a fair punishment. If they got into a fight, I wouldn't just go up and say "you get a detention because he has to have one." (*Looks angry.*) I wouldn't do that! If that other kid wasn't in it, he wouldn't get a punishment. Let me make it up. Say if Sam punched Mike and Mike punched Sam. Two wrongs don't make a right. So what I would do is give them both an essay, probably about 250 words, if they were sixth graders.

I: So they would both get the same amount?

K: Same amount, and the one who started the fight, which would be Sam, would be the one to get the detention, if a detention is to be given. I wouldn't give a detention. If it was his first offense, I would give him a warning. If it was his second offense, I would give him a success plan that had to be signed by his parents.

I: What is a success plan?

K: It's a plan where you ask yourself questions, like what are you going to do the next time? What is your success going to be?

I: Sounds like you really find that helpful to write down things in a success plan.

K: (*Nods yes.*)

I: Well, that's helpful to know.

to pretend: "What if you were the principal of the school—what would you do to be fair?" This strategy was successful in eliciting several ideas from Karl that might actually be incorporated into a school-based intervention plan. For example, Karl wanted more of an open-door policy from the principal. And he wanted the principal to listen to a kid's side of the story. He then laid out a series of steps for disciplining kids at school, including requiring them to write a "success plan." It is a good guess that Karl had already done one or more of these success plans.

The end of the interview segment in Box 5.2 provided some good insights into behavioral interventions that might be successful with Karl at school. More information would be needed to determine whether the school staff was already using disciplinary procedures such as the ones Karl suggested in the interview. Even so, Karl's comments about discipline at home versus what he would like at school underscored the importance of establishing clear and consistent rules and consequences that would fit Karl's conventional level of moral reasoning. It was also clear that Karl needed to feel that adults listened to his point of view. However, listening to Karl's side of a story could easily create a tricky situation for authority figures, who must also avoid getting into endless arguments and power struggles with him. Karl's perception of fairer treatment at home further suggested that closer collaboration between home and school could be very beneficial.

The interview segment in Box 5.2 also provides a good example of how you might deal with a child's reluctance to discuss certain sensitive issues, such as Karl's relationship with his biological mother. The interviewer broached the topic of Karl's relations with his mother several times, weaving it in and out of discussion about other family members. At first, Karl tried to paint only a positive picture of his mother (e.g., she helped him with homework). He was reluctant to elaborate on his mother's reactions when she was angry with him ("you don't want to know") and would not elaborate on his statement that she punched him when he did something wrong. Later in the interview, Karl acknowledged that his mother used to give "hitting" punishments, but excused this as a normal reaction ("every kid gets punishments sometimes"). Karl reported that the hitting punishments had ended when his stepfather took on the role of disciplinarian in the home. This change appears to have been a positive turn of events in Karl's mind. After hearing Karl's perception of the home situation, it would be important to learn in the parent interview what disciplinary strategies Mr. and Mrs. Ladd actually used in the home and whether they felt they were successful. It would also be important to learn more about Karl's relations with his biological father, whom Karl hardly mentioned in the child interview.

CHILD ABUSE AND NEGLECT

Both the United States and Canada have legislation mandating that professionals report cases of suspected abuse or neglect to official child protective service (CPS) agencies. In the United States, mandated reporting is required under the Child Abuse Prevention and Treatment Act (CAPTA; Public Law 93-247, 1974), originally passed in 1974, and reauthorized and amended many times since then. Maltreatment includes physical abuse, sexual abuse, psychological maltreatment, and neglect. CAPTA provides definitions of each type of maltreatment. The individual states, in turn, have developed their own legislation and regulations to carry out the requirements of CAPTA.

National and state statistics about child maltreatment are published each year from the data collected by CPS agencies through the National Child Abuse and Neglect Data System (NCANDS) of the Children's Bureau of the U.S. Department of Health and Human Services. For 2009,

NCANDS documented referrals of alleged abuse or neglect of more than 3.6 million children. Of those, 21% (762,940) children were determined by CPS agencies to be victims of abuse or neglect. Seventy-eight percent of child victims were neglected by their parents or other caregivers. An additional 18% were physically abused, 10% were sexually abused, 8% suffered psychological maltreatment, and 2% suffered medical neglect. Approximately 10% experienced other or unknown types of maltreatment, including abandonment, threats of harm to the child, or congenital drug addiction.

> **In 2009, NCANDS documented over 760,000 cases of American children who were victims of abuse or neglect. Over 50% were children under 7 years of age.**

Slightly more girls (51%) than boys (48%) were victims of maltreatment. The youngest children were the most vulnerable to maltreatment. Of all 2009 victims, 33% were younger than 4 years of age. Among older child victims, 23% were ages 4–7, 19% were ages 8–11, and 24% were ages 12–17 (U.S. Department of Health and Human Services, 2010).

Mandated Reporters

Mandated reporters under CAPTA include physicians, nurses, teachers, psychologists, social workers, guidance counselors, and other professional people who have contact with children. In 2009, professional people submitted 60% of reports, including 17% from educational personnel, 16% from legal or law enforcement personnel, 11% from social service workers, and 8% from medical personnel. Nonprofessionals submitted 30% of reports, including 9% from anonymous sources, 7% from parents, 7% from other relatives, and 5% from friends or neighbors. Federal and state laws protect professionals from criminal and

> **Professional people who have contact with children are mandated reporters of abuse and neglect. These include physicians, nurses, teachers, psychologists, social workers, and guidance counselors.**

civil liability in all jurisdictions, unless the report is malicious or without probable grounds. Informant anonymity is also guaranteed in some, but not all, states. State laws vary as to what specific situations require reporting (e.g., ongoing abuse or neglect vs. strong potential for abuse or neglect vs. past abuse or neglect without current risk). Laws also vary as to the degree of certainty necessary for reporting and sanctions for not reporting (Sattler, 1998; Crooks & Wolfe, 2007).

School-based practitioners should be familiar with federal and state laws for mandated reporting as well as with procedures for contacting CPS agencies in their states and local communities. Since the passage of CAPTA, most school districts have established their own procedures to facilitate mandated reports of suspected abuse and neglect. Often groups of school-based practitioners serve on child protection teams within each school or at the district level. Other school-based practitioners who suspect abuse or neglect of a child can bring their concerns to the child protection team. The team supports the practitioner in examining the concerns and filing the mandatory report to the CPS agency. Members of school child protection teams may also assist the child and family during the investigation process and afterward, as appropriate.

Signs of Abuse or Neglect

Wissow (1995) outlined several physical signs and symptoms that should arouse concern about potential child abuse and neglect. These include unexplained subnormal growth; specific types of head injuries (e.g., torn upper or lower lip, bilateral black eyes, unexplained dental injury, retinal hemorrhage, traumatic hair loss); skin injuries (e.g., bruises or burns in the shape of an object, bite marks); multiple lesions or injuries in various stages of healing; and bone or skull fractures and other traumas inconsistent with a given explanation. Some researchers have reported that sexually abused children exhibit sexually inappropriate behavior more often than nonabused children do. Examples are imitating sexual acts, self-stimulation and hyperarousal, exposing themselves, and sexually aggressive or victimizing behavior toward others (Finkelhor, 1988; Friedrich & Grambsch, 1992; McClellan et al., 1996). Other researchers have found no significant relationship between sexual abuse and sexual behavioral problems (Drach, Wientzen, & Ricci, 2001). Although you should be alert to physical or behavioral signs that may suggest abuse, you should also know that abused children can exhibit a vast array of internalizing and externalizing problems similar to clinically referred children who have not been abused. Accordingly, you should use caution in relying only on physical signs or behavioral problems as indicators of abuse. A child's direct report is a better indicator of potential abuse or neglect than are physical signs or behavioral problems alone.

Interviewing about Abuse and Neglect

It is beyond the scope of this book to discuss investigations of child abuse and neglect. Instead, readers are referred to Sattler (1998), who presented extensive guidelines on investigative interviewing techniques and background considerations for child abuse and neglect. Crooks and Wolfe (2007) also reviewed developmental perspectives and assessment of physically abused and neglected children, and Wolfe (2007) reviewed the epidemiology and assessment of sexually abused children. Horton and Cruise (2001) provide a comprehensive and practical discussion of how school staff should respond to reports of child abuse and neglect.

Comprehensive interviews to evaluate child abuse or neglect should be done only by specially trained investigators. Most school-based practitioners and mental health professionals lack such training. More often, professionals who specialize in social service, forensic, and criminal investigations are the ones who assess child maltreatment. Other practitioners may still be among the first to hear disclosures of abuse or neglect from interviews with children or from interviews with parents and teachers.

> **School-based practitioners may be the first to hear children's reports of abuse and neglect. School child protection teams can then file mandated reports.**

Brassard, Tyler, and Kehle (1983) outlined guidelines for responding to children who report sexual abuse. Similar guidelines, listed below, are appropriate for responding to all children who report maltreatment:

- Conduct your interview in a private place.
- Maintain an atmosphere of informality and trust.
- Believe the child (or at least take the child's report at face value).
- Reassure the child that he/she has done nothing wrong and will continue to have your support.
- Do not display negative reactions such as horror, shock, or disapproval of the child or parents.
- Be sensitive to the child's nonverbal cues.
- Ask for clarification if what the child says is ambiguous.

- Use language that the child understands.
- Use the child's terms for body parts and sexual behaviors, but also obtain the child's definition of such terms.
- Do not suggest answers to the child and avoid probing and pressing for answers.
- If it becomes clear that you must make a report to a CPS agency, give the child a clear and understandable reason why such reporting is necessary.
- Do not suggest that the child conceal your interview from the parents.
- Record clear notes of your interview and the child's disclosure statements, as well as your subsequent actions regarding reporting.

The NCANDS data for 2009 showed that 81% of perpetrators of child abuse and neglect were parents: 38% were mothers acting alone, 19% were fathers acting alone, 18% involved both parents, and 6% involved one parent plus another person. Other relatives accounted for 5%, and unmarried partners of parents for 3% of perpetrators (U.S. Department of Health and Human Services, 2010). As Sattler (1998) pointed out, children who are maltreated by parents or caregivers face a terrible dilemma: If they disclose the abuse or neglect, they may lose the very people that they depend on for love and nurturance; if they do not disclose, they face the likelihood of continued suffering. Children may be reluctant to disclose abuse because they fear retribution or violence from the abuser, breaking up the family, and/or rejection by friends and relatives. Very young victims of sexual abuse may not understand that the sexual activity is wrong. Adolescents who view the sexual abuse as wrong may still fear retribution, abandonment, rejection, and embarrassment or shame if their peers or members of the community find out. Many children and adolescents may also fear that no one will believe their report. It takes courage for a child to disclose abuse and neglect. It is not your job to determine whether the child is lying, exaggerating a situation, or has a faulty memory. Reacting with disbelief when the child is telling the truth can be not only devastating, but can also perpetuate the abuse or neglect and reduce the chance of any further disclosures.

When a child reports circumstances or incidents that lead you to suspect abuse or neglect, you must inform him/her of your legal obligation to report the information to a CPS agency. This requires breaking confidentiality. You can explain that the law requires you to report situations wherein children are not safe. You can also repeat the limits of confidentiality stated at the beginning of the interview, such as saying, "Remember what I said at the beginning of our talk? I said that I would have to tell someone if you said you were going to hurt yourself, hurt someone else, or that *someone has hurt you*. The law requires that I tell certain other people about these things that you have told me."

Expect that the disclosure and required reporting will be upsetting and threatening to the child. Take steps to help the child cope with the anxiety that your reporting may create. Reassure the child that you will still be there to support him/her. Explain what steps you must take next, such as talking with persons on a school child protection team and filing a report to the state or local CPS agency. Remember that it is not your job to establish evidence that the suspected abuse or neglect actually occurred. Your responsibility is to make the report that will initiate the investigative process. Do not make any personal promises to protect the child. If you suspect that the child is in immediate danger, you and other appropriate persons (e.g., the school child protection team) must take action to protect the child, such as notifying law enforcement or social service agencies, or notifying parents in cases when they are not suspected perpetrators.

Once a report has been filed with a CPS agency, that agency must determine the likelihood that abuse or neglect has occurred, assess the risk for further abuse, and determine what course of action must be taken to protect the child. This often requires further interviews of the child and family by the CPS investigators. According to the 2009 data from NCANDS, approximately 21% of reports included at least one child who was found to be a victim of maltreatment. In 67% of reports, the CPS investigators determined that there was no child maltreatment (U.S. Department of Health and Human Services, 2010). The majority of reports were found to be unsubstantiated. The remaining reports were closed for other reasons. Although the majority of reports did not result in charges of maltreatment, the 21% that was substantiated underscores the necessity for careful monitoring and reporting of suspected abuse and neglect of children.

SUMMARY

This chapter discussed interviewing children about their home situation and family relations. Relevant data from research and national reports were included to provide a framework for talking about family issues and interpreting children's interview reports. Segments of clinical interviews with Bruce Garcia and Karl Bryant illustrated interview strategies and use of the KFD for discussing the home situation and family relations. This chapter also presented national data on child abuse and neglect and discussed interviewing strategies and responsibilities for reporting suspected abuse and neglect.

CHAPTER 6

Parent Interviews

Communication with parents is an essential component of assessment and intervention planning for children. As Barkley (2006) stated so well, "No other adult is more likely than the parents to have the wealth of knowledge about, history of interactions with, or sheer time spent with a child" (p. 341). This unique relationship affords parents special expertise about their children that cannot be duplicated by any other informants. Interviews with parents are especially useful for the following purposes:

- To establish rapport and mutual respect between the interviewer and parent.
- To learn the parent's current concerns about the child.
- To identify and prioritize the child's specific problems as targets for interventions.
- To identify the child's strengths and competencies that can bolster interventions.
- To learn more about key areas of the child's history and current circumstances relevant to understanding identified problems.
- To learn which interventions, if any, have already been attempted.
- To assess the prima facie effectiveness of previous interventions.
- To assess the acceptability and feasibility of future interventions.

Despite their value, parent interviews can sometimes be challenging due to time constraints, scheduling difficulties, or other factors. Some parents may be reluctant to be interviewed about personal and family issues. These challenges make it all the more important that you use your interview time efficiently to gather key information, while still eliciting parents' concerns and unique perspectives on their children.

As indicated in Chapter 1, clinical interviews are best viewed as one of several assessment methods for gaining knowledge about a child's functioning and need for help. If you routinely use other assessment methods along with interviews, you can tailor your interviews to achieve goals to which interviews are best suited. For example, if parents are asked routinely to complete a background questionnaire prior to being interviewed, you can use interview time to ask for details about key areas of developmental, medical, educational, and family history that affect the child's current functioning. Likewise, if parents complete standardized behavioral rating scales prior to the interview, you do not have to waste precious interview time asking about all possible problem areas. Instead, you can focus on parents' main concerns about their child and the specific problems revealed on the rating scales.

This chapter discusses parent interviews with a special emphasis on semistructured formats. The first two sections cover issues regarding confidentiality and questioning strategies for parent interviews. Appendix 6.1 provides a reproducible format for the Semistructured Parent Interview (McConaughy, 2004a), which is the main focus of the chapter. Later sections discuss other assessment methods that can dovetail with parent interviews, child psychiatric disorders, and interviewing culturally and linguistically diverse parents.

DISCUSSING CONFIDENTIALITY AND PURPOSE WITH PARENTS

With the exception of certain emergency situations (e.g., abuse, suicide risk), assessment of children younger than 18 requires informed consent from parents or other legal guardians. IDEA 2004 delineates requirements for informed consent to conduct comprehensive evaluations of students with suspected disabilities. Each state also has its own regulations for interpreting and carrying out the mandates of the IDEA. State regulations usually include specific formats for obtaining informed consent from parents. The Family Education Rights and Privacy Act of 1974 (FERPA; 1974, Public Law 93-830) and its modifications also define confidentiality and parental rights regarding release of information from school records. Briefly, FERPA grants parents rights to access their children's official educational records and requires parental consent for release of records to other agencies, except in limited circumstances, such as school transfer, subpoenas, or requests by state educational agencies or accrediting agencies. The Health Insurance Portability and Accountability Act of 1996 (HIPAA, Public Law 104-191) defines rules to protect the privacy and security of patients' physical and mental health information in hospitals and other health care settings. Psychologists who work in health care settings and in private practice typically use specific consent forms to comply with the requirements of HIPAA. However, the U.S. Department of Health and Human Services and the U.S. Department of Education have jointly determined that FERPA provides adequate privacy protection for elementary and secondary school records. Thus school psychologists and other school-based practitioners are required to comply with FERPA, but not HIPAA (for more detailed discussion of FERPA and HIPAA, see Jacob et al., 2011). Respect for client privacy is also a mandate in the ethical codes of most mental health professional organizations, including the ACA, APA, NASP, and NASW.

All mental health practitioners should be familiar with federal and state laws, as well as their own professional ethical codes, regarding privacy and release of information about children and families. School-based practitioners should also be familiar with FERPA and their school district's policies and procedures. Armed with this knowledge, discussion of purposes and limits of confidentiality can become the entrée for the parent interview. If a parent interview is part of a comprehensive special education evaluation, then written informed consent must be obtained, by law, prior to any assessment of the child, including the parent interview. Parents' written consent should also be obtained prior to any other formal assessment of the child.

> **Informed parental consent must be obtained prior to assessment of the child. Begin the parent interview discussing the purposes of assessment and limits of confidentiality.**

As Jacob (2002) pointed out, informed consent involves three key elements: It is knowing, competent, and voluntary. Parents must have a clear understanding of what they are consenting to; they must be legally competent to give such consent; and the consent must be given without coercion or undue enticement. If a parent has already signed a written consent prior to the interview appointment, you should still review the consent form to make sure that the parent understands to what he/she has agreed. If a parent has not signed a written consent form, then you should obtain a signature prior to asking questions about the child. In either case, you need to review the legal limits of confidentiality in a clear and concise way and explain how information from the interview will be released to any other parties. You should also explain that you will be including information from the parent in your written evaluation reports.

As discussed in Chapter 3, exceptions to confidentiality occur when there is a clear and imminent danger to another individual or to the child directly. Under state statutory law and case law, school personnel also have a legal obligation to take steps to ensure the safety of students under school supervision. Jacob et al. (2011) and Sattler (1998) are excellent sources for detailed discussions of legal and ethical issues regarding confidentiality and disclosure. As they recommend, any written consent form should contain some statement that outlines the limits of confidentiality. An example is the following:

> I understand that there may be circumstances under which the law requires school personnel or clinician(s) to disclose confidential information. These circumstances include: (a) abuse or neglect of minors and (b) situations which may pose a danger to my child or others.

The Semistructured Parent Interview (McConaughy, 2004a; Appendix 6.1) begins with a standard introduction about confidentiality and the purpose of the interview. The phrasing of the introduction assumes that parents have already received and signed a written consent form, and have completed a background questionnaire and standardized rating scales prior to their interview appointment. (The questionnaire and rating scales are discussed in a later section of this chapter.) You can adapt this introduction to fit the particular circumstances of your interview:

> "Thank you for taking your time to meet with me today and for completing the various questionnaires that you received before our meeting. I have reviewed the information that you provided on these forms. In this interview, I would like to hear more about your concerns about [child's name]. Your perspective as a parent is very important for understanding him [her].
>
> "To begin, let's talk about confidentiality issues. You have already voluntarily consented to have [child's name] receive an evaluation. This interview is part of my evaluation of [child's name]. The information you provide will be summarized in a written evaluation report. My usual practice is not to include direct quotations of parents' comments in written reports. I will try to respect your privacy by not reporting information that is not relevant to understanding [child's name] functioning and planning appropriate interventions/treatment. We can discuss what information will and will not be included in a written evaluation report at the end of this interview, if you wish.
>
> "There are circumstances under which the law requires clinicians to disclose confidential information. These circumstances include when there is reason to suspect child abuse or when the child poses a danger to self or a danger to other persons. Do you understand these limits to confidentiality?"

STRATEGIES FOR INTERVIEWING PARENTS

The ideal interview fosters open and responsive collaboration between the interviewer and parent, with each party showing respect for the other. However, as pointed out in Chapter 1, clinical interviews are not like ordinary conversations. Because their purpose is essentially information gathering, clinical interviews can arouse considerable anxiety in many parents. Some parents may be reluctant to discuss personal matters because they are afraid of what the information might reveal about themselves, their children, or their family, or what may happen next. Some parents may actually fear you as an interviewer, because they feel socially inferior or ignorant or think that you blame them for their children's difficulties. Other parents may view you as some kind of "miracle worker" who has all the answers for dealing with their children's problems. Parents from different ethnic or cultural backgrounds may feel that you are not capable of understanding their views and attitudes about their children, or may feel, for some reason, that you are insensitive to their ethnic or cultural views. Some parents themselves may have had unpleasant experiences in their parents' homes or in school, which have made them leery of dealing with any mental health or school-based practitioners.

Any one of the above parental perspectives can raise a barrier to good clinical interviewing. Being sensitive to these potential negative perspectives is the first step toward ameliorating their impact. It is important to take time to establish rapport with parents, while also using interview time efficiently. Addressing parents as experts on their children is a good way to show respect. You can start by stating that they, the parents, probably know their child better than anyone else. Then assure parents that their perspective is important for understanding their child. Be careful to phrase questions in ways that do not assign blame to parents (or teachers) for the child's problems. Also avoid starting the interview with reports of teachers' concerns or a litany of other people's negative comments about the child. Instead, explain that you want to hear the parents' views on their child's functioning and what they think might help to address their concerns about their child.

> **Acknowledging parents as experts on their children and not assigning blame for their children's problems can foster rapport and cooperation in parent interviews.**

Many of the interviewing strategies discussed in Chapter 2 for clinical interviews with children also apply to parent interviews. As a general strategy, interviews with parents can be built around a series of open-ended questions to introduce a topic, followed by more focused questions about specific problems or areas of concern. As the interview progresses, you can use several strategies to facilitate effective communication. Busse and Beaver (2000) used the acronym PACERS for the following strategies: paraphrasing, attending, clarifying, eliciting, reflecting, and summarizing.

Paraphrasing means restating or summarizing the content of what has been said by the interviewee. To paraphrase what the parent has said without restating every word exactly, use key words or phrases. This shows that you heard what was said and gives the parent the opportunity to agree or correct misconceptions.

Attending means making comments that show the interviewee that you are paying attention. These include "minimal encouragers" or extenders (e.g., "Uh-huh") and repeating one or two key words (e.g., "You're feeling discouraged . . . ") to encourage the parent to say more about something.

Clarifying means paraphrasing or restating comments or asking questions to ensure that you have understood what the interviewee said. You can also ask more specific questions to elicit examples of a problem (or competency) that the parent reported about the child. Section II of the Semistructured Parent Interview gives examples of clarifying probes for specific problems: "When [child's name] has this problem(s), what exactly does he [she] do? What does he [she] say? Give me some examples of this problem." These kinds of questions help to define the problem in concrete, observable terms.

Eliciting means asking questions or stating direct requests to gather more information or to obtain specific details. Polite direct requests in the form of a "soft command" (e.g., "Tell me more about _____") make it clear that you want more information. However, you should use these requests sparingly, especially when interviewing anxious or angry parents. You can also ask specific questions to gather details about antecedents, consequences, and circumstances surrounding specific problems of concern, as outlined in Section II of the Semistructured Parent Interview. One caveat is not to disguise judgmental statements in the form of clarifying questions (e.g., "Don't you think that Andy would do better if you supervised his homework?")

Reflecting means rephrasing affect or the emotional aspects of the interviewee's statements. This is different from paraphrasing because instead of focusing on the content of what was reported, reflecting validates or clarifies the parent's reactions to the problem (e.g., "Sounds like it is pretty frustrating for you to always have to remind Andy to do his homework"). Reflecting can help maintain rapport by showing empathy for and concern about the difficulties faced by the parent. It is also important to pay attention to nonverbal cues, such as facial expressions, gestures, and tone of voice, to ascertain the emotional aspects of what parents report. Another caveat, however, is to avoid letting reflective statements turn the interview into a rant or diatribe of negative feelings or complaints about the child or other people. Too much negativity can undermine constructive problem solving later on. You also run the risk of sounding patronizing if you seem too sympathetic.

Summarizing means stating the key issues and themes that have been covered on a topic. This is different from paraphrasing because it covers more information and a longer time span of the interview. Summarizing is a good way to end one topic and move onto another. It is also a good strategy for moving the interview along when a parent is getting off track or is going into excessive detail about some topic. At the end of the entire interview, you should summarize the key themes and concerns that were discussed in order to provide closure. Concluding the interview with a summary is also a good way to move into discussing the information you want to highlight in your written evaluation reports and/or any follow-up meetings with other people.

Many of the dos and don'ts listed in Table 2.2 for child clinical interviews also apply to parent interviews, with appropriate modifications for speaking to adults. Among these, several don'ts are especially good to keep in mind:

- Don't ask too many factual questions that make the interview seem like an interrogation or fact-finding mission.
- Avoid questions with obvious right answers or desirable responses.
- Don't ask "why" questions that may seem accusatory to parents.
- Avoid using psychological or educational jargon, especially if it may not be understood, may seem demeaning, or make you appear to be superior to the parent.

TOPIC AREAS FOR SEMISTRUCTURED PARENT INTERVIEWS

The Semistructured Parent Interview (McConaughy, 2004a) in Appendix 6.1 is organized in a modular fashion for the six topic areas listed in Table 6.1. You can pick and choose topic areas and questions, depending on the referral concerns about a particular child. You can also skip certain topics or questions because of time constraints, parental sensitivities, or school policies regarding

TABLE 6.1. Topic Areas for Semistructured Parent Interviews

  I. Concerns about the child

 II. Behavioral or emotional problems
    Specific nature of the problems
    Priorities for interventions
    Antecedents and consequences of priority problem(s)
    Other possible problem areas

III. Social functioning
    Friends
    Social problems
    Fights/aggression
    Anxiety/depression
    Regarding adolescents
        Dating/romances
        Trouble with the law
        Alcohol/drugs

 IV. School functioning
    Subjects/grades/activities
    Special help/school services
    Teachers
    Homework
    Learning problems
    Retention
    School behavior problems
    Other school concerns

  V. Medical and developmental history
    Medical history
    Developmental history and temperament

 VI. Family relations and home situation
    Family composition
    Home environment
    Family relations
    Rules/punishments
    Chores/rewards
    Home environment

subject matter for interviews. The interview protocol in the appendix lists sample questions for each topic area in the left-hand column; you should feel free to adapt these questions to fit your own style or the flow of the interview. The right-hand column provides space to record notes of parents' responses.

Concerns about the Child

After explaining confidentiality and purpose, it is usually good to begin the interview by asking parents to describe their current concerns about the child (Section I). This gives parents the message that you are there to hear what they have to say first. It also validates their unique expertise on their child. After hearing their major concerns, you can ask more specific questions about when they first became concerned about each problem area and how long the problem(s) has existed.

If parents' concerns are primarily about academic problems, you can move to questions in Section IV about school functioning, and later ask questions from other sections of the protocol, as appropriate. If the parents' concerns are mostly about behavioral or emotional problems, you can move directly to questions in Section II.

Behavioral or Emotional Problems

The questions in Section II follow the general format for *behavioral interviewing* that has been discussed by many other authors (e.g., Busse & Beaver, 2000; Hughes & Baker, 1990; Merrell, 2008a; Kratochwill & Shapiro, 2000; Shapiro & Kratochwill, 2000; Sheridan et al., 1996; Zins & Erchul, 2002). Behavioral interviewing was developed in the context of behavioral consultation models (e.g., Bergan & Kratochwill, 1990; Sheridan et al., 1996), which involve four general stages of assessment and intervention planning: (1) identifying a problem; (2) analyzing the problem; (3) developing an intervention plan; and (4) evaluating the intervention plan. You can use the questions from Section II of the Semistructured Parent Interview, shown in Table 6.2, to accomplish the first two stages of the behavioral consultation process.

The first step in identifying a problem is to obtain descriptions of the specific nature of the problem and the conditions under which the problem occurs. To do this, ask the parent to describe specific behaviors that can be observed and recognized by other people (e.g., "What exactly does the child do? What does he/she say?"). Then ask about the duration and frequency of each identified problem and the circumstances under which it occurs (e.g., "How long has he/she been having this problem? How often does this problem occur? Where and when does this problem usually occur?"). If the parent identifies more than one problem, ask for a description of each problem, and then ask the parent to prioritize the problems for planning interventions. Prioritizing may be hard for some parents who want to fix everything immediately. However, you can explain that it works better to select only a few problems on which to focus at any one time, because this will allow you to collaborate better on appropriate interventions.

> **Behavioral interviewing strategies can be used in parent interviews to identify a child's specific problems and the conditions and circumstances under which problems occur.**

TABLE 6.2. Sample Questions about Behavioral or Emotional Problems

Specific nature of the problems

When [child's name] has this problem, what exactly does he/she do? What does he/she say? Give me some examples of this problem.
Ask the parent to give specific descriptions of the problem. If there is more than one problem, ask about each one.

How long has he/she been having this problem?

How often does this problem occur?

Under what circumstances does this problem occur? Where and when does this problem usually occur?
Ask for specific descriptions of where and when each problem occurs at home and/or school.

Priorities for interventions

Which of the problems we have discussed are you most concerned about now? Which do you think is the most important to address now?

How would you rank the other problems in terms of your concerns and their importance for interventions?

Antecedents and consequences of priority problem(s)

Let's talk about the problem(s) you think are of most concern. What usually happens before this problem occurs? What seems to set it off?
If more than one area of concern, ask about the top two or three problems.

What usually happens after this problem occurs?
What do you do? What do other people do?

How do you usually deal with this problem at home?
How do you feel/react when this problem occurs?
What usually happens at school if this problem occurs?
How does [child's name] feel/react when this happens?

Replacement behaviors

What would be acceptable or alternative behavior related to this problem? What would you like to see [child's name] do instead?

What does [child's name] do well? What do you see as his/her strengths that might help address this problem(s)?

Note. From McConaughy (2004a). Copyright 2004 by Stephanie H. McConaughy. Reprinted by permission.

Functional Behavioral Assessment

After selecting two or three key problems, you can move to identifying antecedents and consequences of each specific problem, using questions such as those listed in Table 6.2. Identifying antecedents and consequences is important for obtaining a *functional behavioral assessment* (FBA) of each problem. Through FBA, you can develop hypotheses about why the problem is occurring and identify circumstances in the environment that are maintaining the problem. An underlying assumption of FBA is that problem behaviors serve some function or purpose for a child. Though there may be various reasons for problem behaviors, an FBA distills these down to three basic functions: (1) to increase social attention; (2) to escape or avoid aversive (unpleasant) tasks or situations; or (3) to serve as self-reinforcement (pleasure). The FBA can then be used to develop a *behavioral intervention plan* (BIP). IDEA 2004 and its precursors require an FBA and a BIP for children with disabilities under certain circumstances, such as changes in educational placement or school exclusion. Other authors have given detailed accounts of the steps for conducting FBAs and developing BIPs (e.g., see Fisher, 2003; McComas, Hoch, & Mace, 2000; Steege & Watson, 2009). Although these uses tend to be reactive applications, FBA and BIPs can also be used as proactive strategies to develop positive behavioral support systems for children in special education and general education settings (Crone, Horner, & Hawkin, 2004; Lane, Kalberg, & Menzies, 2009). Positive behavioral supports and interventions are especially important in the three-tiered service delivery models now being used in many schools. The U.S. Office of Special Education Programs website provides information to assist practitioners in developing positive behavioral supports and interventions *(www.pbis.org)*.

A key strategy for developing a good intervention plan is to identify acceptable alternative behaviors that might "replace" a child's problem behaviors. You should also look for strengths and competencies that can be marshaled in interventions. Table 6.2 lists additional questions that interviewers can ask about replacement behaviors and strengths (e.g., "What would be acceptable or alternative behavior related to this problem? What would you like to see [child's name] do instead? What does [child's name] do well?"). These questions turn the focus toward the child's positive characteristics, which can become important building blocks for intervention plans. Focusing on the positive can also strengthen rapport with parents, who may have heard nothing but negative reports about their children.

> **Identifying a child's strengths and competencies, along with acceptable replacement behaviors for problems, can help create positive intervention plans.**

Standardized Parent Rating Scales

The last part of Section II of the Semistructured Parent Interview includes space for recording problem areas that have been reported by parents on standardized parent rating scales. This section is built on the assumption that the parent has completed a standardized rating scale prior to the interview. When this is done, interviewers can examine the scoring profiles to identify areas in which the child exhibits severe problems compared to normative samples. Table 6.3 summarizes characteristics of several standardized parent rating scales that can be incorporated easily into multimethod assessment procedures. The table lists the number of items and scales for each instrument, characteristics of the normative samples, and contact information for the publisher of each instrument.

Each of the instruments listed in Table 6.3 provides a scoring profile of scales that assess different patterns of problems and/or competencies. Standard scores for each scale help you identify areas in which a parent has reported unusual problems or strengths for the child, compared to normative samples of boys or girls of the same age range. For example, the ASEBA CBCL/6–18 (Achenbach & Rescorla, 2001) includes scales measuring empirically derived patterns of problems (Withdrawn/Depressed, Somatic Complaints, Anxious/Depressed, Social Problems, Thought Problems, Attention Problems, Rule-Breaking Behavior, Aggressive Behavior), plus problems consistent with child psychiatric disorders

> **Standardized rating scales can be used to identify parent-reported problems and competencies that are unusual compared to normative samples of children.**

TABLE 6.3. Examples of Published Standardized Parent Rating Scales

Instrument	Items and scales	Normative samples	Publisher
ASEBA Child Behavior Checklist for Ages 1½–5 (CBCL/1½–5; Achenbach & Rescorla, 2000)	100 items *Problem Scales* Total Problems, Internalizing, Externalizing; Emotionally Reactive, Anxious/Depressed, Somatic Complaints, Withdrawn, Sleep Problems, Attention Problems, Aggressive Behavior, Stress Problems, Affective Problems, Anxiety Problems, Pervasive Developmental Problems, Attention Deficit/Hyperactivity Problems, Oppositional Defiant Problems *Competence Scales* Language Development Survey	Combined norms for boys and girls, ages 1½–5 Multicultural norms	Research Center for Children, Youth, and Families, Inc. One South Prospect Street Burlington, VT 05401-3456 802-656-5130 *www.aseba.org*
ASEBA Child Behavior Checklist For Ages 6–18 (CBCL/6–18; Achenbach & Rescorla, 2001)	20 competence and 120 problem items *Problem Scales* Total Problems, Internalizing, Externalizing; Withdrawn/Depressed, Somatic Complaints, Anxious/Depressed, Social Problems, Thought Problems, Attention Problems, Rule-Breaking Behavior, Aggressive Behavior, Obsessive Compulsive Problems, Post Traumatic Stress Problems, Sluggish Cognitive Tempo, Affective Problems, Anxiety Problems, Attention Deficit/Hyperactivity Problems, Oppositional Defiant Problems, Conduct Problems *Competence/Adaptive Scales* Total Competence, Activities, Social, School	Separate norms for boys and girls, ages 6–11 and 12–18 Multicultural norms	Research Center for Children, Youth, and Families, Inc. One South Prospect Street Burlington, VT 05401-3456 802-656-5130 *www.aseba.org*
Behavior Assessment System for Children–2 Parent Rating Scales (BASC-2 PRS; Reynolds & Kamphaus, 2004)	134–160 items *Problem Scales* Behavioral Symptoms Index, Externalizing, Internalizing, Hyperactivity, Aggression, Conduct Problems (ages 6–18), Anxiety, Depression, Somatization, Attention Problems, Atypicality, Withdrawal	Separate norms for boys and girls, ages 2–5, 6–11, 12–18	Pearson 19500 Bulverde Road San Antonio, TX 78259 800-627-7271 *www.psychcorp.com*

Measure	Scales/Content	Norms	Publisher
(continued from previous page)	*Content Scales* Anger Control, Bullying, Developmental Social Disorders, Emotional Self-Control, Executive Functioning, Negative Emotionality, Resiliency *Competence/Adaptive Scales* Adaptive Skills Composite, Adaptability, Social Skills, Leadership (ages 6–18), Activities of Daily Living, Functional Communication		
Behavioral and Emotional Rating Scale (2nd edition)—Parent Rating Scale (BERS-2-P; Epstein, 2004)	57 items *Competence/Adaptive Scales* Total Strengths Score, Interpersonal Strengths, School Functioning, Intrapersonal Strengths, Family Strengths, Affective Strengths, Career Strengths	Separate norms for boys and girls, ages 5–18	PRO-ED 8700 Shoal Creek Boulevard Austin, TX 78757-6897 800-879-3202 *www.proedinc.com*
Child and Adolescent Symptom Inventory—4R—Parent Checklist (CASI-4R-P; Gadow & Sprafkin, 2005)	163 items *Problem Scales* 18 DSM-IV-TR Disorders *Screening Items* 6 DSM-IV-TR Disorders	Separate norms for boys and girls, ages 5–11 and 12–18	Checkmate Plus P.O. Box 696 Stony Brook, NY 11790-0696 800-779-4292 *www.checkmateplus.com*
Conners Comprehensive Behavior Rating Scales—Parent (CBRS-P; Conners, 2008)	203 items *Problem Scales* Emotional Distress, Academic Difficulties, Defiant/Aggressive Behaviors, Hyperactivity/Impulsivity, Perfectionistic and Compulsive Behaviors, Violence Potential Indicator, Physical Symptoms, 14 DSM-IV-TR Disorders *Validity Scales* Positive Impression, Negative Impression, Inconsistency Index	Separate norms for boys and girls, ages 6–11 and 12–18	MHS P.O. Box 950 North Tonawanda, NY 14120-0950 800-456-3003 *www.mhs.com*
Devereux Behavior Rating Scale—School Form (DBRS-SF; Naglieri, LeBuff, & Pfeiffer, 1993)	40 items *Problem Scales* Total Problems, Interpersonal Problems, Inappropriate Behaviors/Feelings, Depression, Physical Symptoms/Fears	Separate norms for boys and girls, ages 5–12 and 13–18	Pearson 19500 Bulverde Road San Antonio, TX 78259 800-627-7271 *www.psychcorp.com*

(cont.)

TABLE 6.3. (cont.)

Instrument and scales	Items and scales	Normative samples	Publisher
Early Childhood Inventory–4R—Parent Checklist (ECI-4R-P; Gadow & Sprafkin, 2010)	133 items *Problem Scales* 13 DSM-IV-TR Disorders *Screening Items* 6 DSM-IV-TR Disorders *Developmental Rating Scale*	Separate norms for boys and girls, ages 3–5	Checkmate Plus P.O. Box 696 Stony Brook, NY 11790-0696 800-779-4292 *www.checkmateplus.com*
Home and Community Social Behavior Scales (HCSBS; Merrell & Caldarella, 2001)	64 items *Problem Scales* Antisocial Behavior Total, Defiant/Disruptive, Antisocial/Aggressive *Competence/Adaptive Scales* Social Competence Total, Peer Relations, Self-Management/Compliance	Combined norms for boys and girls, ages 5–11 and 12–18	Assessment–Intervention Resources 2285 Elysium Avenue Eugene, OR 97401 541-338-8736 *www.assessment-intervention.com*
Preschool and Kindergarten Behavioral Scales—Second Edition Parent Form (PKBS-2-P; Merrell, 2002a)	76 items *Problem Scales* Total Problem Behavior, Internalizing, Externalizing *Competence/Adaptive Scales* Total Social Skills, Social Cooperation, Social Interaction, Social Independence	Combined norms for boys and girls, ages 3–6	PRO-ED 8700 Shoal Creek Boulevard Austin, TX 78757-6869 800-879-3202 *www.proedinc.com*
Social Skills Improvement System—Parent Form (SSIS-P; Gresham & Elliott, 2008)	79 items *Problem Scales* Total Problems, Internalizing, Externalizing, Bullying, Hyperactivity/Inattention, Autism Spectrum *Competence/Adaptive Scales* Total Social Skills, Communication, Cooperation, Assertion, Responsibility, Empathy, Engagement, Self-Control	Separate norms for boys and girls, ages 3–5, 6–12, 13–18	Pearson 19500 Bulverde Road San Antonio, TX 78259 800-627-7271 *www.psychcorp.com*

Note. ASEBA = Achenbach System of Empirically Based Assessment; DSM-IV-TR = *Diagnostic and statistical manual of mental disorders–fourth edition, text revision* (American Psychiatric Association, 2000).

134

(Affective Problems, Anxiety Problems, Somatic Complaints, Attention Deficit/Hyperactivity Problems, Oppositional Defiant Problems, Conduct Problems). The CBCL/6–18 also has scales for measuring children's competencies (Activities, Social, School).

The BASC-2 Parent Rating Scale (Reynolds & Kamphaus, 2004) includes problem scales (Hyperactivity, Aggression, Conduct Problems, Anxiety, Depression, Somatization, Attention Problems, Atypicality, Withdrawal) and adaptive scales (Adaptability, Social Skills, Leadership, Activities of Daily Living, Functional Communication). The Behavioral and Emotional Rating Scale— Second Edition (BERS-2; Epstein, 2004) assesses patterns of behavioral and emotional strengths (Interpersonal Strengths, School Functioning, Intrapersonal Strengths, Family Strengths, Affective Strengths, and Career Strengths). The Child and Adolescent Symptom Inventory–4R—Parent Checklist (CASI-4R; Gadow & Sprafkin, 2005) and Conners Comprehensive Behavior Rating Scales—Parent version (CBRS-P; Conners, 2008) assess problems consistent with DSM-IV-TR psychiatric disorders. The CBRS-P includes seven additional problem scales. Other rating scales listed in Table 6.3 assess problems, competencies, and/or social skills.

After examining the scoring profile of a standardized parent rating scale, you can list problem scales with deviant scores in the spaces provided in Section II of the Semistructured Parent Interview protocol. This list can prompt you to ask parents about problem areas that have not already been discussed. If a parent acknowledges concerns about these problem areas, you can ask further questions about circumstances surrounding the problems and whether anything has been done to address them. You can also ask about situations outside the home that might affect the child's behavior. It is usually good to avoid going into much detail in this part of the interview so as not to overwhelm the parent or prolong the interview. However, questions about other possible problems can broaden the focus for formulating a comprehensive picture of the child.

Social Functioning

Section III of the Semistructured Parent Interview contains questions about children's social functioning, as shown in Table 6.4. Section III questions are modeled on similar questions for child clinical interviews, as discussed in Chapters 3 and 4. The similarity between parent and child interview questions makes it easier to compare the two perspectives on the child's social functioning.

Section III begins with open-ended questions about the child's friendships (e.g., "How many close friends does [child's name] have?") and social activities (e.g., "Do other kids come to your house to play/do things with [child's name]? Does he/she belong to any clubs or social groups?"). Additional questions ask about social problems, fights, aggressive behavior, anxiety, and depression. Each of the latter three topic areas begins with a structured question, asking whether the child has exhibited that type of problem. Interviewers can check boxes on the interview protocol to indicate the parent's responses to each lead-in question ("Yes," "No," "Don't know"). If a parent answers "yes," then you can ask more specific questions to learn about the nature of the problem.

When parents report problems of depression for their child, it is important to follow up with questions about suicidal thoughts or attempts (e.g., "Has he/she ever made comments about wanting to harm or kill him/herself? Has he/she ever attempted to harm or kill him/herself?"). In cases where parents report that the child has had suicidal thoughts or has made suicidal attempts, you should ask more specific questions regarding plans, how many attempts, access to methods (e.g., guns in the house, lethal pills), and deterrents to suicide. When there is sufficient cause to indicate

TABLE 6.4. Sample Questions about Social Functioning

Friends

How many close friends does [child's name] have? Do you think that is enough friends?
How do you feel about his/her choice of friends?

Do other kids come to your house to play/do things with [child's name]?
Does he/she go to other kids' houses?

Does he/she belong to any clubs or social groups (e.g., Scouts, YMCA, teams)?
Does he/she go to church/belong to any church or spiritual groups?

Social problems

Does [child's name] have any problems getting along with other kids (e.g., not liked, teased/picked on, feels left out)?
☐ Yes　☐ No　☐ Don't know

(*If yes*) Tell me more about his/her social problems.
Has anything been done to try to help him/her with social problems (e.g., see a counselor, social skills group, friendship group)?

Fights/aggression

Does [child's name] ever get into physical fights with other kids?
☐ Yes　☐ No　☐ Don't know

(*If yes*) How often?
What usually starts the fights?
How do they usually end?
Has anything been done to try to help him/her avoid fighting?

Do you think he/she has trouble controlling his/her temper?
Has he/she ever used a weapon or object (e.g., stick, stone) to hurt other kids?
Does he/she belong to a gang?

Anxiety/depression

Does [child's name] seem unusually anxious or worried about things?
☐ Yes　☐ No　☐ Don't know

(*If yes*) Tell me more about that.
What does he/she worry about?
Has [child's name] ever seemed very sad or depressed for a long period of time?
☐ Yes　☐ No　☐ Don't know

(*If yes*) Tell me more about that.
Has he/she ever made comments about wanting to harm or kill him/herself?
Has he/she ever attempted to harm or kill him/herself?
If yes, probe more regarding plans, attempts, access to methods, etc. Review confidentiality and legal reporting requirements. Discuss need for intervention.

Note. From McConaughy (2004a). Copyright 2004 by Stephanie H. McConaughy. Reprinted by permission.

risk for suicide, then you will need to discuss limits to confidentiality and legal reporting requirements, as well as the need for intervention. Chapter 9 provides more detailed discussion and guidelines for assessing suicide risk.

Section III provides a format for querying parents about potential problems that is different from the behavioral interviewing format in Section II. If you do not want to conduct an FBA in the parent interview, you can skip Section II and use Section III to ask parents about behavioral and emotional problems. You can also select questions from Section III to cover potential problems that were not discussed in Section II. If a parent has not completed a standardized rating scale prior to the interview, Section III provides a structure for asking about potential problems of both an internalizing and externalizing nature.

The last part of Section III includes questions for parents of adolescents modeled on similar questions discussed in Chapter 4 for directly interviewing adolescents. These cover dating and romances, trouble with the law, and alcohol and drug use. Interviewers can check boxes on the form to indicate parents' responses to lead-in questions about trouble with the law and alcohol or drug problems. When parents report that an adolescent does have problems in these areas, you can ask questions about the nature of the problems, whether there have been any interventions or treatment for the problems, and whether the parent thinks the adolescent needs treatment.

School Functioning

Section IV of the Semistructured Parent Interview provides questions about children's school functioning, as shown in Table 6.5. Some of the questions about school subjects, teachers, and homework parallel similar questions in the child clinical interview. However, parents are asked about these areas in more detail. The initial questions are useful for all parents, to obtain their views on their child's school performance and relationships with school staff.

Section IV also includes questions about learning problems, special help or school services, retention, school behavior problems, and other school concerns. A structured lead-in question asks whether the child has exhibited problems in each of these areas. Because these questions focus more specifically on school problems, they may not be necessary or appropriate for parents of children who function well in school. The lead-in questions about learning problems, special help or school services, retention, and school behavior problems are tied to similar questions listed on the Child and Family Information Form (McConaughy & Achenbach, 2004a) in Appendix 6.2. This background questionnaire covers demographic information, the child's school history, medical and developmental history, family history, and current living situation. As a routine practice, parents can be asked to complete the Child and Family Information Form prior to appointments for the parent interview and assessment of their child. You can then review the questionnaire prior to your parent interview to learn about particular areas of concern. On the protocol form for the Semistructured Parent Interview, you can check boxes ("Yes," "No," "Don't know") in Section IV to indicate how parents responded to each corresponding question on the Child and Family Information Form. During your interview, you can then ask parents to elaborate on areas reported as problems. If parents have not completed the

> **Background questionnaires are efficient methods for obtaining demographic data, plus the child's school, medical, developmental, and family history, and current living situation.**

TABLE 6.5. Sample Questions about School Functioning

Subjects/grades/activities

What are [child's name]'s best subject areas in school? What does he/she like best?
What are [child's name]'s worst subject areas, if any? What does he/she like the least in school?

What kind of grades does he/she get? *Ask about each subject area.*
Have his/her grades changed remarkably in any area?

What are his/her extracurricular activities (e.g., sports, clubs, school play, band, choir)?
Does [child's name] have any problems with school attendance/skipping classes?

Teachers

How many teachers does [child's name] have?
How does he/she get along with each teacher?
How does he/she get along with the principal and other school staff?
Is there anyone at school who is especially important to him/her?

Homework

How much homework does [child's name] typically have? How do you feel about the amount of homework he/she has?

Does he/she have any trouble with homework?
(*If yes*) Tell me more about that.
When and where does he/she usually do homework?
How long does homework usually take?
How much time do you think he/she should spend on homework?
Does he/she get any help with homework?
(*If yes*) How does that work out?

Learning problems

Does [child's name] have learning problems?
☐ Yes   ☐ No   ☐ Don't know
[*See Child and Family Information Form*]

(*If yes*) What kind of learning problems?
Why do you think [child's name] is having learning problems right now?
How long has he/she had these problems?
What has been done to address these problems?

Special help/school services

Does [child's name] receive any special help/special services in school?
☐ Yes   ☐ No   ☐ Don't know
[*See Child and Family Information Form*]

(*If yes*) What kind of help?
Probe for special education, IEP, remedial instruction/Title I services, Section 504 plan, peer tutoring, individual aide, behavior plan, guidance services, school psychologist.

How long has he/she had this special help?
How often does he/she get this help?
What kinds of help has he/she had in the past?

Do you think this is enough help/the right kind of help?
What else would you like to have happen for [child's name] at school?

(continued)

TABLE 6.5. *(continued)*

Retention

Has [child's name] ever been retained/held back a grade?
☐ Yes   ☐ No   ☐ Don't know
[*See Child and Family Information Form*]

(*If yes*) When? For what reason?
How did [child's name] feel about being retained/held back?
How did you feel about his/her being retained/held back?

School behavior problems

Does [child's name] have behavior problems at school?
☐ Yes   ☐ No   ☐ Don't know
[*See Child and Family Information Form*]

(*If yes*) What kind of problems?
What usually happens at school when he/she has these problems?
What has been done to address these problems?

Other school concerns

Do you have other school concerns?
☐ Yes   ☐ No   ☐ Don't know
[*See Child and Family Information Form*]

(*If yes*) What kind of concerns?
What has been done to address these concerns?
If you could change something about school, what would it be?
What would you especially like to see happen for [child's name] at school?

Note. From McConaughy (2004a). Copyright 2004 by Stephanie H. McConaughy. Reprinted by permission.

Child and Family Information Form ahead of time, you can ask about each school problem area, as appropriate.

When parents report that their child has learning problems in school, it is important to elicit their perspectives on these problems and how they feel about any special help that has been provided to address the problems. When asking about school services, you should probe for several possibilities (e.g., special education, IEP, remedial instruction/Title I services, Section 504 plan, peer tutoring, individual aide, behavior plan, guidance services, school psychologist), because parents may not think some of these constitute "special help." Teachers may or may not report similar problems and may have more detailed information on school interventions (see Chapter 7). In my experience, lack of sufficient or appropriate services has often been a key parental complaint and sometimes a source of tension between parents and school staff.

It is also good to ask whether the child has repeated a grade, because grade retention can be a marker for past, current, and future learning or behavioral problems. It has been estimated that as many as 15% of U.S. students are held back each year, even though research has indicated that retention is not an effective strategy for improving educational success (National Association of School Psychologists, 2003a). Retention is often a key worry for elementary school children and may have negative effects on their self-confidence. Section IV also includes questions about school behavior problems. However, if these have already been covered in earlier parts of the parent interview (e.g., Sections I and II), it is not necessary to ask parents about such problems again. In interviews with parents, school-based practitioners, in particular, should make a special effort to maintain a neutral stance regarding children's school problems and any special help they receive so as to encourage parents to express their views openly. Appearing too closely aligned with school staff can undermine rapport and become a barrier to obtaining parental cooperation in intervention efforts.

Medical and Developmental History

Section V of the Semistructured Parent Interview covers aspects of the child's medical and developmental history. Learning about the child's history is important for understanding the nature of current problems. Interviewers in mental health and medical settings often devote considerable time to taking medical and developmental histories (e.g., Barkley, 2006; Barkley & Murphy, 2006). However, asking detailed questions about the child's history can become very tedious and unnecessarily prolong parent interviews for school-based assessments. To reduce time requirements, the questions in Section V are tied to similar questions on the Child and Family Information Form (McConaughy & Achenbach, 2004a; Appendix 6.2). If parents have completed this background questionnaire prior to the interview, you can take the same approach as you did for questions about school problems. That is, review the Child and Family Information Form ahead of time and ask for elaboration only on medical and developmental problems reported by parents as present. If parents have not completed the Child and Family Information Form, you can briefly review each area listed in Section V of the parent interview.

Family Relations and Home Situation

Section VI of the Semistructured Parent Interview asks about the child's family and the home environment. This section was placed last in the protocol because it can be a very sensitive topic

> Information about family relations and the home environment is important for understanding children's functioning and planning appropriate interventions for identified problems.

for many parents. As indicated earlier, some parents may be reluctant to discuss what transpires at home because they consider home life a private matter. Parents may also worry that an interviewer blames them and the home situation for their child's problems. If you begin your interview with such sensitive topics, parents may be unwilling to continue or may be less forthcoming when discussing other issues.

Some of the questions in Section VI are tied to the Child and Family Information Form (Appendix 6.2). With this in mind, you can use that background questionnaire as an entrée for asking about family composition and the home environment. If the parents are divorced or separated, it is important to learn who has legal and physical custody and what visiting arrangements have been made for the child. In cases without joint custody arrangements, you should ask what information, if any, may be shared with the noncustodial parent. The Child and Family Information Form contains specific questions about family history of medical, mental health, and learning problems as well as the child's current living situation. After reviewing this information, you can ask about specific problems that parents reported on the questionnaire. If parents have not completed the Child and Family Information Form, you can ask more general questions about the family and home environment (e.g., "Is there anything about your home or living situation that is a problem for you or the family? Have there been any recent changes or stresses in your living situation or family? Do any family members have medical or mental health problems that might affect [child's name]?").

Other questions in Section VI parallel questions about the home situation and family in the child clinical interview (see Chapter 5). These concern family relations, rules and punishments, and chores and rewards for the child, as shown in Table 6.6. Answers to these types of questions can be very helpful for planning interventions for children with behavioral and emotional problems. For example, some parents may resort to harsh or excessive punishments (e.g., frequent spanking; no TV for the rest of the year; "grounding" for long periods of time) that are ineffective in changing children's behavior. Other parents may report few or no rules or punishments in the home and poor supervision of their children's whereabouts. Research has shown strong associations between children's externalizing problems and poor parental supervision and/or harsh discipline strategies (McMahon & Frick, 2007; McMahon & Forehand, 2003). Asking about reward

---

TABLE 6.6. Sample Questions about Family Relations and Home Situation

Family relations

How does [child's name] get along with members of the family/people in your home?
Ask about the child's relationship with each member of the family, as appropriate: father, mother, stepparents, other adults in home, other caregivers, siblings, stepsiblings.

Who does [child's name] get along with best?
Who does [child's name] get along with least?

Do members of the family have trouble getting along?

Do you have any problems getting along with members of the family (e.g., spouse/partner, your children, relatives, other adults or children in the home)?

Rules/punishments

What are the rules/expectations about behavior in your home? Who makes the rules?
How do you think [child's name] feels about the rules?
What kinds of punishments/discipline procedures are used in your home?
Do children ever get spanked/physically punished for bad behavior?

Who usually gives the punishments/disciplines children in the family?
Do you and your spouse/partner agree on punishments/discipline?
How do you think [child's name] feels about the punishments/discipline?

Have you ever talked with someone else about punishment/discipline (e.g., counselor, teacher, friend, relative)? Would you like help in discipline or behavior management?

Chores/rewards

What happens when a child does something good or special?
Do you give out any special rewards or treats for good behavior/accomplishments?
Does this ever happen for [child's name]?

Does [child's name] have any special chores/jobs at home?
Does he/she get an allowance? (*If yes*) What does he/she have to do for it?
Does he/she have a paying job outside the home?

Note. From McConaughy (2004a). Copyright 2004 by Stephanie H. McConaughy. Reprinted by permission.

systems in the home can also elicit clues to positive incentives for the child that might be incorporated into intervention plans. Asking about chores can give some indication of whether the child has age-appropriate responsibilities and opportunities to earn monetary rewards, such as an allowance. Some parents may report no use of rewards in the home, which could exacerbate problems arising from ineffective discipline and harsh punishments.

As indicated earlier, it is important to frame questions about family issues in ways that do not imply that parents have caused their children's problems. Instead, the challenge is to recruit parents' cooperation in identifying problems and developing appropriate interventions. Helping parents feel respected and treating them as equal partners with you, and with school staff when appropriate, can go a long way toward building effective interventions for children with learning and behavior problems (Miller, Arthur-Stanley, & Lines, 2012). The Achieving–Behaving–Caring program is one example of a home–school collaboration effort built on mutual respect and equal partnership between parents and teachers (Kay, Fitzgerald, & McConaughy, 2001; McConaughy, Kay, Welkowitz, Hewitt, & Fitzgerald, 2008).

CHILD PSYCHIATRIC DISORDERS

Epidemiological studies have estimated that between 3 and 18% of children, ages 5–17, meet criteria for a psychiatric diagnosis that causes significant functional impairment (Costello, Egger, & Angold, 2005). Prevalence rates have varied across studies depending on diagnostic criteria, definitions of impairment, and survey methodology (e.g., structured diagnostic interviews vs. rating scales or questionnaires). Costello et al. (2005) estimated a median prevalence rate of 12% across studies they reviewed, suggesting that at any time, one child in eight has an impairing psychiatric disorder. In an earlier review of 12 epidemiological studies published after 1986, Doll (1996) reported prevalence rates up to 18–22%. Based on those prevalence rates, Doll estimated that a hypothetical school of 1,000 students could be expected to have between 180 to 220 students with diagnosable psychiatric disorders. The high prevalence rates from epidemiological studies suggest that large percentages of school-age children exhibit behavioral and emotional problems severe enough to warrant mental health services.

Utility of Psychiatric Diagnoses

Given the high prevalence rates of psychiatric disorders identified in research studies, new efforts are underway to forge links between community mental health clinics and schools to provide services to children with mental health problems (Doll & Cummings, 2007; Nastasi, 1998; National Association of School Psychologists, 2003b). Psychiatric diagnoses are especially useful in referrals for mental health services in or outside of school. For such cases, psychiatric diagnoses may facilitate communication between school-based practitioners and professionals in mental health and hospital settings (e.g., psychiatrists, clinical psychologists, social workers). In addition, psychiatric diagnoses are often required for reimbursements by third-party payers, including Medicaid, private insurance companies, and health maintenance organizations (HMOs).

> To qualify for a psychiatric disorder, an individual must have the requisite number of symptoms over a specified period of time and show clinically significant impairment.

To guide clinical assessment and research on child psychiatric disorders, the DSM-5 lists specific features, or symptoms, for disorders of childhood and adolescence. Several adult disorders can also be used for children and adolescents. Table 6.7 lists examples of DSM-5 diagnoses that apply to children and adolescents. For each disorder, practitioners must decide whether the child exhibits the requisite number of specified symptoms over a particular period of time (e.g., the past 6 or 12 months). They must then determine whether symptoms reported as "present" produce clinically significant impairment in social, academic, or occupational functioning, and, for some diagnoses, impairment in different settings (e.g., home, school, or work). Some diagnoses require that at least some of the symptoms occur before a certain age (e.g., prior to age 12 for ADHD). Practitioners must also rule out other diagnoses that might account for the symptoms. An individual qualifies for the diagnosis if he/she exhibits the requisite number of symptoms, shows clinically significant impairment, and meets other specified criteria (e.g., age of onset).

In the organizational structure for DSM-5, disorders of infancy, childhood, and adolescence are listed under several different broad categories. For example, the broad category of neurodevelopmental disorder includes intellectual disability, communication disorders, autism spectrum disorder, ADHD, specific learning disorder, and motor disorders. The broad category of disruptive, impulse control, and conduct disorders includes some adult disorders and the childhood disorders of ODD and CD, plus a new callous and unemotional specifier for CD and a diagnosis of disruptive behavior disorder not elsewhere classified for individuals who exhibit symptoms of ODD and/or CD but do not meet diagnostic thresholds for the two diagnoses. The broad category of depressive disorders includes a newly defined diagnosis of disruptive mood dysregulation disorder for individuals between ages 6 and 18 who show severe recurrent temper outbursts that are grossly out of proportion to the intensity or duration of a situation. Diagnoses of non-suicidal self injury disorder and suicidal behavior disorder are listed under the category of other disorders. The DSM-5 also includes revisions to criteria for certain childhood disorders, such as age of onset before age 12 (not age 7) for ADHD and a coding note regarding the frequency of symptoms for ODD (American Psychiatric Association, 2012, 2013).

Although some experts have questioned the utility of psychiatric diagnoses for planning school-based interventions (Gresham & Gansle, 1992), they can be useful for identifying children who are eligible for certain types of services. For example, children with certain diagnoses may be eligible for a Section 504 plan under the Rehabilitation Act of 1973 (Rehabilitation Act, 1973)

TABLE 6.7. Examples of DSM-5 Diagnoses Applied to Children and Adolescents

Adjustment Disorder	Major Depressive Episode
Attention-Deficit/Hyperactivity Disorder	Motor Disorders
Autism Spectrum Disorder[a]	Non-suicidal Self Injury Disorder[a]
Communication Disorders[a]	Obsessive–Compulsive Disorder
Conduct Disorder	Oppositional Defiant Disorder
Callous and Unemotional Specifier for Conduct Disorder[a]	Separation Anxiety Disorder
Disruptive Behavior Disorder Not Elsewhere Specified[a]	Social Communication Disorder[a]
Disruptive Mood Dysregulation Disorder[a]	Social Anxiety Disorder (Social Phobia)
Dysthymic Disorder	Specific Learning Disorder[a]
Generalized Anxiety Disorder	Specific Phobia
Intellectual Disability[a]	Suicidal Behavior Disorder[a]

[a]New or substantially revised DSM-5 diagnoses.

and its revisions in the Americans with Disabilities Act of 1990 (Americans with Disabilities Act, 1990). A psychiatric diagnosis is one form of "disability" covered in these federal civil rights statutes. Section 504 plans outline accommodations in the general education setting, which can serve as alternatives to special education services. Use of Section 504 plans is often the route taken for children with ADHD. Children with diagnoses of mood disorders (depression or anxiety) and some children with CD or ODD may also qualify for Section 504 plans. The key determinant is whether the child's disability has a negative impact on "learning" or "alertness" and interferes with life functioning.

Psychiatric diagnoses are not required for eligibility for special education services under IDEA 2004. Instead, IDEA 2004 has its own definitions of disabilities, including mental retardation (MR), specific learning disabilities (LD), emotional disturbance (ED), and seven other categories. However, a psychiatric diagnosis may provide additional assessment information that is helpful in deciding whether a child meets the IDEA 2004 criteria for a disability. For example, children with diagnoses of mood disorders may qualify as having ED. Some children with diagnoses of disruptive disorders (ADHD, CD, ODD) may also qualify as having ED, though this usage has generated controversy among school-based practitioners and administrators (Skiba & Grizzle, 1991, 1992). Children with ADHD (but no ED or LD) may be eligible for special education under the IDEA 2004 disability category of "other health impairment," which also covers other chronic health conditions (e.g., seizure disorders, cerebral palsy).

Structured Diagnostic Interviews with Parents

Interviews with parents are key assessment procedures for making psychiatric diagnoses. The American Academy of Pediatrics (2000) has also stressed the importance of parent interviews in its guidelines for assessment of ADHD. Since the 1970s, much effort has been devoted to developing structured diagnostic interviews to assess symptoms and other defined criteria for psychiatric diagnosis. Many of the parent structured diagnostic interviews have parallel forms for children. However, research has shown much higher reliability and validity for structured diagnostic interviews with parents than with children (for reviews, see McConaughy, 2000b; Saigh, 1992).

The Diagnostic Interview for Children and Adolescents–IV (DICA-IV; Reich, 2000; Reich, Welner, Herjanic, & MHS Staff, 1999) and the NIMH Diagnostic Interview Schedule for Children—Version IV (NIMH DISC-IV; Shaffer et al., 2000) are two examples of highly structured diagnostic interviews. A computerized version of DICA-IV is distributed by Multi-Health Systems (*www.mhs.com*). A computerized version of the NIMH DISC-IV is distributed by the Columbia University Department of Psychiatry (*www.c-disc.com/disc.htm*). The DICA-IV covers 28 psychiatric diagnoses applicable to children. The NIMH DISC-IV covers approximately 30 diagnoses. Both of these interviews employ a standard set of questions and probes with specific response criteria. Questions are organized into a branching hierarchy with skip functions. A modular format allows interviewers to focus on subsets of specific diagnoses. The Child and Adolescent Psychiatric Assessment (CAPA; Angold & Costello, 2000) and Schedule for Affective Disorders and Schizophrenia for School-Age Children (K-SADS; Ambrosini, 2000) are other examples of structured diagnostic interviews. The CAPA and K-SADS are somewhat less structured than the DICA-IV and NIMH DISC-IV, but they still follow a standard set of questions and probes.

The structured diagnostic interviews were developed primarily for mental health assessment and research. Though it is good to be aware of these interview protocols, their length and detail render them impractical for most child clinical assessments, particularly school-based assessments. For example, the full DICA-IV has approximately 1,600 questions, and the full NIMH DISC-IV has as many 3,000 questions. Administration time can vary from about 1 hour to 2 or 3 hours, depending on the number of diagnoses selected by the interviewer and the number of symptoms endorsed by parents. All of the above published structured diagnostic interviews require special training to administer.

Practitioners can consult the DSM-5 to familiarize themselves with diagnostic criteria for psychiatric diagnoses. They can then incorporate additional questions into parent interviews regarding symptoms and other criteria to screen for psychiatric disorders.[1] Practitioners who do this must have appropriate training in theory and practice for making psychiatric diagnoses. They must also remember that no diagnosis should be based on only one source of information, including the parent interview. Instead, as with other forms of assessment, diagnoses of childhood psychiatric disorders should make use of multiple data sources, such as those outlined in Table 1.2 in Chapter 1.

INTERVIEWING CULTURALLY OR LINGUISTICALLY DIVERSE PARENTS

Interviewing parents with different ethnic or cultural backgrounds presents additional challenges. We discussed interviewing culturally and linguistically diverse children in Chapter 2. Many of the issues and recommendations in that chapter also apply to interviewing parents. Sattler (1998) provided a good summary of demographics and special issues to consider when interviewing African Americans, Hispanic Americans, Asian Americans, Native Americans, and refugees. Rhodes et al. (2005) provided an extensive discussion of interviewing strategies for non-English-speaking parents and parents from diverse cultures. Drawing from Rhodes et al., Table 6.8 outlines specific steps to be taken ahead of time to prepare for the parent interview.

After learning the referral concerns and reviewing records, two key steps are to determine who is the legal guardian of the child and what is the preferred language of the parent or guardian. You should then determine whether an interpreter will be needed. As noted in Table 6.8, if the parent speaks English, do not assume that he/she has sufficient English skills for a clinical interview or that English is the preferred language. Chapter 2 discussed use of interpreters for clinical interviews with children. The same recommendations and precautions apply to using interpreters in interviews with parents. An interpreter may also be needed to help the parent complete questionnaires, such as the Child and Family Information Form in Appendix 6.2 or English versions of one of the standardized parent rating scales listed in Table 6.3. Many of the rating scales in Table 6.3 have been translated into Spanish. The ASEBA CBCL/1½–5 and CBCL/6–18 have been translated into over 85 languages, including Spanish, and profiles for both parent forms can be scored according to multicultural norms for different cultures or societies (Achenbach & Rescorla, 2007).

As stipulated in Chapter 2, interpreters should be fluent in both the language of the interviewer and the language of the parent, should have expertise in translating, and have a basic

---

[1] The first edition of this book offered a Structured Diagnostic Interview for Parents to screen for DSM-IV-TR disgnoses. This second edition does not include that interview protocol because the publication of DSM-5 renders it obsolete.

TABLE 6.8. Steps to Prepare for Interviewing Culturally and Linguistically Diverse Parents

1. Determine the exact referral concerns about the child. Clarify any immediate questions or concerns with the referral source.

2. Review available records, including all previous assessment information, language scores, and reported language spoken in the home.

3. Determine who is the child's legal guardian and who has authority to give permission for educational and psychological assessments.

4. Determine the parent's or guardian's preferred language. If the parent or guardian speaks English, do not assume that English is the preferred language.

5. Determine whether an interpreter is needed. Ask the parent if he or she would prefer to have an interpreter.

6. Contact the parent or guardian to briefly discuss the purpose of the interview, preferred location, and possible times. You may need an interpreter for this initial contact.

7. Ask the parent or guardian if he/she wants any other adult (e.g., friend, family member, family advocate) to be included in the interview. If other adults are to be included, they will be bound by the same confidentiality guarantees as all other participants.

8. Schedule a convenient time and location for all parties, including the interpreter, if needed.

9. Provide a courtesy reminder to the parent or guardian and interpreter prior to the meeting.

10. Examine your own presuppositions or beliefs about the family and its racial, ethnic, or cultural background. If you have strong negative views, prejudices, or stereotypes, seek additional education and/or supervision prior to the interview, or ask to have someone else conduct the interview.

Note. Adapted from Rhodes, Ochoa, and Ortiz (2005). Copyright 2005 by The Guilford Press. Adapted by permission.

> **Interpreters should be fluent in the languages of the interviewer and the parent, have expertise in translating, and understand the assessment process.**

understanding of the assessment process. It is also worth repeating that interpreters should not be friends or family members, and certainly not other children in the family. Unfortunately, children have sometimes been used as interpreters for lack of an immediate alternative, but this is strongly discouraged because of breaches of confidentiality for the referred child and parent and the inappropriate role reversals this entails.

If the family members are recent immigrants to the United States or have some kind of temporary status, such as migrant workers, then it would be good to try to determine their level of acculturation, as discussed in Chapter 2. Assessing acculturation may require a separate interview with the parent prior to the interview focusing on the child. When done with respect, asking questions about acculturation can help establish rapport by showing parents that you are interested in their experiences and cultural beliefs and traditions. Drawing from the recommendations of Rhodes et al. (2005), Table 6.9 provides a series of sample questions for evaluating parents' degree of acculturation. The questions cover language preference, social affiliation, daily living habits, cultural traditions, communication style, cultural identity and pride, perceived prejudice or discrimination, generational status, family socialization and cultural values. Rating scales and questionnaires have also been developed to assess acculturation and cultural self-identity (see Chun, Organista, & Morin, 2003).

Having adequately prepared ahead of time and determined whether an interpreter is needed, the next steps are to contact the parent to discuss the purpose of the interview and to pick a location and time. If parents do not have a phone, try sending them a brief note or consider a home visit

TABLE 6.9. Sample Questions Regarding Acculturation

Domain	Questions
Language use or preference	What language do you use most during your day?
	What language do you feel most comfortable using in social situations?
	What language do you speak to your children?
	What language(s) do your children speak?
Social affiliation	Do your friends speak your language?
	Do your friends share your background or culture?
	Do your child's friends have similar or different backgrounds or culture?
Daily living habits	What kinds of foods do you cook most often?
	Who usually takes care of the house and jobs at home?
	What jobs or chores do your children have?
Cultural traditions	Do you observe any cultural traditions or holidays?
	Do you observe any new traditions or holidays here in the United states?
	Are you teaching your children your cultural traditions?
Communication style	Do you feel you express yourself better in your native language or English?
	Do you feel your style of communication has changed?
	Has your children's style of communication changed?
Cultural identity or pride	What do you consider your culture now?
	Do you participate in any activities to show pride in your native culture?
	Do your children participate in any activities to show pride in your culture?
Perceived prejudice or discrimination	Have you ever felt put down or ridiculed because of your background or practices?
	Do you think people from your culture are discriminated against in the United States or in your community?
	Has your child had any problems with discrimination?
Generational status	Where were you born? If not in the United States, when did you come to the United States?
	Where were your parents born? If not in the United States, when did they come to the United States?
	Where was your child born? If not in the United States, how old was he/she when he/she came to the United States?
Family socialization	Does your family participate in any cultural traditions with other families?
Cultural values	What are your current religious beliefs and practices?
	Are your religious beliefs the same as those in your native culture?
	Does your child share your religious beliefs and traditions?
	If not, how are your child's beliefs different?

Note. Adapted from Rhodes, Ochoa, and Ortiz (2005). Copyright 2005 by The Guilford Press. Adapted by permission.

by yourself or an appropriate member of the school staff (e.g., home–school coordinator or social worker). Use an interpreter for these initial contacts as you would for the actual interview. Also ask the parent or guardian if he/she wants any other adult (e.g., friend, family member, family advocate) to be included in the interview. Some parents may feel more comfortable having someone else there for support. If other adults are to be included, explain that the parent needs to give express permission for their inclusion and that the other adults will be bound by the same guarantees of confidentiality as all other participants. Siblings of the referred child or other children in the family should not be included during the parent interview. Otherwise, it is not your role to determine who is, or is not, appropriate to include along with the parent.

Schedule a convenient time and location for all parties, including the interpreter. If the parent or guardian cannot attend a meeting at school, consider another safe location, such as a neutral place in the community or the home, unless there are specific school administrative policies that require that meetings with parents must take place on school grounds. Some parents may need assistance with transportation or child care to attend meetings at school. If a parent cannot participate in a face-to-face meeting, then consider conducting the interview by telephone. However, because of the impersonal nature of telephone interviews, they should be done only as a last resort in unusual circumstances. As stated in Chapter 2, you also need to examine your own presuppositions or beliefs about the family and its racial, ethnic, or cultural background. If you have strong negative views, prejudices, or stereotypes, seek additional education and/or supervision prior to the interview, or ask to have someone else conduct the interview.

Interviewers can follow the format of the Semistructured Parent Interview shown in Appendix 6.1. As stated earlier, it is not necessary to cover all sections of the Semistructured Parent Interview. Instead, you can choose sections that are most appropriate depending on the concerns of the referral source and the parent. You may also want to ask direct questions about the child's developmental history if the parent has not completed questionnaires ahead of time. As an alternative, some practitioners might prefer to use the reproducible interview protocols provided by Rhodes et al. (2005), which are printed in English and Spanish. Their interview protocols are more structured than the Semistructured Parent Interview. They include specific questions covering the child's birth; developmental, language, health, educational, and behavioral history; plus family history, acculturation status, and the parent's concerns and aspirations for the child (see Rhodes et al., 2005, pp. 113–118).

Drawing on other authors (e.g., Merrell, 2008a; Rhodes et al., 2005) and my own experiences, the following are general recommendations for interviewing culturally and linguistically diverse parents or guardians:

- Choose a neutral place that is private and comfortable. Avoid using offices of authority figures (e.g., the principal's office) or the child's classroom. Provide chairs appropriately sized for adults. Avoid sitting behind a desk because this can seem intimidating.
- Provide a clear, concise explanation of privacy and confidentiality. Tell the parent that you plan to take notes to remember the details of the interview, and that you will keep your notes in a confidential, secure place. If you want to tape-record the interview, ask the parent's permission ahead of time. (Tape recording may be very intimidating to some parents.)
- Explain the purpose of the interview and specific ways that the information will, and will not, be used.
- Speak clearly and avoid idioms, slang expressions, and statements with double meanings.

- Allow time for both parties to participate in the interview without feeling rushed. If an interpreter is used, allow adequate time for translation.
- Treat the parent with respect. Do not talk down to the parent or simplify statements in a way that suggests that he/she has low intelligence.
- Try to be sensitive and respectful of the parent's cultural perspectives and value systems, even if they are different from your own. Try to see the strengths of different cultural coping mechanisms that can be marshaled for interventions.
- Try to avoid making judgments about children and families based on stereotypes or preconceived notions regarding ethnic and cultural backgrounds, socioeconomic status, or child-rearing practices.

Rhodes et al. (2005) offered the following additional advice to guard against the negative influence of preconceived notions or stereotypes about the child and family. "Unless proven otherwise . . . begin the assessment process with the belief that:

- The parent is equally or more concerned than the practitioner about the problem or difficulty his or her child is facing.
- The parent desires to be involved in each step of the assessment process.
- The parent has information that is critical for accurate assessment of his or her child.
- The parent has already worked to address the areas of concern or difficulty at home or through other resources" (p. 106).

The above assumptions are good starting points for successful interviews with all parents, as well as those who come from different ethnic, cultural, or linguistic backgrounds.

CONCLUDING THE PARENT INTERVIEW

To conclude the parent interview, thank the parent for sharing his/her perspectives and feelings about the child. Then briefly summarize what you learned about the child's current functioning: major problem areas, environmental and family circumstances surrounding the problems, and the child's competencies and strengths. Make sure that the clause indicating "release of information to other parties" is clearly marked on the parental consent form. You should also review the limits of confidentiality discussed at the beginning of the interview. Then discuss what family information you plan to report to other parties. Be open to excluding information that parents may not want to share with others. For school-based assessments, in particular, it may not be necessary to include sensitive family history or circumstances in the home that are not directly relevant for placement decisions or intervention planning. Jacob et al. (2011) provide specific guidelines for protecting the confidentiality of sensitive physical and mental health information about students. They wisely advise school-based practitioners to limit the focus of their reports to "communicating the student's functional health, academic, and behavioral difficulties and how to respond" (Jacob et al., 2011, p. 72).

If you plan to write a report, summarize the type of information that will be included and inform parents who will receive copies of your written reports. You should also tell parents about any follow-up meetings you will have with other parties, such as teachers. Whenever possible, arrange a subsequent meeting with parents to discuss the results of your evaluation, plans for any additional data collection, and potential interventions for the child.

SUMMARY

This chapter discussed clinical interviews with parents to obtain their perspectives on their children's functioning. It offered guidelines for questioning strategies with parents, including suggestions for interviewing culturally and linguistically diverse parents. The Semistructured Parent Interview (McConaughy, 2004a; Appendix 6.1) provides a framework for questioning parents about a variety of issues that may be relevant for intervention planning. The Semistructured Parent Interview first addresses parents' concerns about their children and then moves to more specific behavioral and emotional problems. Practitioners can use this part of the interview protocol to obtain an FBA of specific problems of concern. Interview questions about social functioning, school functioning, family relations, and home environment mirror similar inquiries in child clinical interviews. This parallel format facilitates comparisons between parents' and children's perspectives on these topics. More structured questions review medical and developmental history that may impinge upon a child's current functioning. The modular format of the Semistructured Parent Interview allows practitioners to select topics and questions to fit their assessment purposes. Practitioners are also encouraged to use other procedures for obtaining parent reports, including standardized parent rating scales and background questionnaires. The Child and Family Information Form (McConaughy & Achenbach, 2004a; Appendix 6.2) is a background questionnaire directly tied to the Semistructured Parent Interview. Table 6.9 provides sample questions regarding acculturation that can supplement interviews with linguistically and culturally diverse parents.

Semistructured Parent Interview

Child's name _____   Age _____   Gender _____
                        First   Middle   Last

                                                                Relationship
Parent's name _____   to child _____
                        First   Middle   Last

Interviewer's name _____   Date _____/_____/_____
                        First   Middle   Last   Month   Day   Year

CONFIDENTIALITY AND PURPOSE OF THE INTERVIEW

Thank you for taking your time to meet with me today and for completing the various questionnaires that you received before our meeting. I have reviewed the information that you provided on these forms. In this interview, I would like to hear more about your concerns about [child's name]. Your perspective as a parent is very important for understanding him/her.

To begin, let's talk about confidentiality issues. You have already voluntarily consented to have [child's name] receive an evaluation. This interview is part of my evaluation of [child's name]. The information you provide will be summarized in a written evaluation report. My usual practice is not to include direct quotations of parents' comments in written reports. I will try to respect your privacy by not reporting information that is not relevant to understanding [child's name]'s functioning and planning appropriate interventions/treatment. We can discuss what information will, and will not, be included in a written evaluation report at the end of this interview, if you wish.

There are circumstances under which the law require clinicians to disclose confidential information. These circumstances include when there is reason to suspect child abuse or when the child poses a danger to self or a danger to other persons. Do you understand these limits to confidentiality?

I. CONCERNS ABOUT THE CHILD	RESPONSES/COMMENTS
What concerns you most about [child's name]? *If the parent has more than one concern, list each area of concern.*	
When did you first become concerned about this? *If the parent has more than one concern, note when first concerned for each.*	
How long has this been a problem? *If the parent has more than one concern, note duration for each area of concern.* *If the parent's main concerns are about academic problems, ask questions in Section IV first and then return to Sections II and III. If the main concerns are about behavioral or emotional problems, continue with Section II.*	

(continued)

II. BEHAVIORAL OR EMOTIONAL PROBLEMS	RESPONSES/COMMENTS
Does [child's name] currently have behavioral or emotional problems? ☐ Yes ☐ No ☐ Don't know (*If yes*) What kinds of problems? **Specific Nature of the Problems** When [child's name] has this problem, what exactly does he/she do? What does he/she say? Give me some examples of this problem. *Ask the parent to give specific descriptions of the problem. If there is more than one problem, ask about each one.* How long has he/she been having this problem? How often does this problem occur? Under what circumstances does this problem occur? Where and when does this problem usually occur? *Ask for specific descriptions of where and when each problem occurs at home and/or school.* **Priorities for Interventions** Which of the problems we have discussed are you most concerned about now? Which do you think is the most important to address now? How would you rank the other problems in terms of your concerns and their importance for interventions? **Antecedents and Consequences of Priority Problem(s)** Let's talk about the problem(s) you think are of most concern. What usually happens before this problem occurs? What seems to set it off? *If more than one area of concern, ask about the top two or three problems.* What usually happens after this problem occurs? What do you do? What do other people do? How do you usually deal with this problem at home? How do you feel/react when this problem occurs? What usually happens at school if this problem occurs? How does [child's name] feel/react when this happens?	

(continued)

Replacement Behaviors	RESPONSES/COMMENTS

Replacement Behaviors

What would be acceptable or alternative behavior related to this problem? What would you like to see [child's name] do instead?

What does [child's name] do well? What do you see as his/her strengths that might help address this problem(s)?

Other Possible Problem Areas

If behavior rating scales (e.g., ASEBA Child Behavior Checklist or BASC-2 Parent Rating Scale) have been completed and scored prior to the interview, list all problem scales with scores in the borderline or clinical ranges (compared to the relevant normative sample). Summarize the results for the parent. Ask about problem areas that were not discussed as major concerns.

Before our meeting, you completed a questionnaire about [child's name]'s behavior. The questionnaire listed behaviors that can be scored on scales describing different problem areas. Your ratings produced scores indicating severe problems in:

_____

_____

_____

_____

_____

_____

_____

We have already discussed some of these problem areas. What about the problem areas we have not discussed. How much are you concerned about these problems?

Under what circumstances do these problems occur?

What is currently being done to address these problems?

Are there any other areas where you think [child's name] has behavioral or emotional problems?

Do you have concerns about situations outside of your home that might affect [child's name]'s behavior or emotional functioning?

(continued)

III. SOCIAL FUNCTIONING	RESPONSES/COMMENTS

III. SOCIAL FUNCTIONING

Now, let's talk about [child's name]'s social relationships and social behavior.

Friends

How many close friends does [child's name] have?
Do you think that is enough friends?
How do you feel about his/her choice of friends?

Do other kids come to your house to play/do things with [child's name]?
Does he/she go to other kids' houses?

Does he/she belong to any clubs or social groups (e.g., Scouts, YMCA, teams)?
Does he/she go to church/belong to any church or spiritual groups?

Social Problems

Does [child's name] have any problems getting along with other kids (e.g., not liked, teased/picked on, feel left out)?
☐ Yes ☐ No ☐ Don't know

(*If yes*) Tell me more about his/her social problems. Has anything been done to try to help him/her with social problems (e.g., see a counselor, social skills group, friendship group)?

Fights/Aggression

Does [child's name] ever get into physical fights with other kids?
☐ Yes ☐ No ☐ Don't know

(*If yes*) How often?
What usually starts the fights?
How do they usually end?
Has anything been done to try to help him/her avoid fighting?

Do you think he/she has trouble controlling his/her temper?
Has he/she ever used a weapon or object (e.g., stick, stone) to hurt other kids?
Does he/she belong to a gang?

Anxiety/Depression

Does [child's name] seem unusually anxious or worried about things?
☐ Yes ☐ No ☐ Don't know

(*If yes*) Tell me more about that.
What does he/she worry about?

(continued)

154

Anxiety/Depression *(cont.)*

Has [child's name] ever seemed very sad or depressed for a long period of time?
☐ Yes   ☐ No   ☐ Don't know

(If yes) Tell me more about that.
Has he/she ever made comments about wanting to harm or kill him/herself?
Has he/she ever attempted to harm or kill him/herself?
If yes, probe more regarding plans, attempts, access to methods, etc. Review confidentiality and legal reporting requirements. Discuss need for intervention.

REGARDING ADOLESCENTS:

Dating/Romances

Does he/she date? Have a boyfriend/girlfriend?
Do you think he/she is sexually active? Does he/she know about safe sex practices?

Trouble with the Law

Has [child's name] ever been in trouble with the law or police?
☐ Yes   ☐ No   ☐ Don't know

(If yes) For what?
What happened when [child's name] got in trouble with the law/police?

Has [child's name] ever been in any traffic accidents? Had any traffic tickets?
☐ Yes   ☐ No   ☐ Don't know

Alcohol/Drugs

Does [child's name] smoke or chew tobacco?
☐ Yes   ☐ No   ☐ Don't know

Has [child's name] ever drunk beer, wine, or liquor?
☐ Yes   ☐ No   ☐ Don't know

Has [child's name] ever been drunk from alcohol?
☐ Yes   ☐ No   ☐ Don't know

(If yes) When and how often?
Do you think he/she has a problem with alcohol?

Has he/she ever received any help/treatment for alcohol problems?
Do you think he/she needs help/treatment for alcohol problems now?

RESPONSES/COMMENTS

(continued)

	RESPONSES/COMMENTS
Alcohol/Drugs *(cont.)* Has [child's name] used drugs/been high on drugs? ☐ Yes ☐ No ☐ Don't know	

(If yes) When and how often?
What kind of drugs?
Do you think he/she has a problem with drugs?

Has he/she ever received any help/treatment for drug problems?
Do you think he/she needs help/treatment for drug problems now?

IV. SCHOOL FUNCTIONING
Now let's discuss how [child's name] is doing in school.

Subjects/Grades/Activities
What are [child's name]'s best subject areas in school? What does he/she like best?
What are [child's name]'s worst subject areas, if any? What does he/she like the least in school?

What kind of grades does he/she get?
Ask about each subject area.
Have his/her grades changed remarkably in any area?

What are his/her extracurricular activities (e.g., sports, clubs, school play, band, choir)?

Does [child's name] have any problems with school attendance/skipping classes?

Teachers
How many teachers does [child's name] have?
How does he/she get along with each teacher?
How does he/she get along with the principal and other school staff?
Is there anyone at school who is especially important to him/her?

Homework
How much homework does [child's name] typically have? How do you feel about the amount of homework he/she has?

(continued)

	RESPONSES/COMMENTS

Homework *(cont.)*
Does he/she have any trouble with homework?
(*If yes*) Tell me more about that.
When and where does he/she usually do homework?
How long does homework usually take?
How much time do you think he/she should spend on homework?
Does he/she get any help with homework?
(*If yes*) How does that work out?

Learning Problems
Does [child's name] have learning problems?
☐ Yes   ☐ No   ☐ Don't know
[*See Child and Family Information Form*]

(*If yes*) What kind of learning problems?
Why do you think [child's name] is having learning problems right now?
How long has he/she had these problems?
What has been done to address these problems?

Special Help/School Services
Examine the parent's responses on the Child and Family Information Form prior to your parent interview. Check "Yes," "No," or "Don't know" for the parent's reports about problems in each area listed below. Ask for more detail about problems marked "yes," as appropriate. If the parent has not completed the Child and Family Information Form, then ask about each problem area.

Does [child's name] receive any special help/special services in school?
☐ Yes   ☐ No   ☐ Don't know
[*See Child and Family Information Form*]

(*If yes*) What kind of help?
Probe for special education, IEP, remedial instruction/Title I services, Section 504 plan, peer tutoring, individual aide, behavior plan, guidance services, school psychologist.

How long has he/she had this special help?
How often does he/she get this help?
What kinds of help has he/she had in the past?

Do you think this is enough help/the right kind of help?
What else would you like to have happen for [child's name] at school?

(continued)

	RESPONSES/COMMENTS
Retention Has [child's name] ever been retained/held back a grade? ☐ Yes ☐ No ☐ Don't know [See *Child and Family Information Form*] (*If yes*) When? For what reason? How did [child's name] feel about being retained/held back? How did you feel about his/her being retained/held back? **School Behavior Problems** Does [child's name] have behavior problems at school? ☐ Yes ☐ No ☐ Don't know [See *Child and Family Information Form*] (*If yes*) What kind of problems? What usually happens at school when he/she has these problems? What has been done to address these problems? **Other School Concerns** Do you have other school concerns? ☐ Yes ☐ No ☐ Don't know [See *Child and Family Information Form*] (*If yes*) What kind of concerns? What has been done to address these concerns? If you could change something about school, what would it be? What would you especially like to see happen for [child's name] at school? **V. MEDICAL AND DEVELOPMENTAL HISTORY** *Examine the parent's responses on the Child and Family Information Form prior to your parent interview. Check "Yes," "No," or "Don't know" for the parent's reports about problems in each area listed below. Ask for more detail about problems marked "Yes," as appropriate. If the parent has not completed the Child and Family Information Form, then ask about each problem area.* Now, I would like to talk about [child's name]'s medical and developmental history. I have reviewed the information that you reported on the *Child and Family Information Form*. I would like to hear a little more about the problems you marked "Yes."	

(continued)

	RESPONSES/COMMENTS

Medical History
Current medications for behavior problems
☐ Yes ☐ No ☐ Don't know
[*See Child and Family Information Form*]

Current medications for other purposes
☐ Yes ☐ No ☐ Don't know
[*See Child and Family Information Form*]

Illnesses, accidents, operations, medical problems
☐ Yes ☐ No ☐ Don't know
[*See Child and Family Information Form*]

Allergies
☐ Yes ☐ No ☐ Don't know
[*See Child and Family Information Form*]

Problems with pregnancy and newborn period
☐ Yes ☐ No ☐ Don't know
[*See Child and Family Information Form*]

Developmental History and Temperament
Developmental delays
☐ Yes ☐ No ☐ Don't know
[*See Child and Family Information Form*]

Problems in temperament
☐ Yes ☐ No ☐ Don't know
[*See Child and Family Information Form*]

Problems in early behavior
☐ Yes ☐ No ☐ Don't know
[*See Child and Family Information Form*]

VI. FAMILY RELATIONS AND HOME SITUATION
Now I would like to talk about [child's name]'s family relations and home situation. I have reviewed the information you provided on the *Child and Family Information Form*. I want to hear your perspective on the family and home situation.

Family Composition
Who does [child's name] live with most of the time?
If the parents are divorced or separated, ask about visiting arrangements with each family.

Does he/she go to day care/have a day care provider other than the family? How well does that work out?

(continued)

159

	RESPONSES/COMMENTS
Home Environment Is there anything about your home or living situation that is a problem for you or the family (e.g., other persons living in the home, work situation, financial problems, neighborhood violence)? Do any family members have medical or mental health problems that might affect [child's name]? Have there been any recent major changes or stresses in your living situation or family? Has anything happened to [child's name] that was very upsetting for him/her? *Probe further in cases of possible abuse or neglect: What happened, when, was it reported to authorities? Review confidentiality and legal reporting requirements in cases of suspected abuse.* **Family Relations** How does [child's name] get along with members of the family/people in your home? *Ask about the child's relationship with each member of the family, as appropriate: father, mother, stepparents, other adults in home, other caregivers, siblings, stepsiblings.* Who does [child's name] get along with best? Who does [child's name] get along with least? Do members of the family have trouble getting along? Do you have any problems getting along with members of the family (e.g., spouse/partner, your children, relatives, other adults or children in the home)? **Rules/Punishments** What are the rules/expectations about behavior in your home? Who makes the rules? How do you think [child's name] feels about the rules? What kinds of punishments/discipline procedures are used in your home? Do children ever get spanked/physically punished for bad behavior?	

(continued)

160

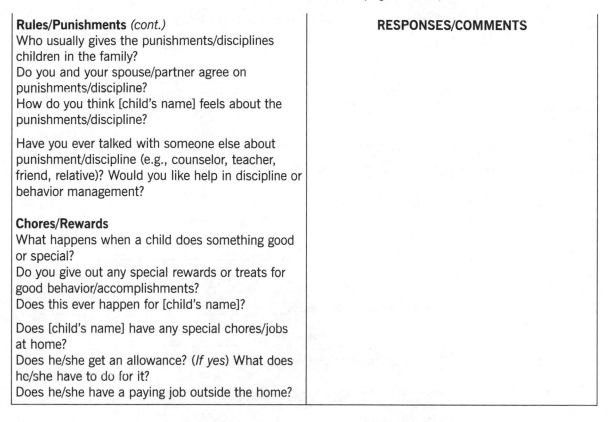

Rules/Punishments *(cont.)*	**RESPONSES/COMMENTS**
Who usually gives the punishments/disciplines children in the family? Do you and your spouse/partner agree on punishments/discipline? How do you think [child's name] feels about the punishments/discipline? Have you ever talked with someone else about punishment/discipline (e.g., counselor, teacher, friend, relative)? Would you like help in discipline or behavior management? **Chores/Rewards** What happens when a child does something good or special? Do you give out any special rewards or treats for good behavior/accomplishments? Does this ever happen for [child's name]? Does [child's name] have any special chores/jobs at home? Does he/she get an allowance? *(If yes)* What does he/she have to do for it? Does he/she have a paying job outside the home?	

CONCLUSION OF THE PARENT INTERVIEW

Conclude the interview by thanking the parent for sharing his/her perspective and feelings about the child. Briefly summarize the interview information about the child's current functioning: major problem areas, circumstances surrounding the problems, and the child's competencies and strengths. Tell the parent what family information will be included in a written evaluation report.

Review the limits of confidentiality. Discuss any concerns the parent may have about reporting information from the interview and/or parent questionnaires. Tell the parent who will receive copies of any written evaluation reports, as agreed upon in prior informed consents. Inform the parent of any follow-up meetings with school staff or other parties to discuss the evaluation results. If possible, arrange a follow-up meeting with the parent to discuss results of the evaluation and appropriate interventions or treatments, if needed.

Child and Family Information Form

Today's date ___/___/___   Filled out by _____   Relationship to child _____
Mo. Day Year

Child's name _____
               First   Middle   Last

Child's birthdate ___/___/___   Age ___   ☐ Boy   ☐ Girl   Child's ethnic group/race _____
               Mo. Day Year

Child's address _____
                  Street   City   State   Zip code

Health insurance for child: ☐ None   ☐ Medicaid   ☐ Private company (specify): _____

PERSONS WITH LEGAL CUSTODY OF CHILD

1. Name _____   Relationship to child _____
        First   Middle   Last

Address _____
            Street   City   State   Zip code

Home phone _____   Work phone _____   Cell phone _____

Birthdate ___/___/___   Highest education completed _____   Ethnic group/race _____
     Mo. Day Year

Type of work _____   Place of work _____

Work day/hours _____   OK to contact at work? ☐ No   ☐ Yes—when? _____

2. Name _____   Relationship to child _____
        First   Middle   Last

Address _____
            Street   City   State   Zip code

Home phone _____   Work phone _____   Cell phone _____

Birthdate ___/___/___   Highest education completed _____   Ethnic group/race _____
     Mo. Day Year

Type of work _____   Place of work _____

Work day/hours _____   OK to contact at work? ☐ No   ☐ Yes—when? _____

                              Whom does the child live with
Is the child adopted? ☐ No ☐ Yes   on a regular basis? _____

OTHER ADULTS AND CHILDREN LIVING IN THE CHILD'S HOME

Please list all other adults and children living with the child, if not listed above. Include stepsiblings, foster children, and related and unrelated adults.

Name	Age	Gender	Relationship to child
_____	_____	_____	_____
_____	_____	_____	_____
_____	_____	_____	_____

(continued)

_____

CHILD'S FULL OR HALF SIBLINGS NOT LIVING IN THE CHILD'S HOME

Name   Age   Gender   Relationship to child

_____   _____   _____   _____

_____   _____   _____   _____

_____   _____   _____   _____

BEST PERSON TO CONTACT FOR APPOINTMENTS FOR CHILD (if different from persons with legal custody)

Name _____   Relationship to child _____
        First   Middle   Last

Address _____
                           Street   City   State   Zip code

Home phone _____   Work phone _____   Cell phone _____

CHILD'S BIRTH PARENTS IF NOT PERSONS WITH LEGAL CUSTODY

1. Father's name _____   Birthdate ___/___/___
                    First   Middle   Last   Mo. Day Year

Address _____
                           Street   City   State   Zip code

Type of work _____   Highest education completed _____

Living? ☐ Yes   ☐ No—year of death _____   Cause of death _____

Reason not living with child? _____   How often does he see the child? _____

2. Mother's name _____   Birthdate ___/___/___
                    First   Middle   Last   Mo. Day Year

Address _____
                           Street   City   State   Zip code

Type of work _____   Highest education completed _____

Living? ☐ Yes   ☐ No—year of death _____   Cause of death _____

Reason not living with child? _____   How often does she see the child? _____

Because we occasionally do follow-up evaluations of our services or need to contact families for other reasons, we would appreciate having the names of two people who would know where to contact you if we are unable to reach you.

1. Name _____   Phone _____
        First   Middle   Last

Address _____
                           Street   City   State   Zip code

2. Name _____   Phone _____
        First   Middle   Last

Address _____
                           Street   City   State   Zip code

(continued)

CONCERNS ABOUT CHILD

What are your concerns about the child? _____

_____

_____

What are the child's strengths? _____

_____

_____

What would you like to see happen for the child? _____

_____

_____

CHILD'S SCHOOL HISTORY

Child's school _____ Grade _____ Teacher _____

OK to contact school staff about the child? ☐ No   ☐ Yes—best person to contact _____

School address _____ Phone _____
                        Street   City   State   Zip code

If yes, please describe:

1. Has the child had learning problems?   ☐ No   ☐ Yes   _____
2. Has the child had behavior problems in school?   ☐ No   ☐ Yes   _____
3. Has the child had social problems in school?   ☐ No   ☐ Yes   _____
4. Is the child receiving any special help in school   ☐ No   ☐ Yes   _____
   (e.g., tutoring, special education, Section 504
   plan, guidance counselor)?
5. Has the child ever been held back a grade?   ☐ No   ☐ Yes   _____
6. Other school problems?   ☐ No   ☐ Yes   _____

CHILD'S MEDICAL HISTORY

Child's physician/pediatrician _____ Phone _____

Physician's address _____
                              Street   City   State   Zip code

Date of last complete check-up ___/___/___ Outcome _____
                               Mo. Day Year

1. Does the child take any medication for behavioral or emotional problems?   ☐ No   ☐ Yes—please
   describe below:

Name of medication:	Dose	Purpose	Effect	Doctor
_____	_____	_____	_____	_____
_____	_____	_____	_____	_____
_____	_____	_____	_____	_____

(continued)

2. Does the child take any medication now for any other purpose?   ☐ No ☐ Yes—please describe below:

Name of medication:	Dose	Purpose	Effect	Doctor
_____	____	_____	_____	_____
_____	____	_____	_____	_____
_____	____	_____	_____	_____

3. Has the child experienced any severe illnesses, accidents, operations, disabilities or handicaps, or repeated medical problems?   ☐ No ☐ Yes—please describe below:

Type of problem	Age	Treatment	Doctor
_____	____	_____	_____
_____	____	_____	_____
_____	____	_____	_____

4. Does the child have allergies (e.g., dust, pollen, pets, certain foods)?   ☐ No ☐ Yes—please describe below:

_____

_____

5. Are you concerned about any aspect of the child's health?   ☐ No ☐ Yes—please describe below:

_____

_____

_____

_____

PREGNANCY AND NEWBORN PERIOD

Birthweight: ___/___
       Pounds Ounces

Please indicate if any of the following occurred during the pregnancy or the newborn period for your child:

If yes, please describe:

1. Medical problems during mother's pregnancy with this child (e.g., bleeding, infections, high blood pressure, diabetes, convulsions, large weight gain, injuries, operations)?   ☐ No ☐ Yes _____

2. Did the mother take medications during the pregnancy?   ☐ No ☐ Yes _____

3. Did the mother smoke during the pregnancy?   ☐ No ☐ Yes _____

4. Did the mother drink alcohol during the pregnancy?   ☐ No ☐ Yes _____

5. Did the mother use drugs during the pregnancy?   ☐ No ☐ Yes _____

(continued)

If yes, please describe:

6. Did the mother experience unusual stress during the pregnancy (e.g., marital problems, job, financial, problems with living situation, problems with other people)? □ No □ Yes _____

7. Were there any problems with labor or the delivery (e.g., prolonged labor, bleeding, breech birth, forceps used, Cesarean section)? □ No □ Yes _____

8. Was the child born prematurely? □ No □ Yes _____

9. Did the child have any problems during the newborn period (e.g., born blue, birth defects, yellow jaundice, seizures, infections, injuries, feeding or sleep problems)? □ No □ Yes _____

10. Was the child difficult to care for as a baby? □ No □ Yes _____

DEVELOPMENTAL DELAYS

If yes, please describe:

1. Have you noticed any problems in the child's development? □ No □ Yes _____

2. Were any of the following difficult or slow to develop for the child? □ No □ Yes _____
   a. Walking alone □ No □ Yes
   b. Speaking □ No □ Yes
   c. Bowel training □ No □ Yes
   d. Bladder training □ No □ Yes
   e. Staying dry at night □ No □ Yes
   f. Tying shoes □ No □ Yes
   g. Riding bike □ No □ Yes
   h. Reading □ No □ Yes
   i. Writing □ No □ Yes

CHILD'S TEMPERAMENT

If yes, please describe:

1. Is the child overactive? □ No □ Yes _____

2. Does the child have trouble paying attention? □ No □ Yes _____

3. Does have trouble staying with one activity? □ No □ Yes _____

4. Does the child go from happy to sad quickly, without any little apparent cause? □ No □ Yes _____

5. Does the child get frustrated easily? □ No □ Yes _____

6. Does the child get upset by abrupt changes? □ No □ Yes _____

(continued)

7. Are the child's emotional responses unpredictable?   ☐ No   ☐ Yes

8. Does it take the child a long time to warm up to new situations or new people?   ☐ No   ☐ Yes

9. Does the child react strongly to physical pain?   ☐ No   ☐ Yes

10. Does the child react strongly to other things?   ☐ No   ☐ Yes

If yes, please describe:
_____
_____
_____
_____
_____
_____
_____

CHILD'S EARLY BEHAVIOR

1. Has the child had any problems in the following areas: If yes, please describe: ☐ No   ☐ Yes
   a. Discipline   ☐ No   ☐ Yes
   b. Temper   ☐ No   ☐ Yes
   c. Fighting   ☐ No   ☐ Yes
   d. Moods   ☐ No   ☐ Yes
   e. Relationships with others   ☐ No   ☐ Yes
   f. Other behaviors   ☐ No   ☐ Yes

If yes, please describe:
_____
_____
_____
_____
_____
_____
_____
_____

FAMILY HISTORY

Has any relative of the child had any of the following problems?

1. Neurological disease (e.g., seizures, fits or spells, weaknesses)   ☐ No   ☐ Yes

2. Chronic disease (e.g., diabetes, thyroid, heart disease, stroke)   ☐ No   ☐ Yes

3. Mental illness (e.g., schizophrenia, bipolar or manic–depressive disorder, depression, anxiety, nervous breakdown)   ☐ No   ☐ Yes

4. Mental retardation   ☐ No   ☐ Yes

5. Learning problems   ☐ No   ☐ Yes

6. Behavior problems   ☐ No   ☐ Yes

7. Excessive use of alcohol   ☐ No   ☐ Yes

8. Drug problems, drug addiction   ☐ No   ☐ Yes

9. Trouble with the law   ☐ No   ☐ Yes

10. Trouble holding a job   ☐ No   ☐ Yes

11. Suicidal behavior   ☐ No   ☐ Yes

12. Violent behavior   ☐ No   ☐ Yes

13. Other problems   ☐ No   ☐ Yes

14. Has anyone in the child's family seen a psychologist, psychiatrist, or other mental health worker?   ☐ No   ☐ Yes

If yes, please describe:
_____
_____
_____
_____
_____
_____
_____
_____
_____
_____
_____
_____
_____
_____
_____
_____
_____
_____

(continued)

CURRENT LIVING SITUATION

Do any of the following problems apply to the child's current living situation?

If yes, please describe:

1. Marital or relationship problems between the child's major caregivers ☐ No ☐ Yes _____

2. Problems with siblings or other persons living in the home ☐ No ☐ Yes _____

3. Problems with work situation ☐ No ☐ Yes _____

4. Problems with present living situation or neighborhood ☐ No ☐ Yes _____

5. Recent major changes or stresses in the child's living situation or family ☐ No ☐ Yes _____

6. Violence in the home or neighborhood ☐ No ☐ Yes _____

7. Alcohol or drug problems in the home or neighborhood ☐ No ☐ Yes _____

8. Other problems ☐ No ☐ Yes _____

PLEASE WRITE DOWN ANYTHING ELSE YOU THINK WE SHOULD KNOW

_____

_____

_____

_____

_____

_____

_____

_____

_____

_____

_____

_____

_____

_____

_____

_____

_____

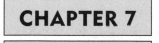

CHAPTER 7

Teacher Interviews

Few child assessments would be complete without a teacher's report about school functioning. In fact, teachers are often the ones who initiate referrals for assessments and interventions, particularly school-based assessments. Over the course of the school year, teachers have many opportunities to observe children's academic performance, behavior, and social interactions. As teachers become more experienced, they accumulate knowledge about patterns of behavior and academic progress that they regard as "typical" for children of different ages. From this knowledge base, teachers become attuned to individual children who seem to be "atypical" compared to other children. Teachers are also likely to know about school-based services available to children in their community. Interviews with teachers are especially useful for the following purposes:

- To learn about the teacher's current concerns regarding the child.
- To identify and prioritize the child's specific problems as targets for school-based interventions.
- To identify the child's strengths and competencies that can bolster interventions.
- To learn about aspects of the child's educational history relevant to understanding identified problems.
- To learn what interventions, if any, have already been attempted.
- To assess the prima facie effectiveness of previous interventions.
- To assess the acceptability and feasibility of future interventions.

Other authors have described specific formats and strategies for interviewing teachers. For example, Shapiro (2011) developed the Teacher Interview Form for Academic Problems to obtain teachers' reports of children's academic problems in reading, mathematics, spelling, and writing. The Academic Intervention Monitoring System (AIMS; Elliott, DiPerna, & Shapiro, 2001) also includes formats for teacher interviews and teacher rating scales for developing, monitoring, and evaluating classroom interventions for academic difficulties. Other authors have written about teacher interviews in the context of school behavioral consultation (e.g., Bergan & Kratochwill, 1990; Knoff, 2002; Kratochwill et al., 2002; Zins & Erchul, 2002) and "conjoint behavioral consultation" (Busse & Beaver, 2000; Sheridan et al., 1996). Conjoint behavioral consultation involves interviewing teachers and parents together to assess problems and develop cooperative interventions.

This chapter discusses teacher interviews within the context of the multimethod assessment model discussed in Chapter 1. It also mirrors the discussion of parent interviews in Chapter 6. The first two sections cover confidentiality issues and questioning strategies for interviewing teachers. Subsequent sections describe the Semistructured Teacher Interview (McConaughy, 2004b; Appendix 7.1), which is the main focus of the chapter. Standardized teacher rating scales are also discussed as assessment methods that can dovetail with teacher interviews.

DISCUSSING CONFIDENTIALITY WITH TEACHERS

All mental health and school-based practitioners should be fully aware of federal and state laws regarding need for parental consent, limits of confidentiality, and release of information about students, as discussed in the previous chapter on parent interviews. School-based practitioners should also be familiar with specific school district policies regarding confidentiality and release of student information. As a general rule, you should obtain informed parental consent before in-depth interviewing of teachers as part of a formal assessment of a child. If the teacher interview is part of a special education evaluation, IDEA 2004 and state regulations govern the timing and format for obtaining parental consent. You should also obtain parental consent before interviewing teachers as part of other formal assessment procedures, such as psychological evaluations, behavioral consultation, and referrals of children and families for mental health services or services from other agencies outside of school.

In other cases, you may want to talk with teachers for screening purposes or as part of team-based support services in school. For example, school psychologists and guidance counselors may participate in "prereferral" teams to discuss student needs and potential interventions in general education classrooms. Or school psychologists and guidance counselors may work with teachers to develop positive behavioral interventions and supports for entire classrooms or small groups of children in three-tiered service delivery models, as discussed in a later section. For these broader purposes, prior informed parental consent is usually not necessary. However, you should be thoroughly familiar with the school district's policies regarding such procedures. As best practice, it behooves school administrators to inform all parents about the support services available in their school. This way, parents will not be surprised or upset when they learn that a school psychologist or guidance counselor has discussed concerns about their child with the teacher. When screening or prereferral discussions lead to requests for more formal assessment, then you must obtain the required parental consent before gathering teacher reports through interviewing and other assessment procedures.

Even when parents have given prior consent to obtain information from teachers, you should explain clearly to teachers what information will be reported to others. For example, teacher reports are especially important to include in written psychological evaluations. You may also want to share teachers' perspectives with parents or other parties in follow-up discussions of a child. To protect confidentiality of teacher reports, a good practice is to refrain from naming individual teachers or quoting teachers' exact words, particularly in written reports. Exceptions are circumstances that require reports of suspected child abuse or neglect (see Chapter 5), suicide risk (see Chapter 9), or when a child poses a threat to other persons (see Chapter 10). In other circumstances, teachers may view naming or quoting their specific comments as a violation of trust, which can lead to reluctance to share their observations and true opinions in future interviews. Some parents may also react negatively when they learn exactly what a teacher said about their child. Bad feelings from either party can undermine future problem solving and collaboration between parents and teachers.

As a general practice, you can inform teachers that you will summarize or paraphrase their comments in reports to other parties. If a child has only one teacher, then of course it will be obvious which teacher provided the information. Still, omitting the teacher's name in a written report will make the information seem less personally tied to that teacher. If a child has more than one teacher, you can cite each

> **Summarizing or paraphrasing teachers' comments in written reports can help to protect confidentiality for teachers, except in special circumstances where more specific information is required.**

teacher's position (e.g., language arts teacher, math teacher, special educator), summarize the general consensus among the teachers, and then indicate certain classes or subject areas in which the child has problems or does particularly well. These reporting practices are especially important for written evaluations because such reports often become part of the student record and may be read again long after particular teachers have had contact with the child.

The Semistructured Teacher Interview (McConaughy, 2004b) in Appendix 7.1 begins with the following standard introduction:

"Thank you for taking your time to meet with me today and for completing the various questionnaires that you received before our meeting. I have reviewed the information that you provided on these forms. In this interview, I would like to hear more about your concerns about [child's name]. Your perspective(s) is important for evaluating [child's name]'s functioning.

"The information you provide will be summarized in a written evaluation report. My usual practice is not to include direct quotations of teachers' comments in written reports. However, I may have to report information to appropriate legal authorities or others (such as parents) if there is reason to suspect child abuse or when the child poses a danger to self or a danger to other persons. In such cases, I may have to quote what you said directly, but I will try to confer with you about that ahead of time."

As indicated in previous chapters, Jacob et al. (2011) and Sattler (1998) provide more detailed discussions of ethics and legal requirements regarding confidentiality and disclosure of information.

STRATEGIES FOR INTERVIEWING TEACHERS

As a general rule, it is best to conduct interviews with teachers who know a child well or who spend a lot of time with the child. For children in preschool or elementary grades, there is usually one lead teacher who will be the best informant on behavioral and academic functioning. If the child has other teachers for "special" classes (e.g., art, music, gym), interviewing some of them may also be appropriate to obtain additional perspectives. You should also interview teachers who provide special services to the child (e.g., remedial instruction, special education). Children in middle, junior, or high school settings usually have multiple teachers. One approach for these children is to interview one (or more) teachers who know the child well, and then gather additional information from other teachers using other methods, such as teacher rating scales. Due to time constraints, it may not be practical to conduct individual interviews with multiple teachers.

An alternative approach is to interview several teachers simultaneously. To do this, you can ask each teacher to give his/her perspective on the child in a round-robin fashion. However, this method takes more time than interviewing one teacher and runs the risk of missing information if certain teachers fail to express their views in a group. Interviewing several teachers at once also runs the risk of reinforcing negative views of the child if the interview degenerates into a mutual complaint session. If this starts to happen, try to move the discussion toward a problem-solving process that involves open exchange of information without pejorative judgments about the child or other adults involved with the child.

Many of the questioning strategies for parent interviews and child clinical interviews also apply to teacher interviews. Semistructured interviews with teachers can start with open-ended questions followed by more specific probes about identified problems or concerns. Interviewers can also use the PACERS strategies (Busse & Beaver, 2000) described in Chapter 6: paraphrasing, attending, clarifying, eliciting, reflecting, and summarizing.

It is particularly important to convey respect toward teachers for their special expertise about children and curricula. By virtue of their work with many children, teachers can provide unique perspectives on a particular individual's learning and behavior compared to other children. Teachers also have knowledge about academic requirements for their different subject areas and grade levels. Teachers may or may not agree on their perspectives about a child. However, each teacher's viewpoint can add important information for understanding the child's functioning and his/her relationship with that teacher. Some teachers may blame parents for a child's problems. Some parents, in turn, may blame teachers. To be an effective interviewer, you need to maintain a neutral stance and avoid aligning yourself with either parents or teachers. Instead, you can acknowledge each person's point of view and seek additional information as needed.

Given the demands and routines of the typical school day, teachers are likely to have limited time to participate in interviews. It is important to respect their time constraints in order to obtain their cooperation. Whenever possible, let the teacher choose the time for the interview. Tell the teacher about how much time the interview will take and stick to the time limit. In some cases, you and the teacher may decide to break the interview into several sessions. Choose a place that provides privacy for teachers and the child concerned. Many school buildings have private conference rooms for such purposes. Another staff member's empty office may be a choice. If you interview the teacher in a classroom, choose a time when no children or other adults are present (e.g., a free period or before or after school).

TOPIC AREAS FOR SEMISTRUCTURED TEACHER INTERVIEWS

The Semistructured Teacher Interview (McConaughy, 2004b; Appendix 7.1) is organized in a modular fashion for the six topic areas listed in Table 7.1. You can select topic areas and questions to fit concerns about a particular child, as well as skip certain topics or questions to save time or to abide by school policies regarding subject matter for interviews. The Semistructured Teacher Interview

TABLE 7.1. Topic Areas for Semistructured Teacher Interviews

    I. <u>Concerns about the child</u>

   II. <u>School behavior problems</u>
       Specific nature of the problems
       Priorities for interventions
       Antecedents and consequences of priority problem(s)
       Other possible problem areas

  III. <u>Academic performance</u>
       Subjects/grades/activities
       Teachers
       Homework

  IV. <u>Teaching strategies</u>
       Strategies
       Retention

   V. <u>School interventions for behavior problems</u>

  VI. <u>Special help/services</u>

---

is modeled on the format used for the Semistructured Parent Interview discussed in Chapter 6 (Appendix 6.1). The interview protocol lists sample questions for each topic in the left-hand column and provides space for notes in the right-hand column. You can adapt questions to fit your own style and the flow of conversation.

Concerns about the Child

Section I begins by asking teachers to describe their current concerns about the child. If several teachers participate in the interview, ask each teacher to articulate his/her concerns. You can list each area of concern in the space in the right-hand column. Then ask the teachers when they first became concerned about each problem and how long the problem has been going on. If the teachers' main concerns are about academic problems, you can move to questions in Section III. If their main concerns are about school behavioral and emotional problems, then move directly to Section II. Many teachers may be concerned about both academic and school behavior problems. In these cases, you can decide which area to address first.

School Behavior Problems

Section II of the teacher interview focuses on school behavior problems. It follows the general format of behavioral interviewing as did Section II in the parent interview. The first step is to ask teachers to describe each problem in specific, observable terms and to give examples of the behavior. The next step is to ask teachers about the duration and frequency of each problem and the circumstances surrounding the problem.

When teachers have concerns about several problems, it is important to prioritize them. You can then choose which specific problems to address first for additional data collection and interventions. As in the case with parents, some teachers may want to address all of their concerns at once. When this happens, you can explain that behavioral interventions work best when you focus on only a few key problems at any one time. After selecting two or three problem behaviors that concern teachers most, ask them to identify antecedents and consequences surrounding the behaviors. Answers to these questions help to develop hypotheses for an FBA, as discussed in Chapter 6. You can also ask teachers how they usually deal with the identified problems in their classrooms and what would be acceptable replacement behaviors. Gathering this information will help you learn what strategies have already been tried and what behaviors teachers usually expect from children in their classrooms. In a later section of the teacher interview, you can ask more specific questions about teaching strategies and potential interventions. It is also important to ask teachers about children's strengths and competencies so that you can build upon positive traits in developing school-based intervention plans.

> **Behavioral interviewing with teachers can identify a child's problems and the conditions under which they occur. Then determine which problems to address first.**

Standardized Teacher Rating Scales

The last part of Section II includes spaces for recording problem areas reported by teachers on standardized teacher rating scales. As in the parent interview, this part of the teacher interview assumes that teachers have been asked to complete standardized rating scales prior to the interview. When this has been done, you can examine the scoring profiles to identify areas where teachers have reported severe problems, compared to normative samples. Table 7.2 lists examples of standardized teacher rating scales that can be incorporated easily into multimethod assessment. The table summarizes the number of items and scales for each instrument, characteristics of the normative samples, and contact information for the publisher.

> **Standardized teacher rating scales provide an efficient way to obtain teacher reports on students' problems and to compare them to other children.**

The instruments listed in Table 7.2 provide standard scores that compare an individual child's scores to normative samples of boys or girls of the same age range. The scoring profiles consist of scales for different patterns of teacher-reported problems and/or competencies. For example, the Academic Competence Evaluation Scales (ACES; DiPerna & Elliott, 2000) provides scales measuring teachers' reports of children's academic skills plus behaviors that "enable" good academic performance (interpersonal skills, engagement, motivation, study skills). The ASEBA TRF (Achenbach & Rescorla, 2001) includes problem scales corresponding to those on the ASEBA CBCL/6–18 for parents, plus scales for adaptive functioning and academic performance. The BASC-2 Teacher Rating Scale (Reynolds & Kamphaus, 2004) has problem and adaptive scales similar to the BASC-2 Parent Rating Scale, plus an additional adaptive scale for study skills. The BERS-2-Teacher Rating Scale (Epstein, 2004) assesses patterns of behavioral and emotional strengths similar to the BERS-2-Parent Rating Scale. The CASI-4R-Teacher Checklist (Gadow & Sprafkin, 2010) and CBRS-Teacher version (CBRS-T; Conners, 2008) assess psychiatric disorders, similar to the parent versions. The CBRS-T has seven additional problem scales. Other rating scales focus on teachers' reports of social behaviors and social skills, paralleling similar forms for parents.

TABLE 7.2. Examples of Published Standardized Teacher Rating Scales

Instrument	Items and scales	Normative samples	Publisher
Academic Competence Evaluation Scales/Teacher Form (ACES; DiPerna & Elliott, 2000)	73 items *Competence/Adaptive Scales* Academic Enablers Total Score, Interpersonal Skills, Engagement, Motivation, Study Skills, Academic Skills Total Score, Reading/Language Arts, Mathematics, Critical Thinking	Combined norms for boys and girls, grades K–2, 3–5, 6–8, and 9–12	Pearson 19500 Bulverde Road San Antonio, TX 78259 800-627-7271 *www.psychcorp.com*
ASEBA Caregiver–Teacher's Report Form for Ages 1½–5 (C-TRF; Achenbach & Rescorla, 2000)	100 items *Problem Scales* Total Problems, Internalizing, Externalizing, Emotionally Reactive, Anxious/Depressed, Somatic Complaints, Withdrawn, Attention Problems, Aggressive Behavior, Stress Problems, Affective Problems, Anxiety Problems, Pervasive Developmental Problems, Attention Deficit/Hyperactivity Problems, Oppositional Defiant Problems	Separate norms for boys and girls, ages 1½–5 Multicultural norms	Research Center for Children, Youth, and Families, Inc. One South Prospect Street Burlington, VT 05401-3456 802-656-5130 *www.aseba.org*
ASEBA Teacher's Report Form (TRF; Achenbach & Rescorla, 2001)	6 adaptive items and 120 problem items *Problem Scales* Total Problems, Internalizing, Externalizing, Withdrawn/Depressed, Somatic Complaints, Anxious/Depressed, Social Problems, Thought Problems, Attention Problems, Rule-Breaking Behavior, Aggressive Behavior, Obsessive Compulsive Problems, Post Traumatic Stress Problems, Sluggish Cognitive Tempo, Affective Problems, Anxiety Problems, Attention Deficit/Hyperactivity Problems, Oppositional Defiant Problems, Conduct Problems, Inattention and Hyperactivity–Impulsivity subscales *Competence/Adaptive Scales* Total Adaptive Functioning, Working Hard, Behaving Appropriately, Learning, Happy, Academic Performance	Separate norms for boys and girls, ages 6–11 and 12–18 Multicultural norms	Research Center for Children, Youth, and Families, Inc. One South Prospect Street Burlington, VT 05401-3456 802-656-5130 *www.aseba.org*
Behavior Assessment System for Children–2 Teacher Rating Scales (BASC-2 TRS; Reynolds & Kamphaus, 2004)	134–160 items *Problem Scales* Behavioral Symptoms Index, Externalizing, Internalizing, School Problems, Hyperactivity, Aggression, Conduct Problems (ages 6–18), Anxiety, Depression, Somatization, Attention Problems, Learning Problems, Atypicality, Withdrawal	Separate norms for boys and girls, ages 2–5, 6–11, and 12–18	Pearson 19500 Bulverde Road San Antonio, TX 78259 800-627-7271 *www.psychcorp.com*

(continued)

175

TABLE 7.2. (cont.)

Instrument	Items and scales	Normative samples	Publisher
Behavior Assessment System for Children–2 Teacher Rating Scales (*continued*)	*Content Scales* Anger Control, Bullying, Developmental Social Disorders, Emotional Self-Control, Executive Functioning, Negative Emotionality, Resiliency *Competence/Adaptive Scales* Adaptive Skills Composite, Adaptability, Social Skills, Leadership (ages 6–18), Study Skills (ages 6–18), Functional Communication		
Behavioral and Emotional Rating Scale (2nd edition)—Teacher Rating Scale (BERS-2-T; Epstein, 2004)	52 items *Competence/Adaptive Scales* Total Strengths Score, Interpersonal Strengths, School Functioning, Intrapersonal Strengths, Family Strengths, Affective Strengths	Separate norms for boys and girls, ages 5–18	PRO-ED 8700 Shoal Creek Boulevard Austin, TX 78757-6897 800-879-3202 *www.proedinc.com*
Child and Adolescent Symptom Inventory–4R–Teacher Rating Checklist (CASI-4R-T; Gadow & Sprafkin, 2005)	120 items *Problem Scales* 12 DSM-IV-TR Disorders *Screening Items* 6 DSM-IV-TR Disorders *Academic Performance Scale*	Separate norms for boys and girls, ages 5–12 and 12–18	Checkmate Plus P.O. Box 696 Stony Brook, NY 11790-0696 800-779-4292 *www.checkmateplus.com*
Conners Comprehensive Behavior Rating Scales–Teacher (CBRS-T; Conners, 2008)	204 items *Problem Scales* Emotional Distress, Academic Difficulties, Defiant/Aggressive Behaviors, Hyperactivity, Perfectionistic and Compulsive Behaviors, Violence Potential Indicator, Physical Symptoms, 14 DSM-TR Disorders *Validity Scales* Positive Impression, Negative Impression, Inconsistency Index	Separate norms for boys and girls, ages 6–11 and 12–18	MHS P.O. Box 950 North Tonawanda, NY 14120-0950 800-456-3003 *www.mhs.com*
Devereux Behavior Rating Scale–School Form (DBRS-SF; Naglieri, LeBuff, & Pfeiffer, 1993)	40 items *Problem Scales* Total Problems, Interpersonal Problems, Inappropriate Behaviors/Feelings, Depression, Physical Symptoms/Fears	Separate norms for boys and girls, ages 5–12 and 13–18	Pearson 19500 Bulverde Road San Antonio, TX 78259 800-627-7271 *www.psychcorp.com*

Instrument	Items and scales	Norms	Publisher
Early Childhood Inventory-4–Teacher Checklist (ECI-4-T; Gadow & Sprafkin, 1997)	95 items *Problem Scales* 11 DSM-IV-TR Disorders *Screening Items* 6 DSM-IV-TR Disorders *Developmental Rating Scale*	Separate norms for boys and girls, ages 3–5	Checkmate Plus P.O. Box 696 Stony Brook, NY 11790-0696 800-779-4292 *www.checkmateplus.com*
Preschool and Kindergarten Behavioral Scales–Second Edition–Teacher version (PKBS-2-T; Merrell, 2002a)	76 items *Problem Scales* Total Problem Behavior, Internalizing, Externalizing *Competence/Adaptive Scales* Total Social Skills, Social Cooperation, Social Interaction, Social Independence	Combined norms for boys and girls, ages 3–6	PRO-ED 8700 Shoal Creek Boulevard Austin, TX 78757-6869 800-879-3202 *www.proedinc.com*
School Social Behavior Scales–Second Edition (SSBS-2; Merrell, 2002b)	64 items *Problem Scales* Antisocial Behavior Total, Hostile/Irritable, Antisocial/Aggressive, Defiant/Disruptive *Competence/Adaptive Scales* Social Competence Total, Peer Relations, Self-Management/Compliance, Academic Behavior	Combined norms for boys and girls, grades K–6 and 7–12	Assessment–Intervention Resources 2285 Elysium Avenue Eugene, OR 97401 541-338-8736 *www.assessment-intervention.com*
Social Skills Improvement System—Teacher Form (SSIS-T; Gresham & Elliott, 2008)	83 items *Problem Scales* Total Problems, Internalizing, Externalizing, Bullying, Hyperactivity/Inattention, Autism Spectrum *Competence/Adaptive Scales* Total Social Skills, Communication, Cooperation, Assertion, Responsibility, Empathy, Engagement, Self-Control, Academic Competence	Separate norms for boys and girls, ages 3–5, 5–12, 13–18	Pearson 19500 Bulverde Road San Antonio, TX 78259 800-627-7271 *www.psychcorp.com*

Note. ASEBA = Achenbach System of Empirically Based Assessment; DSM-IV-TR = *Diagnostic and statistical manual of mental disorders–fourth edition, text revision* (American Psychiatric Association, 2000).

In the spaces provided in Section II of the Semistructured Teacher Interview, you can record problem areas in which a child has obtained deviant scores on standardized teacher rating scales. This list can serve as a prompt to ask teachers about problems that you have not already discussed in the interview. You can then ask further questions about circumstances surrounding any of these additional problems and whether anything has been done to address them. You can also ask about situations in and outside of school that might affect the child's behavior. It is usually good to avoid going into much detail about other problems, so as not to unnecessarily prolong the interview. However, questions about other possible problems can broaden the focus for formulating conclusions and planning interventions.

Academic Performance

Section III of the Semistructured Teacher Interview provides questions about children's academic performance, as shown in Table 7.3. These questions are similar to questions about school subjects, relationships with teachers, and homework in the Semistructured Parent Interview, as discussed in Chapter 6, and in child clinical interviews, as discussed in Chapter 3. Even if teachers have

---

TABLE 7.3. Sample Questions about Academic Performance

Subjects/grades/activities

What are [child's name]'s best subject areas in school? What does he/she like best?
What are [child's name]'s worst subject areas, if any? What does he/she like the least in school?
What grades has [child's name] received in the most recent marking period?
Ask about each subject area.

Have [child's name]'s grades changed remarkably in any area?
What are his/her extracurricular activities (e.g., sports, clubs, school play, band, choir)?
Does [child's name] have any problems with school attendance/skipping classes?

Teachers

How many different teachers does [child's name] have?
How does he/she get along with each teacher?
How does he/she get along with the principal and other school staff?
Is there anyone at school who is especially important to him/her?

Homework

How much homework does [child's name] typically have?
Ask about homework for each subject area.

How much time do you expect a student to spend on homework?
How much time does [child's name] spend on homework?
Does [child's name] have any trouble with homework?

(*If yes*) What kind of trouble?
Does he/she get any help with homework at school?

(*If yes*) How does that work out?
Are homework assignments for [child's name] modified in any way?

Note. From McConaughy (2004b). Copyright 2004 by Stephanie H. McConaughy. Reprinted by permission.

not reported concerns about a child's academic performance, it is usually good to ask some of these general questions to a get a picture of school functioning. The parallel formats of the parent, teacher, and child interviews facilitate comparisons between different perspectives on these issues.

Teaching Strategies

Section IV of the Semistructured Teacher Interview includes questions about different instructional strategies that teachers might use in their classrooms. For each of the seven strategies listed in Table 7.4, you can ask how often teachers or others (e.g., teacher aides) use that approach in their classrooms and how well the child responds to the strategy. You can check boxes on the interview protocol to indicate the frequency of use (often occurs, sometimes, seldom/never) and teachers' perceptions of how the child responds (responds well, doesn't respond well).

School Interventions for Behavior Problems

School staff may use many different interventions to address school behavior problems. Section V of the Semistructured Teacher Interview protocol lists 14 interventions, as shown in Table 7.5. Versions of these approaches have been discussed widely in the educational and psychological literature. You can use this list to ask teachers whether they think such an intervention might work with a particular child in their classroom or school, and whether they or others are actually using the intervention. The interview protocol provides boxes that you can check to indicate teachers' perceptions of the potential effectiveness of each intervention (will work, might work, won't work) and the acceptability of each intervention (doing now, willing to try, won't try).

TABLE 7.4. Sample Questions about Teaching Strategies

What teaching or instructional strategies do you or other people use in your classroom?

How well does [child's name] respond to this strategy?
Ask the teacher(s) about each strategy and how the child responds to each one that is relevant.

Large-group instruction/teacher lecture
Small-group instruction
One-on-one instruction/individual aide
Independent seatwork
Independent hands-on projects
Peer cooperative learning groups/projects
Peer tutoring

Has [child's name] ever been retained/held back a grade?

(*If yes*) When? For what reason?
Do you think that retention was appropriate?
How do you think he/she felt about being retained/held back?

Note. From McConaughy (2004b). Copyright 2004 by Stephanie H. McConaughy. Reprinted by permission.

TABLE 7.5. Sample Questions about School Interventions for Behavior Problems

Let me ask you about a number of different approaches for dealing with children's school behavior
　　problems.
Which of these do you think might work to address [child's name]'s behavior problem(s)?
Which of these are you already doing or would you be willing to try in your classroom/this school setting?
Ask about each intervention listed below.

Classwide rules/behavioral expectations
Classwide behavior program/token reward system
Individual student behavior plan/contract
Classwide social skills instruction
Individual or small-group social skills instruction
Peer buddy system/peer tutoring
Cooperative learning groups/projects
Individual attention from teacher/teacher aide
In-school suspension
Out-of-school suspension
Self time-out/quiet place to work
Self-monitoring
Special education/IEP
Section 504 plan/accommodations
Other—describe:

Do you want help or support for dealing with [child's name]'s problems in your classroom/your situation?

(*If yes*) What kind of support would work best for you?

Note. From McConaughy (2004b). Copyright 2004 by Stephanie H. McConaughy. Reprinted by permission.

Special Help/Services

Section VI of the Semistructured Teacher Interview surveys teachers about 13 types of special
help or special, as services shown in Table 7.6. You can use this list to ask teachers whether the
child is currently receiving any of these services and then check boxes on the protocol form to
indicate teachers' responses ("Yes, No, Don't know"). You can then ask follow-up questions about
the frequency and duration of each current service, and whether the child has received similar
services in the past. You can also ask teachers whether they think the types of current services
are appropriate ("Do you think this is enough/the right kind of help?") and whether other types of
services are available.

　　The sample questions in Sections IV, V, and VI are more structured than questions in earlier
sections of the Semistructured Teacher Interview. The lists of teaching strategies, school interventions for behavior problems, and special help or services are intended to reduce time and increase
the efficiency of these parts of the teacher interview. However, you should feel free to follow up
with more open-ended questions about each of these areas, as time permits. The checklists can
also serve as prompts to ask about different strategies, interventions, or services that teachers
might not mention spontaneously. If the interview is conducted with more than one teacher at the
same time, you can check the appropriate boxes in Sections IV, V, and VI to indicate the general
consensus about each question and use space in the right-hand columns of the protocol to write
notes about differences in approaches or perceptions.

　　Over the past decade or more, many school districts have begun to employ response-to-
intervention (RTI) methods for identifying and resolving students' academic and/or behavioral

TABLE 7.6. Sample Questions about Special Help or Services

Does [child's name] currently receive any special help/special services in school?
Ask the teacher about each type of special service and note his/her comments.

Special education/IEP
Remedial instruction/Title I services
Speech and language services
Adaptive physical education
Section 504 plan/accommodations
Behavioral consultation/behavioral specialist
Individual aide
Guidance services
School psychology services
Psychotherapy/mental health services
Social skills training
School social worker
Gifted and talented program/enrichment
Other—describe:

How often does he/she receive this special help?
How long has he/she received special help?
What kinds of help has he/she received in the past?
Do you think this is enough/the right kind of help?
Are there any other types of services available?

Note. From McConaughy (2004b). Copyright 2004 by Stephanie H. McConaughy. Reprinted by permission.

difficulties. RTI methods are predicated upon a three-tiered service delivery system. Tier 1 involves universal interventions or conditions for all students, such as schoolwide positive behavioral interventions and supports and evidence-based general education instructional strategies. It is assumed that approximately 80% of students should respond successfully to Tier 1 conditions. Tier 2 involves targeted small-group interventions, such as remedial instruction, with regular progress monitoring. Approximately 15% of students should respond successfully to the combination of Tier 1 and Tier 2 interventions. Tier 3 involves more intensive assessment and interventions for approximately 5% of students who do not respond successfully to Tier 1 and Tier 2 interventions (Brown-Chidsey & Steege, 2010).

> RTI methods include a three-tiered delivery system that moves from prevention strategies for entire classrooms, to small-group interventions, to more intensive individualized interventions.

Teachers' answers to questions in Sections IV and V of the Semistructured Teacher Interview can help you determine which teaching strategies and interventions have already been tried and which approaches are acceptable to teachers. Some of the strategies and interventions in Sections IV and V would be considered Tier 1, intended to promote success of all students in the general education setting. For example, is there a clear set of classroom rules and behavioral expectations for all students? Does the entire class receive some form of social skills instruction from either the teacher or another staff member (e.g., guidance counselor or school psychologist)? Do the students work in cooperative learning groups?

Other teaching strategies and interventions would be considered Tier 2 interventions. Examples include remedial instruction/Title I services, a peer buddy system or peer tutoring, and small-group social skills instruction. Additional interventions in Sections V and VI of the Semistructured Teacher Interview include several that would be considered Tier 3, such as special education/IEP, speech and language services, school psychology services, and psychotherapy/mental health services. For Tier 3 assessment, the Semistructured Teacher Interview should be used as one component of multimethod assessment, along with child clinical interviews, parent interviews, and other forms of assessment, as discussed in previous chapters.

CONCLUDING THE TEACHER INTERVIEW

To conclude the teacher interview, thank teachers for taking time out of their busy schedules to talk with you about the child. Then review any pertinent confidentiality issues discussed at the beginning of the interview. If you plan to write a report, it is usually good to summarize the type of information that will be included (e.g., teacher-reported problems, the child's current academic performance, suggestions regarding interventions, results of teacher rating scales). You can tell teachers again that you will not quote their exact words or name them personally in written reports, unless this is necessary for certain reporting purposes. Teachers may also appreciate hearing about plans for additional data collection and any future meetings with them and/or parents. You may also want to involve certain teachers in additional data collection for progress monitoring. Summarizing the next steps to be taken can assure teachers that their reports are valuable and that the time they devoted to the interview has not been wasted.

SUMMARY

This chapter discussed semistructured interviews with teachers to obtain their perspectives on children's school functioning. Many of the questioning strategies discussed in previous chapters on child and parent interviews also apply to teacher interviews. The Semistructured Teacher Interview (McConaughy, 2004b; Appendix 7.1) provides a protocol for obtaining information from teachers that can assist in the development of school-based interventions. Questions in the first two sections of the teacher interview mirror behavioral interviewing strategies used in the Semistructured Parent Interview (McConaughy, 2004a; Appendix 6.1). After asking teachers to describe their concerns about the child, interviewers ask questions about specific problems that can become targets for an FBA. Other sections of the teacher interview cover the child's academic performance, teachers' instructional strategies, school interventions for behavior problems, and special help or services currently provided to the child. The format of the Semistructured Teacher Interview assumes that practitioners will also use standardized teacher rating scales and other procedures to obtain a multimethod assessment of the child.

Semistructured Teacher Interview

Child's name _____ Age _____ Gender _____
First   Middle   Last

Interviewer's name _____ Date ____/____/____
First   Middle   Last   Month   Day   Year

Teacher's name _____ Role/class _____

CONFIDENTIALITY AND PURPOSE OF THE INTERVIEW

Thank you for taking your time to meet with me today and for completing the various questionnaires that you received before our meeting. I have reviewed the information that you provided on these forms. In this interview, I would like to hear more about your concerns about [child's name]. Your perspective(s) is important for evaluating [child's name]'s functioning.

     The information you provide will be summarized in a written evaluation report. My usual practice is not to include direct quotations of teachers' comments in written reports. However, I may have to report information to appropriate legal authorities or others (such as parents) if there is reason to suspect child abuse or when the child poses a danger to self or a danger to other persons. In such cases, I may have to quote what you said directly, but I will try to confer with you about that ahead of time.

I. CONCERNS ABOUT THE CHILD	RESPONSES/COMMENTS
What concerns you most about [child's name]? *If the teacher has more than one concern, list each area of concern.*	
When did you first become concerned about this? *If the teacher has more than one concern, note when first concerned for each area of concern.*	
How long has this been a problem? *If the teacher has more than one concern, note duration for each area of concern.*	
If the teacher's main concerns are academic problems, ask questions in Section III first and then return to Section II. If the main concerns are behavioral or emotional problems, continue with Section II.	
II. SCHOOL BEHAVIOR PROBLEMS Does [child's name] currently have behavior problems at school? ☐ Yes ☐ No ☐ Don't know (*If yes*) What kind of behavior problems?	

(continued)

	RESPONSES/COMMENTS
Specific Nature of the Problems When [child's name] has this behavior problem, what exactly does he/she do? What does he/she say? Give me some examples of this problem. *If there is more than one problem, ask the teacher to describe each one.* How long has he/she been having this problem? How often does this problem occur now? Under what circumstances does this problem occur? Where and when does this problem usually occur? *Ask for specific descriptions of where and when each problem occurs: e.g., classroom, recess, lunch, transition periods, group situations, independent work, morning, afternoon.* **Priorities for Interventions** Which of the problems we have discussed are you most concerned about now? Which do you think is the most important to address now? **Antecedents and Consequences of Priority Problem(s)** Let's talk about the problem(s) you think are of most concern. What usually happens before this problem occurs? What seems to set it off? *If more than one area of concern, ask about the top two or three problems.* What usually happens after this problem occurs? What do you do? What do other people do? How do you usually deal with this problem in your classroom? How do you react? **Replacement Behaviors** What would be acceptable or alternative behavior related to this problem? What would you like to see [child's name] do instead? What does [child's name] do well? What do you see as his/her strengths that might help to address this problem(s)?	

(continued)

Other Possible Problem Areas

If behavior rating scales (e.g., ASEBA Teacher's Report Form or BASC-2 Teacher Rating Scale) have been completed and scored prior to the interview, list all problem scales with scores in the borderline or clinical ranges (compared to the relevant normative sample). Summarize the results for the teacher. Ask about problem areas that were not discussed as major concerns.

Before our meeting, you completed a questionnaire about [child's name]'s behavior. The questionnaire listed behaviors that can be scored on scales describing different problem areas. Your ratings produced scores indicating severe problems in:

_____

_____

_____

_____

_____

_____

_____

_____

We have already discussed some of these problem areas. What about the problem areas we have not discussed. How much are you concerned about these problems?

Under what circumstances do these problems occur?

What is currently being done to address these problems?

Are there any other areas where you think [child's name] has behavioral or emotional problems?

Do you have concerns about situations outside of school that might affect [child's name]'s behavior or emotional functioning?

RESPONSES/COMMENTS

(continued)

185

III. ACADEMIC PERFORMANCE	RESPONSES/COMMENTS

III. ACADEMIC PERFORMANCE

Does [child's name] currently have academic or learning problems?

☐ Yes ☐ No ☐ Don't know

(If yes) What kind of problems?
Summarize all subject areas in which the teacher reports academic or learning problems.

Why do you think [child's name] is having academic or learning problems now?

How long has he/she had these problems?

Subject Areas/Grades/Activities

What are [child's name]'s best subject areas in school? What does he/she like best?

What are [child's name]'s worst subject areas, if any? What does he/she like least?

What grades has [child's name] received in the most recent marking period?
Ask about each subject area.

Have [child's name]'s grades changed remarkably in any area?

What are his/her extracurricular activities (e.g., sports, clubs, school play, band, choir)?

Does [child's name] have any problems with school attendance/skipping classes?

Teachers

How many teachers does [child's name] have?
How does he/she get along with each teacher?
How does he/she get along with the principal and other school staff?

Is there anyone at school who is especially important to him/her?

Homework

How much homework does [child's name] typically have?
Ask about homework for each subject area.

How much time do you expect a student to spend on homework?
How much time does [child's name] spend on homework?

Does [child's name] have any trouble with homework?
(If yes) What kind of trouble?

(continued)

186

	RESPONSES/COMMENTS

Homework *(cont.)*
Does he/she get any help with homework at school?
(If yes) How does this work out?

Does he/she get any help with homework at home?
(If yes) How does this work out?

Are homework assignments for [child's name] modified in any way?

IV. TEACHING STRATEGIES
What teaching or instructional strategies do you or other people use in your classroom?

How well does [child's name] respond to these strategies?

Ask the teacher(s) about each strategy and how the child responds to each one that is relevant. Check the appropriate boxes to indicate the teacher's responses. If you are interviewing several teachers at once, you can indicate the general consensus among them and write notes regarding any differences about teaching strategies.

Large-group instruction/teacher lecture
☐ Often occurs ☐ Sometimes ☐ Seldom/never
☐ Responds well ☐ Doesn't respond well

Small-group instruction
☐ Often occurs ☐ Sometimes ☐ Seldom/never
☐ Responds well ☐ Doesn't respond well

One-on-one instruction/individual aide
☐ Often occurs ☐ Sometimes ☐ Seldom/never
☐ Responds well ☐ Doesn't respond well

Independent seatwork
☐ Often occurs ☐ Sometimes ☐ Seldom/never
☐ Responds well ☐ Doesn't respond well

Independent hands-on projects
☐ Often occurs ☐ Sometimes ☐ Seldom/never
☐ Responds well ☐ Doesn't respond well

Peer cooperative learning groups/projects
☐ Often occurs ☐ Sometimes ☐ Seldom/never
☐ Responds well ☐ Doesn't respond well

Peer tutoring
☐ Often occurs ☐ Sometimes ☐ Seldom/never
☐ Responds well ☐ Doesn't respond well

Other—describe:

(continued)

Retention

Has [child's name] ever been retained/held back a grade?

☐ Yes   ☐ No   ☐ Don't know

(If yes) When? For what reason?

Do you think that retention was appropriate?

How do you think he/she felt about being retained/held back?

V. SCHOOL INTERVENTIONS FOR BEHAVIOR PROBLEMS

Let me ask you about a number of different approaches for dealing with children's school behavior problems.

Which of these do you think might work to address [child's name]'s behavior problem(s)?

Which of these are you already doing or would you be willing to try in your classroom/this school setting?

Ask about each intervention listed below. Check the appropriate boxes to indicate the teacher's responses. If you are interviewing several teachers at once, you can indicate the general consensus among them and write notes regarding any differences about services.

Classwide rules/behavioral expectations
☐ Will work   ☐ Might work   ☐ Won't work
☐ Doing now   ☐ Willing to try   ☐ Won't try

Classwide behavior program/token reward system
☐ Will work   ☐ Might work   ☐ Won't work
☐ Doing now   ☐ Willing to try   ☐ Won't try

Individual student behavior plan/contract
☐ Will work   ☐ Might work   ☐ Won't work
☐ Doing now   ☐ Willing to try   ☐ Won't try

Classwide social skills instruction
☐ Will work   ☐ Might work   ☐ Won't work
☐ Doing now   ☐ Willing to try   ☐ Won't try

Individual or small-group social skills instruction
☐ Will work   ☐ Might work   ☐ Won't work
☐ Doing now   ☐ Willing to try   ☐ Won't try

RESPONSES/COMMENTS

(continued)

188

V. SCHOOL INTERVENTIONS FOR BEHAVIOR PROBLEMS *(cont.)*

Peer buddy system/peer tutoring
☐ Will work   ☐ Might work   ☐ Won't work
☐ Doing now   ☐ Willing to try   ☐ Won't try

Cooperative learning groups/projects
☐ Will work   ☐ Might work   ☐ Won't work
☐ Doing now   ☐ Willing to try   ☐ Won't try

Individual attention from teacher/teacher aide
☐ Will work   ☐ Might work   ☐ Won't work
☐ Doing now   ☐ Willing to try   ☐ Won't try

In-school suspension
☐ Will work   ☐ Might work   ☐ Won't work
☐ Doing now   ☐ Willing to try   ☐ Won't try

Out-of-school suspension
☐ Will work   ☐ Might work   ☐ Won't work
☐ Doing now   ☐ Willing to try   ☐ Won't try

Self time-out/quiet place to work
☐ Will work   ☐ Might work   ☐ Won't work
☐ Doing now   ☐ Willing to try   ☐ Won't try

Self-monitoring
☐ Will work   ☐ Might work   ☐ Won't work
☐ Doing now   ☐ Willing to try   ☐ Won't try

Special education/IEP
☐ Will work   ☐ Might work   ☐ Won't work
☐ Doing now   ☐ Willing to try   ☐ Won't try

Section 504 plan/accommodations
☐ Will work   ☐ Might work   ☐ Won't work
☐ Doing now   ☐ Willing to try   ☐ Won't try

Other-describe:

Do you want help or support for dealing with [child's name]'s problems in your classroom/your situation?

(If yes) What kind of support would work best for you?

RESPONSES/COMMENTS

(continued)

VI. SPECIAL HELP/SERVICES	**RESPONSES/COMMENTS**
Does [child's name] currently receive any special help/special services in school?	

Ask the teacher(s) about each type of special service and note comments.

Special education/IEP
☐ Yes ☐ No ☐ Don't know

Remedial instruction/Title I services
☐ Yes ☐ No ☐ Don't know

Speech and language services
☐ Yes ☐ No ☐ Don't know

Adaptive physical education
☐ Yes ☐ No ☐ Don't know

Section 504 plan/accommodations
☐ Yes ☐ No ☐ Don't know

Behavioral consultation/behavioral specialist
☐ Yes ☐ No ☐ Don't know

Individual aide
☐ Yes ☐ No ☐ Don't know

Guidance services
☐ Yes ☐ No ☐ Don't know

School psychology services
☐ Yes ☐ No ☐ Don't know

Psychotherapy/mental health services
☐ Yes ☐ No ☐ Don't know

Social skills training
☐ Yes ☐ No ☐ Don't know

School social worker
☐ Yes ☐ No ☐ Don't know

Gifted and talented program/enrichment
☐ Yes ☐ No ☐ Don't know

Other—describe:

How often does he/she receive this special help?
How long has he/she received special help?
What kinds of help has he/she received in the past?
Do you think this is enough/the right kind of help?
Are there any other types of services available?
Do you have any other school concerns?

CHAPTER 8

Interpreting Clinical Interviews for Assessment and Intervention

Previous chapters have discussed child, parent, and teacher interviews for multimethod assessment of children's functioning. In child interviews you can learn children's views of their problems and competencies and at the same time directly observe their behavior, affect, and interaction style. In parent and teacher interviews, you can learn, firsthand, parents' and teachers' views of children's problems and competencies and what situations or life circumstances affect children's functioning. Learning each informant's perspective helps you and others weigh different options for ameliorating problems and boosting competencies. Hearing children's views helps you evaluate their awareness of their own competencies and problems and how receptive they might be to different interventions. Hearing parents' and teachers' views helps you evaluate what each party is able and willing to do on the child's behalf.

RECORDING AND REPORTING INTERVIEW INFORMATION

For semistructured interviewing and behavioral interviewing, practitioners have usually relied on written notes (and sometimes audio- or videotaped recordings) to document information. The SCICA protocol (McConaughy & Achenbach, 2001) and the Semistructured Student Interview (McConaughy, 2012; Appendix 3.1) provide standardized protocols that practitioners can use to record notes during clinical interviews with children. The Semistructured Parent Interview (McConaughy, 2004a; Appendix 6.1) and Semistructured Teacher Interview (McConaughy, 2004b; Appendix 7.1) provide standardized protocols for recording notes during interviews with parents and teachers. Practitioners can then use their notes and recordings to summarize information they judge to be important for clinical records and written evaluation reports.

SCICA Rating Forms and Scoring Profile

Interview notes provide anecdotal, qualitative information for evaluating children's functioning. In addition to its protocol form, the SCICA (McConaughy & Achenbach, 2001) provides two structured rating forms that interviewers can use to rate their observations of children's behavior during the interview and children's self-reported problems. The SCICA Observation Form contains 120 items for rating observations of children's behavior, affect and interaction style. Examples include the following: argues; avoids eye contact; defiant, talks back, or sarcastic; disjointed or tangential conversation; doesn't sit still, restless or hyperactive; limited conversation; sudden changes in mood or feelings; and unhappy, sad, or depressed. The SCICA Self-Report contains 125 items for rating problems that children may report in response to questions about the various topics covered in the interview. Examples include the following: reports acts of cruelty, bullying, or meanness to others, including siblings; reports being disobedient at home; reports deliberately harming self or attempting suicide; reports feeling worthless or inferior; reports not being liked by peers; reports getting into physical fights; and reports worrying. There are also two open-ended items for observations and self-reports not covered by the more specific items.

> Interviewers can use the SCICA Observation and Self-Report Forms to rate specific problems they observed and problems reported by children during child clinical interviews.

After completing the interview, interviewers rate the child on each item of the SCICA Observation and Self-Report Forms using a 4-point scale from 0 (no occurrence) to 3 (definite occurrence with severe intensity or 3 or more minutes duration). The SCICA manual (McConaughy & Achenbach, 2001) provides guidelines for scoring the items 0, 1, 2, or 3. Practitioners can also obtain a training videotape and computer software to practice scoring the SCICA rating forms (McConaughy, Arnold, Jacobowitz, & Achenbach, 1994; *www.ASEBA.org*).

To provide quantitative data from the SCICA, interviewers' ratings are scored on a standardized profile of problem scales similar to profiles of other ASEBA forms. The SCICA Profile (McConaughy & Achenbach, 2001) includes five empirically based syndrome scales for interviewer observations: Anxious, Withdrawn/Depressed, Language/Motor Problems, Attention Problems, and Self-Control Problems. It also includes three syndrome scales for problems reported by the child during the interview: Anxious/Depressed, Aggressive/Rule-Breaking, and Somatic Complaints (scored for ages 12–18). The SCICA syndrome scales were derived from factor analyses to identify groupings of problems that tend to co-occur. Additional factor analyses produced an Internalizing grouping comprising the Anxious and Anxious/Depressed scales and an Externalizing grouping comprising the Aggressive/Rule-Breaking, Attention Problems, and Self-Control Problems scales.

In addition to the empirically based scales, the SCICA Profile has six scales for scoring problems consistent with child psychiatric disorders (Affective Problems, Anxiety Problems, Somatic Problems, Attention Deficit/Hyperactivity Problems, Oppositional Defiant Problems, and Conduct Problems), similar to scales scored from the ASEBA CBCL, TRF, and YSR (Achenbach & Rescorla, 2001). The SCICA Profile also provides separate scores for Total Observations and Total Self-Reports.

The SCICA Profile can be scored by hand or by computer. The profile provides normalized clinical *T*-scores and percentiles for ages 6–11 and 12–18 for the eight syndrome scales, Internalizing, Externalizing, Total Observations, Total Self-Reports, and the six DSM-oriented scales. The clinical *T*-scores indicate how scale scores from an individual child compare to scores obtained from clinical samples of children in each of the two age groups. By examining the pattern of scale scores on the SCICA Profile, you can identify areas where the child exhibited severe problems or fewer problems compared to other clinically referred children. In this way the SCICA Profile enables you to judge the severity of a child's problems in relation to an empirical standard, which is not available from other interview formats.

> **Clinical *T*-scores on SCICA problem scales indicate areas where a child exhibits fewer or greater problems than other clinically referred children of the same age range.**

The SCICA Profile is especially useful for making classification or eligibility decisions that require judgments about the severity of problems. An example is determining whether a child meets IDEA 2004 criteria for special education services under the category of ED. The IDEA 2004 definition of ED states that a child must exhibit one of five specific characteristics to "a marked degree." The clinical *T*-scores from the SCICA provide an empirical standard for judging deviance or "marked degree" compared to other clinically referred children. Moderate-to-high clinical *T*-scores on the SCICA Profile usually indicate more severe problems. Accordingly, McConaughy and Achenbach (2001) consider SCICA clinical *T*-scores of 55 or higher (at or above the 69th percentile) as indicating severe problems. Because standard scores on the SCICA Profile are based on clinical samples, the 69th percentile cut point for severe problems is lower than the 97th percentile cut point on the ASEBA CBCL, TRF, and YSR profiles, which are based on normative samples of nonreferred children.

INTEGRATING CLINICAL INTERVIEWS WITH OTHER ASSESSMENT DATA

Although clinical interviews have considerable value for assessment and intervention planning, they should never serve as the sole source of information for such purposes. Instead, information from clinical interviews must be integrated with other assessment data to make judgments about children's functioning and to decide which, if any, services may be required to meet children's needs.

Table 1.2 in Chapter 1 outlined five data sources to consider in multimethod assessment of children's functioning: parent reports, teacher reports, cognitive assessment, physical assessment, and direct assessment of the child. It is beyond the scope of this book to discuss all aspects of multimethod assessment in detail. Instead, the focus is on how to integrate interview information with other assessment data for decision making and intervention planning. To illustrate this process, the next sections summarize information from multiple sources for the five case examples introduced in previous chapters. To illustrate multimethod assessment, assessment data are summarized for the child clinical interview, parent and teacher interviews, standardized rating scales, cognitive and academic testing, and other procedures relevant to each case. The assessment data were derived from research and clinical work using the SCICA and other ASEBA forms. Some case information has been changed to protect confidenti-

> **Data from child clinical interviews should be integrated with data from self-reports/tests, parent/teacher reports, and physical assessment.**

ality and all names are pseudonyms. Scores on the SCICA Profile are discussed to illustrate quantitative interpretations of child interview data. Assessment of all five cases included the ASEBA CBCL and TRF, and three included the YSR. However, multimethod assessment can incorporate any of the standardized parent and teacher rating scales listed in Tables 6.3 and 7.2 and the standardized self-report scales listed in Table 4.9. For cases involving mostly school problems, practitioners might choose to use the Semistructured Student Interview (McConaughy, 2012; Appendix 3.1) in place of the SCICA, and thus forego quantitative scoring of the child interview. The Semistructured Parent Interview (McConaughy, 2004a; Appendix 6.1) and Semistructured Teacher Interview (McConaughy, 2004b; Appendix 7.1) would be appropriate for interviewing parents and teachers in most cases.

Case Example: Andy Lockwood

As indicated in Chapter 1, 7-year-old Andy Lockwood was referred for evaluation because his mother and teacher were concerned about his slow progress in school, even after repeating first grade. Chapter 3 provided two segments from the child clinical interview with Andy. From these it became clear that Andy was well aware of his academic difficulties. Although he did not seem distressed about repeating first grade, he still thought the work was hard and disliked just about everything in school. He seemed to feel overwhelmed by the amount of work, but liked getting extra help. In another part of the interview, Andy described himself as one of "the kids who are being bad" in school. However, he thought the bad kids were "luckier" than other kids because they got happy faces on a card to help them be good. He said that he only had one more happy face to go to get a treat. However, it was not clear that Andy understood what counted as "good" behavior.

On the SCICA Profile, Andy obtained a score at the 81st percentile on the Aggressive/Rule-Breaking scale, indicating that he reported many more problems of this nature than other clinically referred children. Andy obtained scores at the 79th percentile on the Attention Problems scale and at the 73rd percentile on the Attention Deficit/Hyperactivity Problems scale, reflecting the interviewer's observations of high levels of inattention and restlessness during the interview. Andy also scored at the 79th percentile on the Anxious scale, reflecting his lack of confidence, fear of making mistakes, and frequent requests for feedback on academic screening tasks.

In the parent interview Ms. Lockwood reported that Andy was the younger of two children. The parents had divorced when Andy was 2 years old. Andy's father continued to visit with the children every other weekend. Ms. Lockwood, who was college educated, began work as a secretary when Andy entered first grade. Prior to that, she had worked as a substitute teacher, so she thought she had a good idea of what to expect from school.

Ms. Lockwood acknowledged that Andy was easily distracted and had trouble doing schoolwork:

"Everyday, he brings home worksheets that he hasn't finished in class. Then we have to spend time after dinner getting them done. He complains that they are boring, but I sometimes wonder if he understands what he is supposed to do. When I explain it to him, he gets everything right. But if I'm not sitting right next to him, he starts daydreaming and fooling around and doesn't work. It gets pretty frustrating having to nag him all the time to get things done."

At the end of the last school year, Andy's teacher sent home a pile of worksheets to complete, but Ms. Lockwood decided that all the work was "ridiculous" and told Andy he didn't have to do it. Ms. Lockwood thought that Andy's current teacher didn't like him because she called home frequently complaining about his behavior in school. The teacher seldom had anything nice to say about Andy. Ms. Lockwood said that her older daughter had had similar problems when she was younger, but now was doing fine in fifth grade.

Ms. Lockwood described Andy's early development as normal, although he had some trouble with his fine-motor skills, such as tying shoelaces. He also seemed to depend on others to do things for him. She said that Andy was still a very active child who likes sports and being outdoors. She also said that she had trouble disciplining Andy at times because "he wants to do everything his own way." She reported occasionally resorting to spanking, but mostly she sent him to his room when he disobeyed. Ms. Lockwood said that she would be open to trying a "behavior system" with Andy if someone would help her with it. When she had tried "checklists" in the past, they didn't seem to work very well. When asked about Andy's strengths, Ms. Lockwood said that he seemed very creative; he loved to draw and make things with clay and other crafts materials; he enjoyed building things with Legos; and he had a great sense of humor. Following the general interview, the school psychologist reviewed symptoms for several childhood psychiatric disorders with Ms. Lockwood. She endorsed many symptoms of hyperactivity, impulsivity, and inattention. She also reported oppositional behavior at home.

In her interview with the school psychologist, Andy's teacher reported that he had beginning first-grade skills because he was a "repeater," but at midyear he was falling behind in reading, language arts, and math. He did better in science and social studies. He seemed to like hands-on projects, but did not like writing assignments. The teacher was frustrated with Andy's inability to keep his mind on academic tasks. "In my class, he's in outer space," she said. "He's a bright boy who is severely sidetracked and seems to be in his own world." When asked to give an example of what she meant, the teacher said, "He's distracted by everything. He does not recognize when he is being spoken to. If I give a direction and then ask him to repeat it, he can't do it." When asked about circumstances and types of tasks that were difficult for Andy, the teacher reported:

"He has a lot of difficulty finishing his work without one-to-one supervision. He seems to become more easily distracted if the task he is doing is hard for him—like math papers. Sometimes, incentives work for him and other times, they don't. It is very difficult to find something that works for him consistently."

Through further probing, the school psychologist learned that the teacher put "happy faces" or stickers on Andy's papers when he finished them correctly. But often the work was not done on time, so she made Andy stay in during recess to finish it, and then he would not get a happy face. At the end of each week, if he had done his work, Andy could earn a treat from his mother. However, he seldom earned the treats. The teacher sent a note home each Friday summarizing Andy's performance that week. She did not use any formal method for charting his progress or work completion.

When asked about Andy's social relations, the teacher reported that he had difficulty getting along with other children because he acted immature and silly. He seemed to "gravitate" toward other kids who got into trouble. He clowned around in class to get attention and disturbed other kids when they were supposed to be working quietly. When Andy became too disruptive, she sent him to the principal's office. At recess, Andy sometimes got into fights with other kids, particularly one other boy. Andy always said that the fights were not his fault and that the other kid started it by calling him names or teasing.

On the CBCL and TRF, Andy's mother and teacher both scored him in the clinical range (above the 97th percentile) on the Attention Problems and Attention Deficit/Hyperactivity Problems scales, indicating severe problems compared to nonreferred 6- to 11-year-old boys. The teacher's ratings produced scores above the 98th percentile on the TRF Inattention and Hyperactivity–Impulsivity subscales. Both informants also scored Andy in the borderline to clinical range on the Social Problems and Aggressive Behavior scales. Andy's mother scored him low on the CBCL School scale, and his teacher scored him low on the TRF Adaptive Functioning scale.

The school psychologist observed Andy several times in class under various instructional conditions. Andy showed a consistent pattern of inattention, distractibility, and poor on-task behavior that corroborated the parent and teacher reports. The school psychologist observed that Andy stayed on task when the teacher gave specific directives (e.g., "Get your work out") or stood by his desk to give him help or let him sit next to her desk. Although Andy frequently raised his hand and approached the teacher to ask for help, he did not always get a response from the teacher. When the teacher wasn't paying attention to Andy or wasn't physically near him, he was usually off task, staring out the window or looking around the room, talking to other students, or clowning around to get other students' attention.

On a standardized intelligence test, Andy scored in the high-average range for verbal and nonverbal performance ability. Although he scored in the low-average range on tests of working memory, there were no significant differences among the subtest scores. Standardized achievement tests also produced scores in the average to high-average range.

Andy's high scores on the CBCL, TRF, and SCICA profiles, plus information from parent and teacher interviews and classroom observations, all suggested severe problems of inattention, hyperactivity, and impulsivity consistent with a DSM-5 diagnosis of ADHD. With this information, the school multidisciplinary team referred Andy and his mother to a mental health clinic for further evaluation and treatment for Andy's ADHD. Ms. Lockwood agreed to a trial of methylphenidate for Andy. She also agreed to participate in a parent training group at the clinic that focused on behavioral interventions for children with oppositional behavior (Barkley, 1997).

Results from Andy's multimethod assessment were consistent with research showing that many children with ADHD exhibit academic and social–behavioral problems (McConaughy, Volpe, Antshel, Gordon, & Eiraldi, 2011). The school multidisciplinary team developed a Section 504 plan to address these problems. The interviews and classroom observations were particularly informative for developing classroom accommodations and behavioral interventions. Andy's plan involved several components. First, the teacher and school psychologist created a positive incentive plan to improve on task behavior and reduce his disruptive behavior in class (e.g., clowning around and disturbing others during quiet time). The plan divided each school day into smaller periods that made sense to Andy (e.g., morning to recess, recess to lunch, lunch to end of school day). As Andy met behavioral targets for each time period, he earned points toward a menu of rewards at the end of each day. Andy earned extra points when he avoided fights on the playground. The teacher charted Andy's daily progress

> **Many children with ADHD exhibit academic and social-behavioral problems that warrant school-based interventions in addition to medical treatments for their inattention and hyperactivity.**

toward behavioral goals. She also posted a large chart of classroom rules at the front of the room for all students.

Second, the teacher agreed to break Andy's assignments into smaller components to reduce his feelings of being overwhelmed by schoolwork. She checked routinely to ensure that Andy understood directions and then praised him for his efforts. Andy also received small-group instruction in reading and math.

Third, the teacher created an individual school–home note system (Kelley, 1990) to keep Andy's mother informed of his progress. She sent Ms. Lockwood a copy of Andy's behavior chart at the end of each week, along with notes about his behavior and accomplishments. The teacher also sent home brief homework assignments to reinforce specific skills taught in class (Power et al., 2001). Clear instructions for homework assignments, plus a home-based reward system, helped to reduce conflicts between Andy and his mother over homework.

Fourth, with the support of the school psychologist, Andy's teacher used curriculum-based measures in reading and math to monitor and chart his academic progress. With all of the above educational interventions and mental health services in place for the rest of the school year, Andy successfully moved into second grade the following year.

Case Example: Bruce Garcia

Chapters 3 and 4 provided segments of the child clinical interview with 9-year-old Bruce Garcia. There we learned that Bruce had great difficulty in his social interactions with peers. Though Bruce clearly wanted friends, he seemed not to know how to go about making friends. Arguments over rules of a game often deteriorated into fights. Bruce was also the victim of frequent teasing and physical harassment by peers. With limited coping skills, Bruce felt powerless to deal with these problems and turned to others to defend him. Bruce also reported arguments at home with his mother and stepsister, Barbie. He admitted having difficulty controlling his temper, especially when he felt bossed around. Even small things, such as his mother telling him to do his chores, aroused intense angry feelings.

Bruce's self-reported problems produced a score at the 69th percentile on the SCICA Aggressive/Rule-Breaking scale. He scored at the 92nd percentile on the SCICA Language/Motor Problems scale, reflecting the interviewer's observations of difficulties in expressive language, concrete and tangential thinking, as well as fine-motor problems while producing his KFD (shown in Chapter 3). He also scored at the 69th percentile for observed problems on the SCICA Withdrawn/Depressed scale.

In her interview with the psychologist at the psychiatric clinic, Ms. Garcia reported that Bruce was the middle child in a blended family. She had retained custody of Bruce after divorcing his father when Bruce was age 2. She married Mr. Garcia 2 years later, who then adopted Bruce. Bruce's biological father had been diagnosed with schizophrenia and had been hospitalized several times. Ms. Garcia took Bruce to Florida once to visit his father, but she planned no further visits because of difficulties they had encountered.

Ms. Garcia reported that Bruce was delayed in speech and motor development and seemed socially immature. As a young child, he had displayed odd behaviors, such as rubbing his stomach over and over and rocking and hitting himself, but he no longer did those things at age 9. Ms. Garcia thought Bruce still seemed young for his age and had difficulty getting along with other kids. He often came home complaining about being teased and picked on at school and sometimes was beaten up by older boys. He seldom had other kids over to the house to play. Most of the time, Bruce played with Barbie and her friends. Ms. Garcia thought that Bruce got along best with his 14-year-old stepbrother, Sam, who played football with him and looked out for him. She reported some difficulties disciplining Bruce and Barbie at home, but felt that this was not a big problem, and that her husband was very good at backing her up when she needed it. She also felt that Bruce and Mr. Garcia generally got along well. She said that Bruce considered Mr. Garcia to be his dad.

As indicated in Chapter 1, Bruce had received speech and language services since age 4 and, at age 9, was undergoing a 3-year reevaluation for special education services. Bruce's third-grade teacher reported that he was performing at grade level in most subjects, though he had trouble expressing his ideas orally and in written assignments. Sometimes his answers to questions were "way off topic." By contrast, math was a special strength and Bruce's favorite subject. He was in the top math group, working on multiplication and division. The teacher concurred with Ms. Garcia's concerns about Bruce's social interactions. She thought that other students viewed him as "weird" and sometimes avoided him. She said that he stuck out in a group because of odd mannerisms. When asked to give examples, she said he sometimes sucked his fingers, rocked and hummed while in his seat, and twirled around on tiptoes when in line. She also thought he was a bit odd in appearance and dress. When he did try to interact with other kids, the teacher said, he often talked about topics that were not of interest to the other kids (e.g., his collections of football cards).

Bruce's mother and teacher concurred in their ratings of severe problems on the CBCL and TRF Social Problems and Thought Problems scales, producing scores above the 97th percentile for 6- to 11-year-old boys. They also reported attention problems. Though both mother and teacher noted that Bruce sometimes argued, they did not report temper tantrums or severe problems with aggression or rule-breaking behavior. They reported few problems related to anxiety, depression, or withdrawal.

Cognitive testing produced an overall IQ score in the average range, in sharp contrast to an IQ score in the mentally deficient range when Bruce was age 4. Testing at age 9, however, showed a significant discrepancy between Bruce's high-average verbal ability and his below-average non-verbal performance. His particular strengths were in verbal reasoning and acquired knowledge, in contrast to weaknesses in visual–spatial reasoning and processing speed. He also showed average working memory and attention. Additional testing revealed below-average expressive language skills and poor visual–motor integration.

Achievement tests indicated above-average math skills and average skills in all other areas, consistent with reports of good academic performance from Bruce's teacher. However, when a special education aide observed Bruce in the classroom, he was on task only 45% of the time, compared to 90% for two randomly selected "control" boys.

Bruce's pattern of problems did not appear to qualify for any specific psychiatric diagnosis, although he showed some characteristics that might suggest a mild version of a DSM-5 diagnosis of autism spectrum disorder (what had previously been called Asperger's syndrome in DSM-IV-TR). Although attention problems and some hyperactivity might also suggest ADHD, such a diagnosis would fail to capture Bruce's unusual behavior and thought processes, which might indicate an emerging thought disorder. His biological father's diagnosis of schizophrenia was an important factor to consider as a genetic vulnerability that could account for some of his odd behavior and uneven pattern of cognitive functioning.

The school multidisciplinary team decided that the multimethod assessment results justified continuation of speech and language services, particularly focusing on pragmatic and expressive language. In addition, interviews and high scores on standardized rating scales revealed significant problems in peer relations. To address his social problems, Bruce was enrolled in a social skills program with several other children. *Skillstreaming the Elementary School Child* (McGinnis, 2012) is an example of a program that would be especially good for Bruce. *Skillstreaming* offers lessons in the acquisition of 60 discreet skills that can then be reinforced in the classroom and at home. For each child in the program, parents and teachers complete "skillstreaming checklists" to identify specific deficits that can become targets for instruction. The program includes lessons on classroom survival skills, friendship-making skills, dealing with feelings, alternatives to aggression, and dealing with stress—many of which could be beneficial for Bruce. Regular consultation between the social skills trainer and Bruce's mother and teacher would also help to generalize specific skills from group sessions to other settings.

Case Example: Catherine Holcomb

Parent, teacher, and child interviews were especially important for understanding the different perspectives on Catherine Holcomb's functioning. The clinical interview with Catherine revealed lingering sadness over the death of her father, even though he had died 4 years ago. In the interview segment in Chapter 4, Catherine told the school psychologist that she often had sad thoughts about her father that intruded into her school day. Catherine described most of her school subjects as "boring," but also admitted difficulty understanding math problems.

The SCICA Profile produced an elevated score at the 93rd percentile on the Anxious/Depressed scale, indicating that Catherine reported many more problems related to anxiety and depression than other clinically referred children. Elevated scores on the SCICA Anxious (73rd percentile), Withdrawn/Depressed (98th percentile), and Affective Problems (98th percentile) scales reflected the interviewer's observations that Catherine looked very sad and withdrawn during the interview. She seemed to be very self-consciousness, had low energy and poor eye contact, and was reluctant to talk about feelings.

During the parent interview, Ms. Holcomb acknowledged that Catherine seemed sad and withdrawn, but more often she just seemed "irritable and hard to get along with." Ms. Holcomb said that Catherine often argued with her and had temper tantrums. She also argued and fought with her older brother, though the fights were usually not physical. When Ms. Holcomb tried to "lay down the rules with her," Catherine typically started crying and stomped off to her room. Ms. Holcomb relied mostly on time-outs as punishments, although she did not think they worked very well. She said that she never spanked her kids.

When asked more about the family and home situation, Ms. Holcomb reported that her work as an accountant sometimes required long hours at the office. Over the past years, she had relied on several different housekeepers, who also provided child care when she could not be home. Ms. Holcomb described her late husband as a good man who had enjoyed the outdoors. When he was alive, the family often spent time at their summer camp, hiking, canoeing, and picnicking. Ms. Holcomb said that she was "depressed" for the first year or so after her husband had died, but she had not seen a counselor. Instead, she used her work as a way "to move on." She thought that her son Billy was the one who missed his father the most after his death. But now Billy was in high school and involved with friends and sports activities.

Ms. Holcomb and the fifth-grade teacher both expressed concerns about Catherine's poor school performance, which had prompted the referral for evaluation. Ms. Holcomb told the school psychologist that her arguments with Catherine usually centered on homework. She thought that Catherine "was certainly smart enough," but seemed lazy and not interested in schoolwork. "Sometimes it's like pulling teeth just to get her to finish a math paper," she said. Reading assignments also created difficulties, especially when she had to answer questions or write book reports. However, Catherine did seem to enjoy reading books of her own choosing, especially fantasies and mystery stories.

In her interview with the school psychologist, the teacher described Catherine as "listless and hard to motivate," saying "it was hard to know what was going on with her." The teacher wondered if Catherine had an attention deficit or a learning disability. Catherine often failed to complete assignments, which resulted in poor or failing grades. She sometimes had difficulty understanding directions, but mostly seemed to be daydreaming or not concentrating. When the teacher called on her in class, she often didn't know what was expected and seemed embarrassed. Although Catherine was not disruptive, the teacher had to remind her to do her own work instead of watching what others were doing. She seldom asked for help from the teacher. Catherine left the classroom for 30 minutes of remedial tutoring in math and reading twice a week. When asked about her strengths, the teacher reported that Catherine was good in drawing and seemed to enjoy hands-on activities in art class.

Scores on standardized rating scales supported impressions of withdrawal and depression from interviews. Catherine's mother and teacher rated her in the clinical range on the CBCL and TRF Withdrawn/Depressed and Affective Problems scales, indicating severe problems for 6- to 11-year-old girls. Catherine's teacher also rated her in the clinical range on the TRF Anxious/Depressed scale. Similar to ratings by her mother and teacher, Catherine's self-ratings on the YSR produced high scores for internalizing problems. However, Catherine scored the YSR item "Unhappy, sad, or depressed" as "not true," which was a sharp contrast to her reports of sadness and her sad demeanor during the SCICA. In the clinical interview, Catherine also reported that she had not discussed her sad feelings with anyone prior to the interview. Catherine began to open up about her feelings as the interview progressed, which suggested that she might now be amenable to psychotherapy.

In addition to depression and withdrawal, interviews suggested that Catherine had a very limited social network. In the child clinical interview, Catherine reported that she had no close friends and she seemed not to know how to make friends. For example, she said that she usually played alone at recess because other kids didn't like her and she didn't like the games other kids played. She preferred playing with younger children because they didn't tease her or boss her around. In the parent interview, Ms. Holcomb reported that Catherine had no friends and instead "stuck to herself." She said that Catherine preferred solitary activities, such as reading books and doing crafts. Although she belonged to Girl Scouts, Catherine seldom attended meetings because she didn't like them. On weekends, she spent most of her time in her room. In the teacher interview, Catherine's teacher described her as a "loner." She said that at recess, Catherine wandered around the playground by herself or hung around the playground supervisors.

Low scores on the CBCL and TRF competence and adaptive scales also indicated limited social involvement and poor school performance, compared to other girls Catherine's age. Catherine's mother and teacher both rated her academic performance as below average. Her teacher rated her very low in terms of how hard she was working, how much she was learning, and how happy she was, compared to other students in the class. The teacher reported that Catherine had failing grades in math, social studies, and science. The teacher also scored Catherine in the borderline range on the TRF Attention Problems scale.

In the context of the parent and teacher reports, it was surprising to learn that Catherine's full-scale IQ on an intelligence test was in the superior range and that she showed no significant deficits among subtest scores. Standardized achievement tests revealed average academic skills in all areas.

Based on information from Catherine's multimethod assessment, the school multidisciplinary team concluded that she met IDEA 2004 criteria for ED. There was especially strong evidence of the ED characteristic of "a general pervasive mood of unhappiness or depression." The clinical interviews were especially important in tailoring interventions to meet Catherine's needs. From all perspectives, Catherine appeared to be a good candidate for cognitive-behavioral therapy for anxiety and depression (Merrell, 2008b). Accordingly, Catherine began individual psychotherapy with a clinical psychologist who provided school-based mental health services. The psychologist also held occasional joint sessions with Catherine, her mother, and her brother to address relationship problems at home.

The school multidisciplinary team developed an IEP that focused on reducing Catherine's social withdrawal and improving her organizational skills. The school psychologist conducted classroom observations and additional interviews with the teacher to obtain an FBA of Catherine's academic difficulties. The team then developed a positive behavioral intervention and support plan to improve her productivity and completion of assignments. The plan involved a coordinated effort among the classroom teacher, special educator, school psychologist, and Catherine's mother.

Catherine remained in her fifth-grade classroom for most of her school day, with instructional support in math and study skills. Because several other fifth-grade students also had problems in peer relations, the school psychologist and teacher provided weekly social skills training to the entire class as a Tier 1 intervention, focusing on making friends, coping with social problems, and controlling anger. The fifth-grade teacher and school psychologist consulted regularly on social skills that could be reinforced throughout the school day.

Prompted by what she had learned about her relationship with Catherine, Ms. Holcomb decided to seek individual psychotherapy to address her own symptoms of depression. Ms. Holcomb's psychotherapy, coupled with interventions for Catherine, proved to be very helpful in reducing conflicts at home.

Case Example: Karl Bryant

The interview with 12-year-old Karl Bryant in Chapter 3 offered a vivid picture of his aggressive behavior toward other children at school. Unlike Bruce, Karl was more often the perpetrator than the victim of aggression. A sense of self-righteousness and lack of guilt overlaid his descriptions of fighting and cruelty toward peers. In the interview segments in Chapter 5, Karl hinted at conflicts with his parents, although he viewed their discipline as "fair," unlike what happened at school. He seemed to have a positive relationship with his stepfather and respected him as the "boss of the house." After probing from the interviewer, Karl acknowledged arguments with his mother and having been punched and hit by her in the past when he did something wrong. A striking feature of Karl's interview was his strong desire to be treated fairly by adults and his views of what constituted unfair treatment at school.

On the SCICA Profile, Karl's self-reports produced a score at the 97th percentile on the Aggressive/Rule-Breaking scale, indicating severe problems compared to other clinically referred 12- to 18-year-olds. The interviewer's observations of Karl also produced high scores for Attention Problems (79th percentile) and Self-Control Problems (92nd percentile). Karl's openness about his problems during the clinical interview contrasted sharply with his self-ratings on the YSR, which produced scores below clinical cut points on all scales.

In the parent interview, Mrs. Ladd reported that Karl had had a history of behavior problems from an early age, including temper tantrums, hyperactivity, and aggressive behavior. She said that he had always been difficult to discipline because he insisted on having his own way. When he was 6 years old, the family pediatrician initiated a trial of stimulant medication for hyperactivity. However, Mrs. Ladd discontinued the medication after a year because she felt it was ineffective. When asked about their current discipline strategies, Mrs. Ladd said, "We mostly try to reason with Karl, but this often ends up in long, drawn-out arguments." Since his marriage to Karl's mother, Mr. Ladd had tried to lay down rules at home—for example, when kids had to do homework or chores, when kids could watch TV or use the computer, where Karl could go out at night. When Karl broke the rules, he was sent to his room or grounded. Detentions at school resulted in being grounded for a month. Despite these efforts, Mrs. Ladd reported that "it's a constant struggle to deal with Karl's defiant behavior."

Mrs. Ladd felt that Karl's behavior had deteriorated after agreed-upon visits with his biological father during Christmas and summer vacations. Mrs. Ladd suspected that Mr. Bryant provided very little supervision and instead let Karl do "pretty much whatever he wanted." Mrs. Ladd reported that Mr. Bryant was an alcoholic, as was his own father, and had been physically abusive toward her. Mrs. Ladd said that as a young child, Karl had witnessed several violent episodes between his parents, but he had never been the victim of physical abuse. Karl's parents had divorced when he was 5 years old.

School records indicated that Karl had received several in-school suspensions for aggressive and defiant behavior in the past year. He was also suspended out of school once for smoking on school grounds. Karl's homeroom teacher reported that he was failing three of his sixth-grade subjects, largely due to suspensions and incomplete assignments. The school staff had tried several different behavior plans with Karl, including a point system targeted on homework completion and reducing disruptive behavior in class. Karl occasionally met with the guidance counselor when he got into trouble on the playground. When he got into fights, he was sent to the principal's office and given an in-school suspension. However, the teacher felt that none of these interventions had worked very well. She said:

"Karl wants to please but is often unable to control his temper when things don't go his way. He seeks attention by asking questions constantly and bothering other students. He's very loud in class. He gets into many fights with other kids he doesn't know well and sometimes with his own friends. He seems to have good days and bad days. He really has been trying to improve his behavior, but he has a long way to go. I think he has a hard time with authority figures. He doesn't get along with the principal at all. One good thing is the way he shows great concern for other kids when they have a problem. His energy level is amazing."

Mrs. Ladd and the sixth-grade teacher both rated Karl in the clinical range on the CBCL and TRF Aggressive Behavior scale, and in the borderline to clinical range on the Social Problems scale. Karl's teacher rated him in the borderline clinical range on the Anxious/Depressed, Attention Problems, and Rule-Breaking scales, and Mrs. Ladd rated him in the borderline range for Thought Problems. These high scores indicated severe problems compared to norms for 12- to 18-year-old boys. Mrs. Ladd also rated Karl low on the CBCL Social and School scales. Observations by the school psychologist corroborated the teacher's reports of disruptive and aggressive behavior. The school psychologist also observed that Karl frequently sought the teacher's attention in class.

A high-average score for verbal ability on an intelligence test supported the teacher's impression that Karl was a "bright boy." The intelligence test showed no specific deficits, except a below-average score for auditory attention span. Karl also scored in the average range on standardized achievement tests.

After the school multidisciplinary team examined all the information from multiple sources, they concluded that Karl met IDEA 2004 criteria for ED. The aggressive behavior reported in interviews and on standardized rating scales provided strong evidence of the ED characteristic of "inappropriate types of behavior or feelings under normal circumstances." There was also strong evidence of the ED characteristic of "an inability to build or maintain satisfactory relationships with peers and teachers." The team determined that these

> **Data from clinical interviews, standardized parent/teacher rating scales, and standardized self-report scales can determine whether a child meets IDEA 2004 criteria for ED.**

behavioral and emotional problems had a direct adverse effect on Karl's school performance, leading to failing grades in spite of his high-average intellectual ability and average academic skills. The pattern of Karl's behavioral problems was also suggestive of a DSM-5 diagnosis of CD, but this was not a reason to deny him special education services for ED (for discussion of this issue, see McConaughy & Skiba, 1993; Skiba & Grizzle, 1991, 1992).

The clinical interviews with Karl and his mother and teacher suggested that he was a good candidate for a school-based behavioral contract. It became obvious that Karl needed clear and consistent rules and consequences to fit his conventional level of moral reasoning. Although the school staff had previously tried a point system with Karl, further probing in the teacher interview revealed that the system was loosely defined and limited only to the homeroom setting. The teacher also said that she and other school staff had not always followed through on rewards outlined in the plan. Knowing this, it was certainly worth trying a behavioral contract again. But this time, the plan included clearly defined behavioral goals that applied across all school settings. The plan included a menu of material and social rewards to provide variety, plus a clear warning system regarding unacceptable behavior, steps for time-out procedures, and opportunities for problem solving about future behavior. It also included options for salvaging lost points when Karl demonstrated good anger control. Many published resources are available for helping school staff develop school-based behavioral interventions for students such as Karl. Examples include *Responding to Problem Behavior in Schools* (Crone et al., 2004), *The Tough Kid Book* (Rhode, Jenson, & Reavis, 1993), and *Tough Kid Tool Box* (Jenson, Rhode, & Reavis, 1994).

Karl's description of "success plans" in the child clinical interview suggested that, under the right conditions (e.g., his perception of being treated fairly), he would probably respond positively to a well-structured behavioral contract. Involving Karl directly in negotiating the terms of the contract would address his desire to be heard and thus increase his level of commitment. To maintain consistency, the contract would need to be a coordinated effort among all school staff who had contact with Karl. Ongoing behavioral consultation between the school psychologist and Karl's teacher would provide a venue for developing such a contract and monitoring Karl's progress. Conjoint behavioral consultation (Sheridan et al., 1996) might be especially appropriate in Karl's case to maintain consistency between home and school.

Interventions for Karl also needed to extend beyond school. Although Karl minimized any family problems, Mrs. Ladd reported great difficulty managing his behavior at home. In addition, Karl's aggressive behavior, poor social coping skills, and association with other kids who got into trouble put him at risk for future antisocial behavior. Addressing these problems required interventions involving Karl and his parents. One option was to seek individual psychotherapy for Karl, coupled with parent training in behavior management skills. Good examples are the problem-solving skills training and parent management training programs described by Kazdin (2010). These evidence-based programs involve weekly individual therapy sessions to teach the child a series of problem-solving steps: identifying the problem, generating alternative solutions, evaluating possible solutions, choosing a solution, and evaluating the consequences of the chosen solution. The sessions incorporate a reward system and homework assignments. Parents then meet with a different therapist to learn how to alter their interactions with the child to reduce aggression and to promote prosocial behavior.

Social skills training would be another option for Karl. Social skills programs usually involve groups of children, but practitioners can also select components of programs to use in individual sessions. One caveat would be to avoid grouping Karl with other antisocial peers, because research has shown that this approach actually increases problems instead of reducing them (Dishion, McCord, & Poulin, 1999). Social skills training for Karl should focus on social problem solving and alternatives to aggression, as done in Kazdin's (2010) problem-solving skills training, as well as anger management, perspective taking, and postconventional moral reasoning. The Anger Coping and Coping Power Program (Lockman, Boxmeyer, Powell, Barry, & Pardini, 2010) is an example of one approach that includes separate sessions for children and parents. Parent sessions address social reinforcement and positive attention, the importance of clear house rules, behavioral expectations and monitoring procedures, and effective discipline strategies.

There are now many published social skills programs for use in small-group settings and school classrooms. Some examples are *Aggression Replacement Training* (Goldstein, Glick, & Gibbs, 1998), *Skillstreaming the Elementary School Child* (McGinnis, 2012), *Skillstreaming the Adolescent* (McGinnis, Sprafkin, Gershaw, & Klein, 2012), *The Stop & Think Social Skills Program* (Knoff, 2001), *The Tough Kid Social Skills Book* (Sheridan, 1997), and *The Tough Kid Parent Book* (Jenson, Rhode, & Hepworth, 2003). January, Casey, and Paulson (2011) provided a good review of the effectiveness of classroomwide social skills programs.

Case Example: Kelsey Watson

As we learned in Chapter 4, Kelsey Watson was admitted to a psychiatric hospital at age 13, where she was diagnosed with major depressive disorder and placed on antidepressant medication. At age 14 she was placed in a residential group home in the custody of the state social service agency. She continued to take antidepressant medication and received weekly therapy sessions with a mental health counselor at the group home. When she entered eighth grade in the local school, the school staff referred her for a psychological evaluation to determine if she needed additional school-based services.

It became apparent during the clinical interview with Kelsey that she was experiencing serious emotional and behavioral problems, including depression, suicidal thoughts, alcohol and drug use, and risky sexual activity. Kelsey's openness in discussing her problems was reflected in scores above the 80th percentile on the SCICA Anxious/Depressed and Aggressive/Rule-Breaking scales. Kelsey also appeared nervous and agitated during the interview, as reflected by a score at the 73rd percentile on the SCICA Anxious scale. In addition to the interview, Kelsey completed the YSR and the Reynolds Adolescent Depression Scale—2nd Edition (RADS-2; Reynolds, 2002). Kelsey's self-ratings on the YSR produced a clinical range score (above 97th percentile) on the Rule-Breaking scale, which indicated more antisocial behavior than typically reported by 12- to 18-year-old girls. At the same time, she scored herself in the normal range on other YSR scales, including those measuring anxiety, depression, and withdrawal. She also scored below the clinical cut point on the RADS-2, although she did report suicidal thoughts. These differences between the SCICA versus the YSR and RADS-2 suggested that Kelsey was much more willing to disclose emotional problems in a face-to-face interview than to acknowledge them on self-report questionnaires.

One of the counselors at the group home summarized Kelsey's history and current functioning in a phone interview. The same counselor also completed the CBCL. (Kelsey's mother lived in a different town and refused to provide information for the evaluation.) The counselor reported that Kelsey was still adjusting to her new environment in the group home. Although she followed general routines, she often seemed argumentative and sad. She continued to make comments to the staff about suicide and occasionally cut and picked at her skin, but none of these behaviors appeared to be life-threatening. Kelsey had threatened to run away and twice had left the grounds without permission. She also disobeyed "no smoking" rules at the group home. The counselor said that residential staff kept a close watch on Kelsey's behavior and supervised her activity in the community. Although Kelsey was supposed to visit her mother once a week, her mother seldom arranged visits. Kelsey became agitated and upset whenever her mother missed a visit. Although the CBCL produced scores below clinical cut points on all scales, Kelsey scored near the 90th percentile on the Anxious/Depressed and Rule-Breaking scales.

Ratings by two of Kelsey's eighth-grade teachers produced clinical range scores on the TRF Anxious/Depressed, Social Problems, and Rule-Breaking scales. One of the teachers also scored Kelsey in the borderline clinical range on the TRF Withdrawn/Depressed scale. In a joint interview the teachers expressed particular concerns about Kelsey's emotional state and social interactions. They worried that Kelsey seemed fascinated by drugs and sex. Drugs and sex appeared as recurrent themes in her creative writing assignments, and the teachers had overheard her talking with peers about drugs and sex. The teachers also thought that Kelsey was very flirtatious toward boys and that she tended to gravitate toward fringe groups that got into trouble in the community. Though there was no dress code at the school, Kelsey's typical attire clearly stood out as sexually provocative and different from the mainstream kids.

The teachers did not think that Kelsey was a "behavior problem" in classes. Though she sometimes whined about certain assignments, she was not disrespectful or disruptive. She generally kept to herself and sometimes seemed sad and in her own world. Although the teachers thought that Kelsey had average ability, they felt that she lacked certain basic eighth-grade skills. For example, she had trouble doing math involving fractions or word problems, and she could not organize her ideas for writing assignments. Kelsey also had very poor study skills. When asked about her strengths, the teachers said that Kelsey seemed to be very creative. She also liked doing projects on the computer, which was one way to get her to complete writing assignments.

Consistent with the teachers' impressions, cognitive testing with Kelsey produced scores in the high-average to superior range. Achievement tests produced average scores in reading and written language, but below average scores in math.

Clinical records at the group home indicated that Kelsey had a history of persistent emotional and behavioral problems. This made it all the more surprising that she had never received any special education services for ED. In the clinical interview Kelsey reported persistent feelings of sadness that were consistent with her diagnosis of major depressive disorder and her treatment with antidepressant medication. Scores on parent and teacher rating scales indicated high levels of anxiety and depression, compared to normative samples. Given Kelsey's high-average ability and the absence of evidence of a learning disability, the school multidisciplinary team determined that she was eligible for special education under the ED category. They recommended placement in a districtwide day treatment program for children with severe behavioral and emotional problems.

Because Kelsey had previously attempted suicide, it was important to establish in the child clinical interview that she had no current plans for suicide. Nonetheless, her suicidal ideation, coupled with depression and impulsive behavior, placed her at risk for future suicide attempts. The psychologist emphasized this risk in her written evaluation report and recommended careful monitoring of Kelsey's mood and behavior, especially during and immediately following home visits with her mother. The psychologist also recommended close monitoring for any wrist-cutting behavior. (See Chapter 9 for more detailed discussion of assessing suicide risk and nonsuicidal self-injury.)

The child clinical interview also indicated continued risk for substance abuse. Kelsey's initial alcohol and drug use most likely involved experimentation with peers, which is not uncommon among adolescents. However, the fact that Kelsey began experimenting with alcohol and marijuana at age 12 was worrisome, and her use of heroin was particularly alarming. Kelsey's regular cigarette smoking, coupled with her continued desire to get high on marijuana, suggested that she was moving beyond experimentation. Given this information, the psychologist recommended a more thorough evaluation of Kelsey's substance use by a local alcohol and drug abuse treatment program.

> **Along with her serious emotional/ behavioral problems, Kelsey's case raises serious concerns about adolescent high-risk behaviors, including alcohol/drug abuse and early sexual activity.**

Kelsey's early and continued sexual activity placed her at high risk for teenage pregnancy, as well as for HIV and other STDs. Association with deviant peers and adults could also place her at risk for sexual abuse, rape, and sexual exploitation, including prostitution. Sex education and learning about safe sex practices would be especially important for Kelsey. Along this line, it was encouraging to learn, in the child clinical interview, that Kelsey wanted to talk with a gynecologist or Planned Parenthood staff about safe sex practices. Careful monitoring by the group home staff would also be appropriate.

Finally, Kelsey's association with antisocial fringe groups highlighted the importance of encouraging more involvement with nondeviant, prosocial peers. This was one area in which school-based practitioners could be especially helpful. For example, school staff could encourage Kelsey to participate in sports, clubs, and other activities of interest. In the clinical interview Kelsey reported a special interest in computers. In fact, she thought it was "cool" to do schoolwork on the computer, and she liked belonging to computer chat groups. She also enjoyed writing, music, and theater. These were all strengths that could be cultivated in school-based interventions.

At the same time, adults would need to monitor Kelsey's use of the Internet and social networking sites to guard against sexual exploitation and access to information that could exacerbate suicide risk and cult activities.

SUMMARY

Clinical interviews with children, parents, and teachers provide separate windows on children's behavior, emotions, and life circumstances. Interviews are rich sources of information that cannot be obtained in other ways. The SCICA protocol (McConaughy & Achenbach, 2001), Semistructured Student Interview (McConaughy, 2012; Appendix 3.1), Semistructured Parent Interview (McConaughy, 2004a; Appendix 6.1), and Semistructured Teacher Interview (McConaughy, 2004b; Appendix 7.1) provide standardized formats for organizing interview questions and recording information obtained from children, parents and teachers. The SCICA also utilizes standardized rating scales and a scoring profile to provide a quantitative picture of interviewers' observations and children's self-reported problems.

As emphasized in other chapters, no one data source provides a definitive picture of children's functioning. Instead, practitioners must obtain different perspectives on children and then integrate data across multiple sources. To illustrate how data from clinical interviews can be integrated with other data sources, this chapter summarized findings for the five case examples discussed in previous chapters. Assessment data for all five cases included child, parent, and teacher interviews, standardized rating scales, intelligence and achievement tests, and other procedures appropriate for the case.

Three-tiered school-based interventions were warranted for all five children to improve their academic performance and social functioning. These included Tier 2 small-group and Tier 3 individually targeted interventions, as discussed in Chapter 7. Three children (Catherine Holcomb, Karl Bryant, and Kelsey Watson) were good candidates for Tier 3 special education services for ED. One child (Andy Lockwood) qualified for Tier 2 small-group remedial instruction in reading and math and individual behavioral accommodations as part of a Tier 3 Section 504 plan. Another child (Bruce Garcia) received Tier 3 speech and language services while being monitored for an autism spectrum disorder. Four children were good candidates for social skills training either in Tier 2 small groups or as part of a Tier 1 classroomwide program. One child (Kelsey Watson) received social skills training in a Tier 3 special education day treatment program. Information obtained from child, parent, and teacher interviews was also important for developing mental health and behavioral interventions, including individual behavioral contracts, individual psychotherapy, family therapy, and parent training.

CHAPTER 9

Assessing Risk for Suicide

David N. Miller

Child and adolescent suicidal behavior—including suicidal ideation, suicide-related communication (e.g., suicidal threats, making a suicide plan), suicide attempts, and suicide—is an enormous, worldwide public health problem (Miller, Eckert, & Mazza, 2009). In the United States, suicide is the third leading cause of death among children and young adults, trailing only accidents and homicide (Miller & Eckert, 2009). The risk for suicidal behavior increases as children grow older, with adolescent boys being at highest risk. There is also a "gender paradox" with regard to adolescent suicide. Specifically, although girls attempt suicide at a much higher rate than boys, nearly five times more boys than girls in the 15- to 19-year-old age range die by suicide (Berman, Jobes, & Silverman, 2006). Other groups at proportionally higher risk for suicidal behavior include Native American youth; students who reside in Western states and Alaska; youth with easy access to firearms; and gay, lesbian, and transgender youth (Miller, 2011).

Because children and adolescents spend much of their time in schools, school-based practitioners—particularly mental health practitioners such as school psychologists, counselors, and social workers—can play a key role in identifying and assessing students who may be at risk for suicide. Unfortunately, research suggests that school personnel, including school psychologists, frequently perceive themselves as being inadequately prepared to effectively assess and intervene with potentially suicidal youth (Debski, Spadafore, Jacob, Poole, & Hixson, 2008; Miller & Jome, 2008). Moreover, this problem is exacerbated by the fact that suicidal youth often feel hopeless or view suicide as a form of weakness, and are therefore reluctant to seek help (Miller, 2011). The fact that suicidal behavior is an internalizing problem that is often difficult to observe directly complicates matters even further (Miller, 2010). Despite these challenges, school personnel are obligated to intervene with suicidal youth, and their ability to do so can literally mean the difference between life and death.

David N. Miller, PhD, is Associate Professor of School Psychology at the University of Albany, State University of New York. His primary research and clinical interest is suicidal behavior and related internalizing problems in children and adolescents, particularly school-based suicide risk assessment and prevention.

It is therefore critically important that school practitioners be knowledgeable about a variety of issues regarding youth suicidal behavior, including liability and ethical issues; possible risk factors, warning signs, and precipitants of suicidal behavior; how to conduct effective suicide risk assessments; procedures for intervening with suicidal youth; and how to effectively distinguish between suicidal behavior and nonsuicidal self-injury. This chapter discusses each of these issues and provides practical guidelines for assessing suicide risk in children and adolescents in school settings.

LIABILITY AND ETHICAL ISSUES

School-based practitioners should realize that school personnel can and have been sued for a variety of actions related to student suicide, including failing to notify parents regarding their child's suicidal communications, failing to intervene in situations in which a student communicated a suicide plan, and failing to follow established school policies and procedures regarding youth suicidal behavior (Berman, 2009). Although schools and school personnel have been the recipients of many such lawsuits, a review of published court decisions in which families have attempted to hold school officials liable for student suicides reveals that the vast majority of these cases were found in favor of school officials (Fossey & Zirkel, 2011). Moreover, these lawsuits have seldom, if ever, occurred except under the condition that a student died by suicide and the parents of the deceased youth believed that school personnel could have prevented the suicide but failed to do so. Nevertheless, it is clear that litigation, whether directed toward a school district or a school district employee, should be avoided whenever possible. Regardless of the outcome, the associated costs—not only in terms of personal tragedy and monetary costs but also in time, labor, and bad publicity—are typically substantial (Miller, 2011).

Most court cases involving schools and student suicides have concerned issues of *negligence* and *foreseeability* (Berman, 2009); that is, when school personnel were egregiously negligent in their failure to prevent suicide, or when foreseeability of suicide was evident, but an adequate response was not provided. For example, courts have ruled that schools and individual school personnel can be found negligent when they fail to notify parents of students who are known, or believed, to be suicidal. Similarly, it is considered negligent not to provide close supervision of students considered to be at risk for suicide. Even under conditions in which a particular student denies suicidal intent, if school personnel suspect the student might be suicidal, they are obligated to notify the student's parents (Jacob et al., 2011).

According to Jacob (2009), all school personnel have an ethical duty to protect students "from reasonably foreseeable risk of harm" (p. 243). School personnel should be aware, however, that "foreseeability is not synonymous with predictability" (Berman, 2009, p. 234). That is, to date school personnel have not been held liable by the courts for failing to accurately identify or predict precisely which students may become suicidal (Fossey & Zirkel, 2011). Instead, *foreseeabilty* refers to a "reasonable assessment of a student's risk for potential harm" (Berman, 2009, p. 234). What may be considered "reasonable" is open to interpretation, however, and the courts have generally given schools wide latitude in this regard (Fossey & Zirkel, 2011).

> **When a student is suspected of being suicidal, school personnel must conduct a reasonable assessment of a student's risk for potential harm.**

School personnel, particularly mental health professionals such as school psychologists and counselors, should also be cognizant of their own professional ethical codes with regard to student suicidal behavior, including the fact that ethical codes are typically more stringent than legal mandates (Jacob, 2009). In addition, although school personnel must behave in a manner congruent with legal mandates and their particular code of professional ethics, meeting both sets of requirements should be viewed as the minimum standard expected, and does not necessarily reflect or limit what school-based mental health professionals could or should do (Miller, 2011). For example, Poland (1989) has recommended that all schools should (1) detect potentially suicidal students; (2) assess the severity level of potentially suicidal students; (3) notify the parents of a suicidal student; (4) work with parents to secure the needed supervision and services for the student; and (5) monitor the student and provide ongoing assistance. These recommendations reflect not only an attempt to meet legal and ethical guidelines, but also go beyond them by providing an example of best practices in school-based suicide prevention. Essentially, best practice can and should be *informed* by legal requirements and ethical duties, but need not be *limited* by them (Miller, 2011).

For additional information on school-based ethical and legal issues in the context of youth suicidal behavior, see Berman (2009), Fossey and Zirkel (2011), Jacob (2009), Jacob et al. (2011), and Miller (2011).

RISK FACTORS, WARNING SIGNS, AND PRECIPITANTS

Risk Factors for Suicide

Variables that help to explain or predict youth suicidal behavior can be placed into two categories: risk factors and warning signs. *Risk factors* may predispose an individual to suicidal behavior, whereas *warning signs* indicate the imminent possibility of suicidal behavior. Moreover, risk factors are typically longstanding, relatively unchangeable, and have been derived scientifically from research. Warning signs are more dynamic and have generally been derived from clinical practice rather than empirical studies (Miller, 2011).

Youth suicide is a complex phenomenon that includes many possible risk factors, as outlined in Table 9.1. The two most prominent risk factors for suicide are (1) the presence of at least one mental health disorder, and (2) a history of previous suicidal behavior, particularly suicide attempts. There is strong evidence that the overwhelming majority (over 90%) of children and adolescents who die by suicide experienced one or more mental health disorders (Miller & Eckert, 2009), most commonly mood disorders (e.g., depression, bipolar disorder), substance-related disorders (e.g., alcohol and/or drug abuse), and disruptive behavior disorders (e.g., conduct disorder; Fleischman, Bertolote, Belfer, & Beautrais, 2005). Many individuals who die by suicide appear to have had multiple (i.e., comorbid) mental health disorders at the time of their deaths.

Additionally, Joiner has developed a comprehensive and empirically supported theory of suicidal behavior (Joiner, Van Orden, Witte, & Rudd, 2009) in which particular risk factors play a prominent role. In his theory, suicide is conceptualized as being a function of both *desire* and *capability*. From Joiner's perspective, the *desire* to die by suicide is caused by the emotional distress resulting from perceived burdensomeness (i.e., the perception that one is a burden to others) and failed belongingness (i.e., the perception that one is disconnected from others in his/her environ-

> Young people are at increased risk for suicide if they have both the *capability* to die by suicide and the *desire* to do so.

TABLE 9.1. Risk Factors for Suicide

Child/adolescent risk factors

Previous suicide attempt

Current suicidal ideation (thoughts), intent, and plan (resolve)

Mental disorders—particularly mood disorders (e.g., major depression, dysthymic disorder, bipolar disorder) and disorders of low-impulse control (e.g., conduct disorder)

Co-occurring alcohol and substance abuse disorders

Feelings of hopelessness and helplessness

Sexual-minority status

Unwillingness to seek help because of stigma attached to mental and substance abuse disorders and/or suicidal thoughts

Isolation, a feeling of being cut off from other people

Ineffective coping mechanisms and inadequate problem-solving skills

Cultural and/or religious beliefs—for example, the belief that suicide is a noble resolution of a personal dilemma

Family and environmental risk factors

Easy access to lethal methods, especially guns and medications

Exposure to suicide and/or family history of suicide

Influence of significant people—family members, celebrities, peers who have died by suicide—through direct personal contact or inappropriate media representations

Local epidemics of suicide that have a contagious influence

Barriers to accessing mental health treatment

---

ment). The *capability* to die by suicide results when an individual becomes gradually desensitized and habituated to pain and violence through frequent exposure to both, such as through engaging in self-injury. When both the desire for suicide as well as the capability to carry it out is present, an individual is at high risk for suicide (Joiner, 2005).

Environmental factors and family history are also important variables to consider. For example, easy access to lethal methods is a prominent environmental risk factor in child and adolescent suicides. The presence of firearms in the home, particularly loaded guns, greatly increases the risk for death by suicide, especially for boys. Access to lethal medications (pills) may increase suicide risk as well, especially for girls. Access to Internet websites that encourage and promote suicide may pose additional risks, especially among youth already predisposed to suicidal behavior (Miller, 2011). A family history of suicide and personally knowing someone who died by suicide are additional risks. Young people who are potentially vulnerable to suicide can be influenced by the suicides of family members, friends, and celebrities, as well as by highly publicized suicides

> **Access to firearms in the home (loaded guns) greatly increases suicide risk, especially for boys. Access to lethal medications (pills) increases suicide risk for girls.**

by other youth in their communities, especially if these are covered extensively by the media. Family problems, such as divorce and strained parent–child relationships, may contribute to suicide risk, although it is important to realize that most youth who experience family problems are not suicidal.

Warning Signs for Suicide

As opposed to risk factors, warning signs are more proximal in time and suggest the increased probability of a suicidal crisis (Miller, 2011). Many individuals who are seriously thinking about suicide give signals or display warning signs. Because children and adolescents typically do not refer themselves for treatment, it is critically important for the adults around them to be aware of warning signs of potential suicidal behavior. Table 9.2 lists several possible warning signs of youth suicide.

The American Association of Suicidology (AAS) has also developed a useful mnemonic for remembering possible warning signs of suicide—IS PATH WARM:

- *I* is for suicidal ideation
- *S* is for substance abuse
- *P* is for purposelessness
- *A* is for anxiety and agitation (including being unable to sleep)
- *T* is for trapped (as in feeling trapped)
- *H* is for hopelessness
- *W* is for withdrawal
- *A* is for anger
- *R* is for recklessness
- *M* is for mood fluctuations

Any form of suicide-related communication, such as suicide notes or threats, should be treated seriously. Suicide threats may be direct (e.g., "I want to die," "I'm going to kill myself") or indirect (e.g., "The world/my family would be better off without me"). Suicidal youth may share suicide plans, or hint at plans, to friends or (less likely) adults. They may also show increased interest in guns or other lethal methods, or talk about how to gain access to lethal methods. Sudden changes in behavior might take

> **Suicide notes or threats, and other forms of suicide communication, should be treated seriously.**

TABLE 9.2. Possible Warning Signs for Suicide

Suicide notes

Suicide threats

Suicide plan/method/ access

Sudden changes in behavior, friends, or personality

Changes in physical habits and appearance

Preoccupation with death and suicide themes

Increased inability to concentrate or think clearly

Loss of interest in activities that were previously important or pleasurable

Symptoms of depression

Increased heavy use and abuse of alcohol and/or drugs

Increased interest in guns or other lethal methods

the form of withdrawing from friends or family, increased sadness or apathy, or a sudden switch from negative feelings to feelings of peacefulness. Changes in habits and appearance can include loss of sleep or sleeping too much, sudden changes in weight, or poor personal hygiene.

Preoccupation with death or suicide themes might appear in drawings, journals, poetry, or conversation. Some suicidal youth visit Internet websites that feature themes of death, suicide, or violence, as well as instruction on suicide methods. Although the vast majority of students who are depressed are not suicidal, and not all suicidal students are depressed, the presence of depression can be a risk factor and/or a warning sign for potential suicidal behavior. Similarly, the use of alcohol and/or drugs is not only a key risk factor for suicide, but can also be a warning sign when there is an increase in use or abuse.

Situational Crises, Stressful Events, and Precipitants

The risk for suicidal behavior is increased when acute situational crises or stressful life events, such as some type of interpersonal loss, occur in conjunction with other more chronic risk factors, such as depression, substance abuse, and/or access to lethal methods. Researchers have identified several stressful events that often precipitate suicidal behavior in youth (Gould & Kramer, 2001; Kalafat & Lazarus, 2002). Although these events do not directly cause suicide, they have the potential to trigger suicidal behavior in vulnerable youth. Table 9.3 provides a list of these potential precipitating events. Although no one stressful event is highly predictive of suicide, the risk for suicide rises as the number and emotional intensity of stressful events increase.

TABLE 9.3. Stressful Events That May Trigger Suicidal Behavior

Breakup from boyfriend or girlfriend

Disappointment and rejection, such as a dispute with a boyfriend/girlfriend, failure to get a job, or rejection from college

Bullying or victimization

Getting into trouble with authorities (e.g., school, police); not knowing and being afraid of the consequences of getting into trouble

Death of a loved one or significant other

Conflict with family; family dysfunction

Disappointment with school results; school failure

High demands at school during examination periods

Unwanted pregnancy; abortion

Infection with HIV or other STDs

Anniversary of a death of a friend or loved one

Separation from friends, girlfriends/boyfriends

Relational, social, work, or financial loss

Severe or terminal physical illnesses

Serious injury that may change the individual's life course

Note. Adapted from Kalafat and Lazarus (2002). Copyright 2002 by the National Association of School Psychologists, Bethesda, MD. Adapted by permission of the publisher. *www.nasponline.org.*

Before concluding this section on risk factors, warning signs, and possible precipitants of youth suicidal behavior, a few caveats should be briefly noted. First, despite their utility, many of the warning signs discussed earlier have not been validated specifically for school-age populations. Second, although the giving away of possessions and making final arrangements have frequently been described as warning signs for suicide, there is currently no empirical support for this contention. Third, it is important to realize that no single risk factor, warning sign, or stressful event will predict suicidal behavior with perfect accuracy. Moreover, some youth may exhibit multiple risk factors or warning signs and still not make a suicide attempt. Because suicide is a relatively rare event, it is not possible to predict with a high degree of precision (Miller, 2011).

Fortunately, interviews and other assessment procedures, when used appropriately, can help to identify youth at risk for suicidal behavior. The next sections discuss the purpose of school-based suicide risk assessment, followed by multimethod procedures for assessing suicide risk, with a particular emphasis on the child/adolescent clinical interview.

THE PURPOSE OF SCHOOL-BASED SUICIDE RISK ASSESSMENT

School-based suicide risk assessment has two primary purposes. The first is to determine if a student is potentially suicidal and, if so, to what extent. The second purpose is to link assessment results with interventions that will best meet a particular student's needs. Suicide risk assessment is linked to intervention in the sense that the level of suicide risk will help to determine the level of intervention that is required (Miller, 2011). For example, if the risk assessment suggests that the student should be considered at high risk for suicide, the intervention will typically involve keeping the student safe until he/she can be transported away from the school, probably to an area hospital or mental health clinic, for further assessment and intervention.

> The primary purposes of school-based risk assessment is to determine if a student is suicidal, and what interventions would best meet the student's needs.

Rudd (2006) has identified five possible suicide risk levels based on a continuum from "minimal risk" to "extreme risk." Below is a listing of each risk category, including a brief description of the behavioral markers for each category:

1. *Minimal risk level:* no identifiable suicidal ideation.
2. *Mild risk level:* suicidal ideation of limited frequency, intensity, duration, and specificity.
3. *Moderate risk level:* frequent suicidal ideation with limited intensity and duration; some specificity in terms of plan; no associated intent.
4. *Severe risk level:* frequent, intense, and enduring suicidal ideation; specific plans; no subjective intent but some objective markers of intent (e.g., choice of lethal methods).
5. *Extreme risk level:* frequent, intense, and enduring suicidal ideation; specific plans; clear subjective and objective intent.

Interventions will differ depending on where a student is assessed to be on this continuum. For example, for students determined to be at mild risk, the intervention might include a phone call to the parents to apprise them of the situation, ensuring that the student is not left alone for the remainder of the school day, and frequently monitoring the student to determine if his/her risk for suicidal behavior increases. Interventions for students who are determined to be at severe or extreme risk levels would likely involve hospitalization. Regardless of the level of suicide risk in which a particular student is categorized, each time a suicide risk assessment is conducted the student's parents should be contacted and apprised of the results. Moreover, even if the assessment suggests that a student should be considered to be at low risk for suicide, the student should not be left alone for any time while at school. In such situations, school personnel should also recommend that parents come to the school to pick the student up (Miller, 2011).

MULTIMETHOD RISK ASSESSMENT

Interviewing Children and Adolescents

The clinical interview of the child or adolescent is the single most valuable component of a good suicide risk assessment. Because of its importance and the sensitivity of the topic, interviewing youth who may be suicidal can be an extremely stressful and anxiety-provoking experience for both the interviewer and the youth. It is important that interviewers not become so intimidated by the process of suicide risk assessment that they become immobilized. Having a standard protocol for the interview can greatly reduce anxiety in a suicide risk assessment. Additionally, gaining experience in conducting suicide risk assessments should boost confidence and decrease discomfort and anxiety.

Developmental issues are important to keep in mind when conducting suicide risk assessments with younger children. For example, children under the age of 12 may have difficulty verbalizing or articulating possible suicidal intent (Pfeffer, 2006). In such cases, interviewing the child's parents and teachers becomes especially important. Practitioners should also be aware that children under the age of 8, and older children with cognitive impairments, will often have difficulty reflecting on and reporting their emotions and subjective experiences, including any suicidal thoughts or feelings they may be having (Miller, 2011).

> **An interview with the identified student is the single most important component of a suicide risk assessment.**

When interviewing a child or adolescent about possible suicidal behavior, it is important to remain calm and to proceed in a concerned but relaxed manner. Barrett (1985) identified three important issues that practitioners must consider to effectively assist suicidal youth: (1) They must not let their attitudes toward death, in general, and suicide, in particular, interfere with their ability to be reasonably comfortable with the topic; (2) they must be careful not to exhibit anxiety or irritation to the individuals they are interviewing; and (3) they must deal with feelings of insecurity or lack of confidence and seek out additional training and support, as needed.

To maximize the effectiveness of a suicide risk assessment, it is preferable to have a positive, established relationship between the youth and the individual conducting the interview. If there is no such prior history, the interviewer should endeavor to make the youth as comfortable as possible. For example, if the youth has a good relationship with a particular teacher, that teacher could be asked to sit in (with the youth's permission) on the risk assessment.

It is very important that the interviewer be direct and specific in language and approach when conducting interviews with potentially suicidal youth (Miller, 2011). The school professional conducting the interview should document, as much as possible, exactly what was said by the youth in response to questions (Rudd, 2006). To begin the interview, the youth should be informed as to why the assessment is being conducted. For example: "John, Mrs. Smith was concerned about some of your writings in one of your homework assignments, and she shared them with me. I wanted to meet with you to discuss them." It should be clearly communicated to the youth that many people care about him/her and want him/her to be safe.

Several structured and semistructured interviews focus specifically on child and adolescent suicidal behavior. However, many of these are expensive, difficult to acquire, and vary widely in their reliability and validity (Goldston, 2003). Nevertheless, it is imperative that professionals dealing with potentially suicidal youth have a specific set of questions that will quickly and reliably obtain needed information. I have provided the following examples of specific areas to cover when interviewing youth for possible suicide risk (Miller, 2011):

- How the youth currently feels
- Past and current level of depression
- Past and current level of hopelessness
- Past and current level of suicidal ideation
- Perceptions of burdensomeness and belongingness
- History of drug and alcohol abuse
- Current problems/stressors at home
- Current problems/stressors at school
- History of any previous suicide attempts
- Method(s) used in any previous suicide attempt(s)
- Presence or absence of a suicide plan
- Specificity and potential lethality of method in suicide plan
- Availability of lethal means
- Possibility/probability of rescue
- Current support systems
- Reasons to live

Although all of the above issues are important to address, the most serious indicators of high risk for suicide include *previous suicide attempts, clear plans and methods*, and *access to lethal means*.

Brock and Sandoval's (1997) Student Interview for Suicide Risk Screening (SISRS) is particu-

> **Among many possible indicators of suicide risk, the most serious are previous suicide attempts, clear plans and methods, and access to lethal means.**

larly appropriate for school-based practitioners. Their interview, shown in Appendix 9.1, consists of four components: engagement, identification, inquiry, and assessment. The SISRS is appropriate for comprehensive assessments of youth who appear at moderate to high risk for suicide, such as youth who have experienced an acute crisis or who have given warning signs of being possibly suicidal.

Youth who are seriously contemplating suicide typically experience a high degree of subjective distress and emotional upheaval. Even so, many will respond to interview questions openly and honestly if the questions are posed by a caring, respectful, and empathic adult. Poland (1989) provided the following guidelines for the interview process:

- Calmly gather information to assess lethality of method and identify a course of action.
- Use effective listening skills by reflecting feelings, remaining nonjudgmental, and not minimizing the problem.
- Communicate caring, support, and trust, while providing encouragement for coping strategies.
- Emphasize the youth's worth and previous coping skills; be hopeful.
- Gather information about the youth's and family's history, with emphasis on suicide and substance abuse.
- Emphasize alternatives to suicide.
- Do not make any deals to keep the suicidal thoughts or actions a secret. Explain the limits of confidentiality, and why it is in the youth's best interest to inform parents or guardians so that everyone can work together to assist him/her.
- Keep notes of your interaction with the youth.
- Do not leave high-risk youth alone.
- Get supportive collaboration from colleagues.
- Be familiar with community resources.
- Outline for the youth the steps that will be taken to help him/her.

Finally, although there will often be a high degree of consistency between what a suicidal person says and does, this is not always the case. There may be some instances in which a potentially suicidal youth says one thing but does another (e.g., a youth may deny any suicidal thoughts but display behavior that suggests the contrary, such as engaging in multiple suicide attempts). In this situation, it is important to clarify and resolve any discrepancies by gently but firmly challenging the youth during the interview. For more information on this topic, the reader is referred to Rudd (2006).

Interviewing Teachers and Parents/Caregivers

Research suggests that teachers and parents/caregivers often are unaware of the suicidal behaviors exhibited by children in their care. However, when used in conjunction with child/adolescent interviews, teacher and parent interviews can be helpful, particularly for examining informants' perceptions across multiple environments and contexts. Table 9.4 shows examples of questions for teachers, and Table 9.5 lists questions for parents/caregivers.

TABLE 9.4. Questions for Teachers Regarding a Student's Risk for Suicide

Have you noticed any major changes in your student's schoolwork since school started?

Have you noticed any behavioral, emotional, or attitudinal changes?

Has the student experienced any trouble in school? What kind of trouble?

Does the student appear depressed and/or hostile and angry? If so, what clues does the student give?

Has the student verbally, behaviorally, or symbolically (in an essay or story) threatened suicide or expressed statements associated with self-destruction or death?

TABLE 9.5. Questions for Parents or Caregivers Regarding a Student's Risk for Suicide

Has any serious change occurred in your child's or family's life recently?

(*If yes*) How did your child respond?

Has your child had any accidents or illnesses without a recognizable physical basis?

Has your child experienced a loss recently?

Has your child experienced difficulty in any areas of his/her life?

Has your child been very self-critical, or does he/she seem to think that you or teachers have been very critical lately?

Has your child made any unusual statements to you or others about death or dying? Any unusual questions or jokes about death or dying?

Have you noticed any changes in your child's mood or behavior over the last few months?

Has your child ever threatened or attempted suicide before, or attempted to harm him/herself in any way?

Have any of your child's friends or family, including yourselves, ever threatened or attempted suicide?

How have these last few months been for you? How have you reacted to your child (e.g., with anger, despair, empathy)?

Other Assessment Methods

In addition to interviews, several self-report rating scales are available for assessing suicide risk. Self-report scales can be useful as initial screening measures to identify youth who should be interviewed individually for a more comprehensive assessment of suicide risk. One example of a useful school-based screening measure is the Suicidal Ideation Questionnaire (SIQ; Reynolds, 1988). Reynolds (1991) recommended using the SIQ in a two-step process in which (1) all students in a classroom or school are asked to complete the SIQ, and (2) those students who score at clinically significant levels on it are subsequently interviewed by a mental health professional at the school (e.g., school psychologist or counselor).

Research has shown that this two-step approach can successfully identify youth who are at risk for suicide (Shaffer & Craft, 1999). Unfortunately, other studies also suggest that this approach may meet with some resistance among school personnel (Eckert, Miller, DuPaul, & Riley-Tillman, 2003; Miller, Eckert, DuPaul, & White, 1999; Scherff, Eckert, & Miller, 2005) and students (Eckert, Miller, Riley-Tillman, & DuPaul, 2006). Some school personnel may feel that suicide screening is too intrusive. Others may believe that asking specific questions regarding suicide will lead students who are not suicidal to become suicidal as a result of the screening (i.e., that a screening will "put ideas into their heads"). There is no empirical support for this belief (Gould et al., 2005), however, and ensuring that school personnel understand this point is critical to effective school-based suicide prevention efforts.

Because currently available rating scales for assessing youth suicidality vary in their reliability and validity, it is important to choose an instrument with sound psychometric properties. The choice of instruments should also be based on cultural considerations, the specific needs of the assessor, the purpose for which the instrument will be used, and the outcome the assessor wants to measure (Goldston, 2003; Goldston et al., 2008). Practitioners who use standardized self-report scales

> There is *no empirical evidence* that shows that asking questions regarding suicide will lead students who are not suicidal to become suicidal.

TABLE 9.6. Standardized Self-Report Scales for Assessing Suicide Risk

Adolescent Psychopathology Scale (APS; Reynolds, 1998)

Beck Scale for Suicide Ideation (BSSI; Beck & Steer, 1991)

Children's Depression Inventory–2 (CDI-2; Kovacs, 2010)

Reynolds Adolescent Depression Scale—2nd Edition (RADS-2; Reynolds, 2002)

Reynolds Child Depression Scale–2 (RCDS-2; Reynolds, 2010)

Suicidal Ideation Questionnaire (SIQ; Reynolds, 1988)

should be aware that there is no "gold standard" with regard to these instruments, and that currently no one instrument (or combination of instruments) can predict, with a high degree of accuracy, who will attempt suicide. Keeping this caveat in mind, Table 9.6 lists examples of some popular and commercially available self-report scales that have demonstrated reasonable utility for identifying potentially suicidal youth.

In addition to the instruments listed in Table 9.6, other broad-spectrum assessment measures contain problem items that may indicate suicidal thoughts and suicide attempts. Examples of such measures include the ASEBA CBCL/6–18 and YSR (Achenbach & Rescorla, 2001) and the BASC-2 PRS and SRP (Reynolds & Kamphaus, 2004). Some practitioners also use projective techniques (e.g., human figure drawings, apperception tests) to assess possible depression or suicidal ideation. However, because projective methods have not demonstrated adequate reliability or validity for identifying suicidal youth, their use is not recommended when conducting suicide risk assessments (Miller, 2011). For readers interested in more information in this area, Goldston (2003) provides a comprehensive description and review of a variety of suicide risk assessment instruments.

Immediate Interventions for Suicidal Youth

When a youth appears at risk for suicide, it is especially important to assess the lethality of the intended method and take appropriate steps to protect him/her from carrying out plans for suicide. If an assessment indicates moderate to high risk for suicide, school-based practitioners must take immediate protective action. In such crisis situations, the primary goal is to keep the youth safe and to quickly mobilize resources to provide the youth with necessary supports. The actions school personnel should take in these circumstances are discussed below.

> If an assessment indicates moderate to high risk for suicide, school-based practitioners must take immediate protective action to keep the youth safe and supported.

Breaking Confidentiality

Ethical codes typically require that school personnel report any suicidal behaviors they observe to the youth's parents. When this occurs, it requires breaking the confidentiality of the child/adolescent interview. For this reason, it is important, at some point in the interview with the youth, to state the limits of confidentiality. This should be done in such a way that emphasizes to the youth that many people care about him/her, including his/her parents, and that they want the youth to be safe. At the end of the interview, the interviewer should clearly explain the next steps that will be taken.

Notifying Parents/Caregivers

Parents/caregivers should be notified regarding all suicide risk assessments after their completion, regardless of the degree of assessed risk (Miller, 2011). In their guidelines for suicide interventions, Poland and Lieberman (2002) pose four important questions to consider regarding parent notification: Are the parents available? Are the parents cooperative? What information do the parents have that might contribute to the assessment of risk? What mental health insurance, if any, does the family possess? (The question about insurance is important for assessing access to mental health services outside of school.) If there is an imminent danger of suicide, school personnel should notify the youth's parents immediately, ask them to come to the school to get their child, and advise them to seek admission to an emergency room or hospital for their child.

Making Use of Commitment-to-Treatment Statements Rather Than No-Suicide Contracts

"No suicide" or "safety" contracts are written or verbal agreements commonly negotiated with suicidal individuals in the hope of improving intervention compliance and decreasing the probability of suicidal behavior (Brent, 1997). These "contracts" appear to be popular among many mental health professionals, particularly in outpatient settings (Berman et al., 2006). There is increasing belief, however, that such procedures should not be used, primarily because they provide professionals with a false sense of security and may decrease clinical vigilance (Lewis, 2007). Jobes (2003) has suggested that safety contracts "are neither contractual nor do they ensure genuine safety," because they tend to emphasize what clients "won't do versus what they will do" (p. 3). A literature review on this topic found no empirical support for no-suicide contracts, which led the authors to propose the use of commitment-to-treatment statements as a preferred alternative (Rudd, Mandrusiak, & Joiner, 2006). Practitioners are therefore encouraged to make use of commitment-to-treatment statements rather than no-suicide contracts when intervening with suicidal youth—for example, having the youth sign and agree to a statement such as: "I am committing myself to getting help for my problems, including calling an appropriate person if I ever feel suicidal."

> **Commitment-to-treatment statements are better than no-suicide contracts with suicidal youth because they emphasize what the youth *will do* rather than *won't do*.**

If parents are available and cooperative, school-based practitioners should provide information about mental health services available in the community. If parental permission is obtained, school personnel can contact the service provider to provide pertinent information and then follow up to make sure that the youth arrived at the appropriate agency. It is essential to obtain written consent from parents to release information to other agencies.

If a youth is in immediate danger of suicide and the parents are uncooperative or deny the danger, then school-based practitioners may decide to contact local law enforcement or child protective services (CPS) to take action on the youth's behalf. If the parents are not available, school-based practitioners may have to take action themselves to ensure the safety of a high-risk youth. Usually this action is taken in collaboration with an established school-based crisis team. The team may decide that the level of risk warrants escorting the youth to an emergency room in a hospital, a mental health facility, or other community agency.

If a suicidal youth does not want his/her parents notified, possible reasons for this stance should be elicited from the student. Based on information from the suicide risk assessment, the crisis team must then determine whether the youth would be placed in a more dangerous situation by notifying the parents. If this is the case, then it is usually appropriate to notify CPS or local law enforcement. However, it will still be necessary to notify parents at some point about the youth's suicide risk, and to attempt to gain their support for an immediate intervention.

Removing Access to Lethal Means

For any youth at risk for suicide, it is essential to "suicide-proof" the home and other home-like environments (e.g., frequently visited homes of friends or relatives). This means eliminating access to lethal sources such as guns, poisons, medications, knives, and other objects that could be used to inflict self-harm. Guns, other weapons, and potentially lethal medications should be kept in locked cabinets, without the youth's access to the key, or removed to a safe place unknown to the youth. If a gun cabinet has a glass window, the guns should be moved to a more

> **Eliminating access to lethal methods in the home or other home-like environments is an essential step for protecting suicidal youth.**

secure place. Eliminating access to guns can be especially challenging in some families, especially those who enjoy hunting and other gun sports. Any medications that could be potentially life-threatening should also be kept out of reach from young people who may be suicidal, including (but not limited to) painkillers, antidepressant medication, and aspirin. Parents of suicidal youth should also carefully monitor their child's use of the Internet and be especially watchful of their child's visits to websites that feature death and morbid themes, have suicidal or violent games, or promote suicidal behavior.

Keeping the Youth Safe

A youth who is at risk for suicide, even if it is determined that the risk is minimal, should never be left alone. The youth should always be accompanied by an adult, who should be in close proximity to the youth at all times.

Documentation

Every school district should have protocols for addressing suicide risk in students. The protocols should require documenting information from the assessment process and the steps taken by school personnel to address the problem. School-based practitioners should also carefully record and date all other actions taken on behalf of the at-risk youth, including notification of parents and referrals and reports to mental health professionals or community and mental health agencies.

PREPARING FOR THE YOUTH'S RETURN TO SCHOOL

Young people who are hospitalized as a result of suicidal behavior may not return to school for several weeks, or may return in 1 or 2 days. In preparing and providing services for a youth's return to school, a "wraparound" approach, similar to the one used with children who exhibit disruptive, acting-out behavior problems (Quinn & Lee, 2007), is encouraged. As the term implies, a *wraparound* approach provides comprehensive, multisystemic interventions for troubled youth. Although the effectiveness of wraparound has not been evaluated in the context of suicidal youth, this approach is consistent with what is known about effective interventions for a variety of child and adolescent mental health problems (Miller, 2011).

DIFFERENTIATING SUICIDAL BEHAVIOR FROM NONSUICIDAL SELF-INJURY

The use of firearms is the most common method of youth suicide (Gould & Kramer, 2001; Miller & Eckert, 2009), although other methods may be used as well. One possible method involves the self-destruction of body tissue, such as the cutting of an artery in an attempt to die by suicide through self-inflicted blood loss. Some children and adolescents, however, engage in the intentional self-destruction of body tissue without deliberate suicidal intent. This behavior has been previously described as self-mutilation (Lieberman & Poland, 2006) but now is more commonly referred to as nonsuicidal self-injury (NSSI).

NSSI often begins during early adolescence, although it can begin earlier, and may persist for years or even decades if not effectively identified and treated. It often appears to provide rapid, but temporary, relief from stress and tension, a sense of security or control, and/or decreases in distressing thoughts or feelings (Miller & Brock, 2010). Walsh (2012) outlined nine points of distinction for determining if a self-destructive behavior is suicidal or self-injurious: (1) intent, (2) level of physical damage and potential lethality, (3) frequency of the behavior, (4) multiple methods, (5) level of psychological suffering, (6) constriction of cognition, (7) level of hopelessness, (8) level of helplessness, and (9) psychological aftermath of the self-harming incident.

The relationship between suicidal behavior and NSSI is nuanced and complex, and one is often mistaken for the other (Miller & Brock, 2010). Students who engage in NSSI are at increased risk for a variety of suicidal behaviors, including suicidal ideation and suicide attempts as well as suicide (Jacobson & Gould, 2007). Individuals who engage in NSSI are more likely to attempt suicide if they report being repulsed by life, are highly self-critical and apathetic, have fewer connections to family, and show less fear about suicide in comparison to their peers who do not engage in self-injury (Muehlenkamp & Gutierrez, 2004, 2007). Further, individuals are at increased risk for suicide if they engage in NSSI to escape or avoid highly unpleasant and distressful emotions (Miller & Brock, 2010).

Joiner (2005, 2009) has suggested that engaging in repeated NSSI may serve as "practice" for other potentially lethal behaviors, such as suicide by desensitizing oneself to pain and violence through habituation. There is also evidence suggesting that adolescents who engage in both NSSI and suicide attempts are more impaired than those who do either one or the other (Jacobson & Gould, 2007). Individuals who engage in NSSI may also be more likely to become suicidal if and when their self-injury stops working as an effective emotional regulation technique (Walsh, 2012).

Despite their considerable overlap, research suggests that suicidal behavior and NSSI are two different types of problems with different etiologies (Miller, 2011). Making an accurate distinction between suicidal behavior and NSSI is critical, because despite some similarities in appearance, they serve different functions. Specifically, the individual engaging in suicidal behavior is contemplating or attempting to end all feelings, whereas the individual engaging in NSSI is typically trying to feel better (Miller & Brock, 2010). Consequently, students who engage in NSSI typically do it as a morbid, although often effective, form of coping and self-help (Walsh, 2012).

> **The individual engaging in suicidal behavior is attempting to end all feelings, whereas the individual engaging in NSSI is typically trying to feel better.**

Because youth who engage in NSSI are often secretive and reluctant to refer themselves for treatment, identification and assessment of these individuals can be difficult. This problem is further complicated by the lack of standardized assessment instruments for NSSI (Miller & Brock, 2010). If a youth is suspected of engaging in self-injury, a comprehensive assessment should include both direct observations/examinations (e.g., checking for cuts or burn marks and the presence of unusually heavy or unseasonable clothing designed to mask scars) and individual interviews with the youth, parents/caregivers, and school personnel. When interviewing the youth, school-based mental health practitioners should directly ask the youngster if he/she is engaging in self-injury (e.g., "Some kids cut themselves, not because they want to die, but maybe because the cutting makes them feel better in some way. Have you ever done that?"). If a youth reports engaging in NSSI, an assessment of possible suicide risk should be conducted as well. Other areas should also be assessed, including the following: (1) degree of anger and its expression; (2) degree of self-esteem or self-concept; (3) history of abuse, particularly, sexual abuse; (4) possible cognitive distortions; and (5) family tolerance for expression of feelings (Favazza, 1999).

Additionally, events that precipitate and follow acts of NSSI should be assessed, including determining where it occurs as well as the cognitive and behavioral goals, benefits, and consequences of it (Walsh, 2012). Conducting a functional behavioral assessment (FBA) can be useful for linking assessment to intervention. An FBA involves gathering information about antecedent conditions, behaviors, and consequences of the behaviors to determine the reason or function of NSSI. For example, the function of NSSI for one individual might be escape (e.g., releasing mounting anxiety and unbearable tension), whereas for another individual it might be attention (e.g., a teenage girl who cuts herself to receive attention from a boyfriend). Identical behaviors (e.g., skin cutting) may serve different functions for different individuals and will therefore require different interventions (Miller & Brock, 2010). Walsh (2006) describes a functional approach to NSSI that expands upon the assessment of environmental variables to incorporate the assessment of cognitive and emotional states.

When NSSI is suspected, assessment may need to include a multidisciplinary approach. For example, although a school psychologist or counselor may be involved in interviewing the youth and other adults in the youth's environment, a school nurse may be needed to conduct a physical inspection of the youth in question, particularly if the possible injury is not immediately visible.

Interventions for Youth Who Engage in NSSI

If it has been clearly established that a youth engages in NSSI, his/her parents should be contacted. As with suicidal behavior, school personnel may not be directly involved in treatment, but they can provide support by making appropriate referrals and securing assistance from others. Unfortunately, little information is currently available on effective treatments for youth who engage in NSSI. A form of cognitive-behavioral therapy known as dialectical behavior therapy (DBT) has shown some promise. DBT emphasizes two fundamental and related treatment concepts: acceptance and mindfulness. It was originally developed for use with individuals with borderline personality disorder (Linehan, 1993), and more recently has shown to be potentially useful with suicidal adolescents (Miller, Rathus, & Linehan, 2007). DBT focuses on treating faulty problem-solving behaviors, low distress tolerance, and inadequate coping skills (Walsh, 2012). Cognitive-behavioral procedures such as DBT may also be combined with psychopharmacological interventions.

Treatment of youth who engage in NSSI can often be difficult and requires a high level of commitment and skill on the part of treatment providers. For more information on assessing and treating NSSI in schools, the reader is referred to Miller and Brock (2010).

ENHANCING PROFESSIONAL SKILLS IN SUICIDE RISK ASSESSMENT

An extensive discussion of the many complexities and nuances of effective suicide risk assessment is beyond the scope of this chapter. Readers interested in enhancing their professional skills in this area are encouraged to review other resources, including Rudd's (2006) suicide risk assessment system, the Chronological Assessment of Suicide Events (Shea, 2002), the Collaborative Assessment and Management of Suicidality (CAMS; Jobes, 2006), and the Suicide Risk Assessment Decision Tree (Joiner et al., 2009). Although these models of suicide risk assessment were not developed specifically for use with children and adolescents, they can be effectively used with them in school settings. For more information on school-based suicide prevention generally, including assessment issues, see my previous publication (Miller, 2011).

SUMMARY

Assessing youth at risk for suicidal behavior is one of the most anxiety-inducing but often necessary tasks for school-based mental health professionals. Given the critical importance of this problem and its lethal potential, it is imperative that school practitioners acquire the necessary knowledge, ability, and confidence to conduct effective suicide risk assessments. School-based mental health professionals are encouraged to participate in ongoing training and professional development activities to continually update and enhance their skills in this unique and specialized form of assessment.

Student Interview for Suicide Risk Screening (SISRS)

Child's name _____
First   Middle   Last

Child's date of birth ___/___/___ Age _____ Gender _____ Grade _____
Month Day Year

Interviewer's name _____ Date ___/___/_____
Month Day Year

Engagement

It seems things haven't been going so well for you lately. Your parents and/or teachers have said _____. Most teens/children would find that upsetting.

Have you felt upset, maybe had some sad or angry feelings you've had trouble talking about? Maybe I could help you talk about these feelings and thoughts?

Do you feel like things can get better, or are you worried (afraid, concerned) things will just stay the same or get worse?

Are you feeling unhappy most of the time?

Identification

Other teenagers/children I've talked with have said that when they feel sad and/or angry, they thought for a while that things would be better if they were dead. Have you ever thought that?

Is this feeling of unhappiness so strong that sometimes you wish you were dead?

Do you sometimes feel that you want to take your own life?

How often have you had these thoughts?

(continued)

Inquiry

What has made you feel so awful?

What problems/situations have led you to think this way?

Tell me more about what has led you to see killing yourself as a solution.

What do you think it would feel like to be dead?

How do you think your father and mother feel? What do you think would happen to them if you were dead?

Assessment

A. Current Suicide Plan

Have you thought about how you might make yourself die?

Do you have a plan?

On a scale of 1–10, how likely is it that you will kill yourself? When are you planning to, or when do you think you will do this?

Do you have the means with you now, at school or at home?

Where are you planning to kill yourself?

Have you written a note?

Have you put things in order?

(continued)

B. Prior Behavior

Has anyone that you know of killed or attempted to kill him/herself? Do you know why?

Have you ever threatened to kill yourself before? When? What stopped you?

Have you ever tried to kill yourself before? How did you attempt to do so?

C. Resources

Is there anyone or anything that would stop you?

Is there someone to whom you can talk about these feelings?

Have you or can you talk to your family or friends about your feelings of suicide?

Summary:

CHAPTER 10

Assessing Youth Violence and Threats of Violence in Schools

School-Based Risk Assessments

William Halikias

Concerns about youth violence and other forms of aggression remain a pressing problem for schools, communities, and society in general (Borum 2003; Gellman & Delucia-Waack, 2006; Roberts, Zhang, & Truman, 2010). Professionals called upon to conduct assessments of a youth's potential for violence confront many interesting and difficult challenges, including how best to collect, synthesize, understand, and communicate this information in ways that assist the youngster and the community with safety concerns. School shootings resulting in the violent deaths of students and adults have received tremendous media attention and public scrutiny, and have altered perceptions about the presumed threat that children pose to others (Elliott, Hamburg, & Williams, 1998; Ryan-Arredondo et al., 2001). (For brevity, the word *child* in this chapter includes adolescents in middle school and high school.) Reports about terrorist acts and workplace killings helped to reinforce concerns about school safety. For professionals consulting to schools over the past decade, a culture change has been evident in the increased scrutiny given to people entering these buildings along with the presence of police and safety officers, and, in some instances, the use of metal detec-

William Halikias, PsyD, is a forensic and clinical psychologist whose practice includes supervision of mental health professionals, schools, and social services agencies. As a licensed psychologist and board-certified diplomate for the American Board of Assessment Psychology, he consults with human service organizations and conducts evaluations in Massachusetts, New Hampshire, and Vermont. He has taught advanced doctoral-level seminars in psychology and the law, child and family psychology, and advanced psychological assessment. His articles about children and the law and psychological evaluations appear in law and psychology journals. His research interests include development of scientist-practitioner models of psychological assessment and consultation.

A previous version of this chapter appeared in Halikias (2004). Copyright 2004 by the American Psychological Association. Adapted by permission.

tors (Gellman & Delucia-Waack, 2006). Clinicians who work in or with schools have also witnessed an increase in the number of children referred for risk-of-violence assessments.

Compared with other school-based evaluations, the school-based risk assessment (SBRA) is one of the most challenging assessment venues. Questions about a child's potential for violence pose an array of complex predicaments that go to the heart of the assessment enterprise, including dilemmas associated with the prediction of future behavior. Of no small consequence to the child and his/her family, SBRAs help decide whether some children remain part of a school community or lose that right. Although many elements of the SBRA appear consistent with a forensic psychology practice, this chapter addresses all practitioners who work in or with educational institutions, including school, clinical, and counseling psychologists.

The SBRA model described in this chapter emanates from a scientist-practitioner orientation (Stricker & Trierweiler, 1995; Stricker, 2002) and draws heavily from a pragmatic philosophy (Fishman, 1999; Rorty, 1982). Pragmatic psychology attempts to integrate historically opposing camps of positivism—the belief that all germane knowledge falls within the bounds of science—and the idiographic and narrative traditions of naturalistic, case-driven, qualitative inquiry. The scientist-practitioner model also seeks to integrate science with the local culture. The scientist-practitioner model and pragmatic psychology help to shape the philosophy of the SBRA toward solution-focused and case management strategies to prevent school violence.

SOCIAL CONTEXT OF RISK ASSESSMENTS

The increased call for SBRAs is part of a shift in societal attitudes toward juvenile offenders. Over the past 25 years there has been a movement away from protection and rehabilitation of wayward youth toward punishment and retribution (Halikias, 2000). This movement followed dramatic increases in juvenile crime between 1980 and 1994 (Dahlberg, 1998). The shift from rehabilitation to retribution with juveniles was also fueled by retrospective studies of adult criminals with an early offending profile (e.g., Farrington et al., 1990; Piquero & Buka, 2002). Researchers and media commentators voiced alarm about a seeming plague of child and adolescent "super predators," and state legislators reacted by enacting increasingly punitive measures for young lawbreakers (Dodge, 2008). These factors combined to undermine the juvenile court's earlier philosophy of therapeutic jurisprudence. However, juvenile crime has historically fluctuated, rising or falling without evident causes. Nevertheless, public and media attention galvanized on the notion that serious child and adolescent law breaking was legion.

Although school shootings remain relatively rare events, the vivid nature of such crimes influences people to overestimate the chance that such events will occur again. For each incident of a school shooting, the public has experienced repeated exposure to emotional and graphic images of its perpetrators and victims. However, the chance that a person will be murdered at school is less than 1 in a million (U.S. Department of Education & U.S. Department of Justice, 1999).

> **Despite much media attention, school shootings are rare events. The chance that a person will be murdered at school is less than 1 in a million.**

On the other hand, and less dramatic than homicides, aggression, and exposure to violence and victimization are pervasive problems in schools. For example, between July 2008 and June 2009, 24 homicides occurred in schools, while, in 2008, about 1.2 million children, ages 12–18, were victims of nonfatal crimes in schools, including theft, assault, and being threatened or injured with a weapon (Roberts et al., 2010). Thus, clinicians performing SBRAs see an array of aggressive behavior short of mass murder, including peer aggression, bullying (physical and relational), intimidation, and sexual harassment.

Shootings and more common forms of violence in schools can be difficult to predict, and profiling formulas have proven an ineffective way to weed out violent students (American Psychological Association, 1993; Sewell & Mendelsohn, 2000). Consider in this regard the base rate problem of violence forecasting. One rule of Bayes's theorem—a formula that calculates probabilities—is that predictive accuracy increases as the base rate approaches 50% (Kamphuis & Finn, 2002). But the base rate for violence in the general population is quite low. Thus, predicting that all children referred for SBRAs, even those who bring a weapon to school, will not act violently would result in a high accuracy rate but miss the few who will act violently. If 50 people in 1,000 will be violent, the evaluator could predict the null hypothesis—that nobody will be violent—and achieve a 95% accuracy rate. On the other hand, predicting that every child referred for an SBRA will engage in violence would produce a very high and unacceptable false-positive rate. Furthermore, risk assessments with youth involve additional error because of maturation factors: Children's movement through developmental stages makes it harder to chart their future (Dodge & Pettit, 2003). Because of the difficulties in predicting school violence, some have criticized risk-for-violence assessments in schools because of their unacceptably high false-positive rates and their potential to stigmatize students (Mulvey & Cauffman, 2001; National Association of School Psychologists, 2008).

DANGEROUSNESS VERSUS THREATS OF VIOLENCE

Acts of violence take many forms, and aggression exists along a continuum. Interpersonal violence can involve physical aggression that results in bodily harm or, in the case of school shootings, homicide. However, violence in schools more often takes the form of physical attacks or fights, property crimes, verbal harassment, intimidation, bullying, or sexual harassment. Although school shootings and murders in schools are rare events, an alarming proportion of children are victims of other crimes at school (Fitzpatrick, 1999; Roberts et al., 2010) and the rate of school violence is regarded by some as a public health hazard (Gellman & Delucia-Waack, 2006).

One potentially confounding element of SBRAs is distinguishing between *dangerousness* versus *targeted violence* when accepting referrals and conducting evaluations. School shootings fall into the category of targeted violence because these were planned acts of violence with identified targets (Borum, Fein, Vossekuil, & Berglund, 1999). However, many students referred for SBRAs are more suited for dangerousness assessments. These individuals have problems with excessive anger and chronic or intermittent aggression. Many have emotional or conduct problems. The dangerousness assessment considers the risk that a person with a history of aggression will behave that way in the future, whereas a targeted violence or threat assessment focuses more on individuals without a history of aggression but who have made verbal threats or communicated a plan to injure an individual or a group.

> It is important to distinguish between "dangerousness" (history of excessive anger and aggressive behavior) versus "targeted violence" (carefully planning a violent attack against an individual or group).

Children referred for dangerousness evaluations fit the literature on violent juveniles. An important consideration for these youngsters is whether their transgressions occur at a specific phase of development or in a specific context, or whether their behavior is more ongoing and trait-like. Research has shown a strong association between high-frequency offending and the increased likelihood of persistent antisocial acts (Loeber, Farrington, & Waschbusch, 1998; Tremblay et al., 1999). Conduct problems that begin early in childhood appear to be more invariable than those that begin in adolescence (Frick, 2004; Lahey & Loeber, 1994; Moffitt et al., 2008). It seems that some children progress through a series of behaviors that increase or decrease their chances of developing and sustaining chronic criminal behavior (Halikias, 2000; Patterson, Forgatch, Yoerger, & Stoolmiller, 1998). Comorbid factors, including hyperactivity combined with conduct problems (Lahey, Loeber, Burke, Rathouz, & McBurnett, 2002; Lynam, 1996) or low socioeconomic status and conduct problems (Nagin & Tremblay, 2001; National Survey on Drug Use and Health, 2010), exert a compelling influence on the stability of aggression.

The second class of individuals referred for risk-for-violence assessments are best conceptualized as falling within the targeted violence or threat assessment protocol. The threat assessment model was derived from work of the United States Secret Service (USSS) of the Department of the Treasury, an agency whose mandate includes protecting national leaders, candidates, and visiting heads of state from assassination and assassination attempts (Borum et al., 1999; Fein & Vossekuil, 1999). This model focuses on individuals who select a target and plan violent acts. The USSS data base, called the Exceptional Case Study Project (ECSP), helped define targeted violence protocols. The ECSP was a study of people who planned and carried out an attack or near-attack on a prominent person in the United States since 1949 (Fein & Vossekuil, 1998). The ECSP used a pragmatic and case-centered approach to delineate the attacker's history, motivation, thoughts, and behavior before the attack or attempted attack. This same strategy was then applied to targeted violence in schools under the heading of the Safe School Initiative (SSI; Fein et al., 2002; Vossekuil et al., 2002). Since that time, the pragmatic and case-centered approach to targeted violence has become well established (Hoffmann, Meloy, Guldimann, & Ermer, 2011; Meloy, 2004).

The SSI case studies provided practitioners with valuable information about the behavior, thinking, and motives of youngsters who engaged in targeted violence in schools. The data base included 37 school shootings and 41 attackers, ages 11–21, since 1974. All of the subjects were male and all were current students or recent students at the school. The sample showed a mix of racial, ethnic, and sociocultural backgrounds, with 75% White. Behavioral histories ranged from few or no known problems to multiple problems. Few of the attackers had been diagnosed with a mental disorder, and a minority had a known history of substance use or abuse. However, all had deliberate attack plans, often formulated several weeks before the incident. The most frequently used weapons were handguns, rifles, and shotguns. As a group, the attackers knew how to use guns and had access to weapons, usually from home. Most reported that they felt persecuted or bullied. Some experienced a loss or other life crisis prior to the attack. They often voiced thoughts about the attack to a peer, but rarely to the intended target(s). Many performed acts that, in retrospect, produced suspicion: verbal or written statements, drawings about killing and death, or attempts to obtain weapons. As an example, Vossekuil, et al. (2002) cited a case in which a boy frightened peers by telling them that he put rat poison in the cheese shakers at a local restaurant.

For the targeted violence group, planning the attack became an important source of their identity. The plan evolved over time: Getting the idea, thinking about it, maybe telling another person seriously or in jest, practicing or rehearsing, and then executing or trying to execute the attack. Like the ECSP sample, school shooters did not act on a political ideology but had more diverse motives, including gaining notoriety, bringing attention to a grievance, and sometimes creating an elaborate justification for their anticipated death. In short, the attack plan gave them a perceived solution to a seemingly irresolvable conflict.

Although in practice it is sometimes hard to distinguish dangerousness from threat assessments, an example of the former is an assessment of a child who impulsively injured one or more individuals at school. In this hypothetical case, the student had a history of aggression and other conduct problems, became frustrated, and retaliated. Students and staff were not surprised that the student committed the act. Given the history of problematic behavior, this situation conforms to the dangerousness model of assessment. In the threat assessment model, the various school shooting incidents serve as a prototype. In these acts, motivated youngsters across the country had the wherewithal to carefully plan and effectively carry out assaults. Many times these students lacked a well-documented history of violence, school discipline problems, or mental illness.

PREREQUISITES FOR SCHOOL-BASED RISK ASSESSMENTS

As discussed, predicting school violence—and violence, in general—is an inherently problematic undertaking. Practitioners should avoid a false sense of certainty about their ability to make accurate predictions in these matters, and instead adopt a case-centered and risk management philosophy. A good SBRA is discovery driven and inductive; it tries to individualize the reasons that a child came to the evaluation, and it considers the interventions that might decrease a child's willingness to commit violent acts.

Practitioners who conduct SBRAs should have training and expertise in clinical child psychology (Jackson, Alberts, & Roberts 2010), theories of development (Sameroff, 2010), and adolescence (Smetana, Campione-Barr, & Metzger, 2006; Steinberg & Morris, 2001). They must know how to conduct interviews with children and parents, be skilled in intervention and consultation strategies, have knowledge of educational and support systems affecting children and families and be fluent in the ethical and legal issues surrounding minors. Without this training and experience, adult-oriented practitioners lack the requisite "boundaries of competence" to perform SBRAs (American Psychological Association, 2002, p. 1063).

> **Practitioners who conduct SBRAs must have training in clinical child psychology and be knowledgeable of relevant ethical and legal requirements.**

SBRAs also require knowledge of the ethical dilemmas involved in coerced evaluations (Committee on Ethical Guidelines for Forensic Psychologists, 1991; Foote & Shuman 2006). In the SBRA, parents have the option of denying consent for the evaluation. However, this refusal to consent might result in their child facing such consequences as restricted access to school, placement in alternative educational settings, or possibly expulsion from the school.

Practitioners who conduct SBRAs must understand the legal requirements covering regular versus special education students. For example, students in special education cannot be deprived of an education due to behavior that is directly related to their disability, even if those actions constitute a risk to others (Katsiyannis & Smith, 2003). Under the requirements of the Individuals with Disabilities Education Act (IDEA; 2004), the SBRA may be considered a "manifestation determination" (Turnbull, 2005). A *manifestation determination* is an inquiry into whether a student's disability had a relationship to the problematic behavior, or if the disability impaired or diminished the student's sense of consequences for his/her actions. The evaluation might also occur as part of an FBA. Whereas the manifestation determination explores the relationship between a disability and a behavior, the FBA identifies techniques to manage problematic behaviors (Knoster, 2000; Smith, 2005).

When a special education student has been suspended or otherwise excluded from school, IDEA 2004 prohibits the exclusion from exceeding 10 days, by which time the school must allow the student to reenter school or provide some alternative program with the requisite special instruction (Smith, 2005). When working with special education students around issues concerning their violence potential, the SBRA often needs to be completed in a timely manner.

CORE QUESTIONS
INFORMING THE SCHOOL-BASED RISK ASSESSMENT

Practitioners conducting SBRAs need to focus on several critical areas of inquiry. These questions help shape procedures and data collection methods and are crucial to ultimately formulating and communicating a child's level of risk. When conducing an SBRA, the evaluator should avoid relying on dichotomous distinctions (e.g., *violent* vs. *not violent*) and diagnostic labels (e.g., *conduct disorder*). Instead, the goal is to understand and communicate the factors that brought the child to the evaluation and to offer "thick" rather than "thin" descriptions of the their status (Fishman, 1999). A thick formulation is essentially a narrative that describes individuals, including their ways of constructing meaning, their human interactions, and their context. Thin descriptions tend to be summaries, abstractions, or diagnostic labels that try to group people based on presumed shared traits or features. Appendix 10.1 provides a reproducible worksheet with core questions to guide the practitioner in conducting SBRAs (Halikias, 2004).

The use of core questions in SBRAs follows recent trends in assessment psychology called *structured professional judgment* (SPJ; Borum, 2000; Douglas, Cox, & Webster, 1999) that evolved from risk assessment research and assessment protocols. Beginning with Monahan's (1981) research, studies surrounding violence prediction passed through what some described as three generations (Borum, Bartel, & Forth, 2006). In the first generation, practitioners relied on clinical judgment and tended to believe that violence was dispositional or a stable personality trait within an individual. The second generation relied on actuarial methods and empirically derived formulas. The first generation was notoriously unreliable, with predictive accuracy rates hovering around 20–35% (Monahan & Steadman, 2001). The statistical equation methods of the second generation proved more accurate, but had limited generalizability and did not translate well into different referral populations, age groups, and contexts (Borum et al., 1999). SPJ evolved in the third generation as an attempt to reconcile clinical and actuarial methods. Essentially, SPJ methods and instruments focus on salient variables that are empirically or rationally connected to the identification of risk. SPJ imposes a structure on the professional's judgments that helps ensure the inclusion of risk-relevant inquiries and discovery of salient information. The research into the effectiveness and utility of SPJs has produced good

> **Core questions in SBRAs follow the assessment model of structured professional judgment (SPJ): identifying salient risk-for-violence factors and developing appropriate case management strategies.**

results, and the methodology has been applied to a number of risk and case management assessment instruments (McGowan, Horn, & Mellott, 2011).

Core questions for SBRAs concern salient risk for violence factors or address case management strategies. For example, a history of aggression or the presence of a mental illness represents important information about a child's status, the child's potential to act in destructive ways, and the type or intensity of services that may be required. By the end of the assessment, evaluators should be able to answer each question or to designate the question as nonapplicable to a particular child. Answering these questions provides a foundation for conducting a feedback conference with school staff, the child, and parents at the end of the SBRA or writing the report. Information derived from these questions should be used to develop risk-reduction strategies and case management recommendations.

CHARACTERISTICS OF CHILDREN REFERRED FOR SCHOOL-BASED RISK ASSESSMENTS

Children referred for SBRAs comprise a heterogeneous group. In thinking about these youngsters, it is useful to consider the links between the seriousness of the precipitating event, their motivation, and the intensity of case management requirements. Grouping students into risk categories based on motives and actions captures the diversity among students seen in SBRAs. Appendix 10.2 provides a reproducible worksheet for assigning referred students to one or more of five broad groups, according to risk status and case management requirements (Halikias, 2004). Each group is summarized below. Names and details of the case vignettes have been created or altered to protect confidentiality.

> In conducting SBRAs, it is useful to categorize referred students into risk status groups based on their motives, actions, and case management requirements.

Group A (low risk) children come to the SBRA with little or no history of psychological problems, but have done something that violated the school climate or confronted a zero tolerance policy. This may include a child who brought a plastic gun to school or who forgot that he/she had a penknife in his/her backpack. Such children generally require a brief and focused assessment and may benefit from low-intensity interventions, such as a conference with the child, a restitution plan, or apology letter. They generally pose little risk for violence and require the least comprehensive and costly assessment and case management plans.

Children in Group B (low to medium risk) are generally nonviolent students who engaged in a thoughtless and sometimes accidental act that worried others. John, a passive and developmentally delayed 14-year-old, should not have watched a horror flick—the movie scared and stimulated him. The combination of poor judgment and confusion about pronouns found him telling a peer how he killed people. The student reported John's statements to the principal. Group B children, such as John, benefit from direction and support and, like Group A children, need less intensive case management plans. This group may benefit from a behavior contract and/or short-term counseling for problem solving.

Children in Group C (medium risk) may or may not come to the SBRA with a history of psychological problems. For them, the critical incident is often a distress signal that reflects inept problem solving. When Frank transferred to the school, students and teachers noticed that he came to classes dressed in military clothing and made references to guns. An isolated and socially awkward teenager, Frank created elaborate and obviously fanciful stories about his exploits, including telling people that he was a Special Operations soldier assigned to that school. His comportment and stories made him the object of ridicule among some students. Once, after being taunted for telling a tall tale, Frank told the student to "watch your back" because he was going home to get his M-16 rifle. Previous inquiry had indicated that Frank's family owned no firearms and that Frank had no experience with the military or guns. A teacher overheard Frank's statement and reported it to the principal.

A developmental crisis or failure often explains Group C students' behavior and their motivation for engaging in threatening actions. These students profit from focused case management interventions to ameliorate the crisis and their inept problem-solving attempts. Interventions might focus on addressing degrading aspects of a school climate (Brookmeyer, Fanti, & Henrich, 2006) as well as improving the student's problem-solving skills, anger management, and/or status and self-esteem.

Children in Group D (high risk—specific target) best reflect the subjects from the SSI study. They may or may not come to the evaluation with a known history of social–emotional and/or conduct problems. The hallmark of this group is their ongoing interest in injuring or having unwelcome contact with a target. This group also includes children with obsessional fixations and possible delusions about a fantasized attachment figure (Evans & Meloy, 2011). However, the most worrisome behavior is the development of an attack plan. Group D students may spend considerable time thinking about and rehearsing an attack. The perceived enormity of this mission lends a sense of purpose to their life. They often conceive the plan because they have experienced a distressing loss, life change, grievance, or harassment, or have suicidal thoughts and feelings (Meloy et al., 2004). Vossekuil et al. (2002) reported that in the SSI sample, almost 75% of the students had previously threatened to kill themselves, made a suicidal gesture, or tried to commit suicide.

Few students carry out a calculated attack at school, and one would not know how many students in this category actually get referred for evaluations—few in the SSI sample had been previously assessed—or how many change their plans because of the attention they received from an evaluation. Assigning a child to Group D requires credible information about an attack plan and method. When these students get referred to the SBRA, it is usually because they told somebody or did something that brought them to the attention of school authorities.

Richard, age 17, was a small boy who was targeted as effeminate by a group of students at his high school. He also struggled with juvenile diabetes and ongoing grief about the death of his father 2 years ago. Richard called the students who persecuted him "the jocks" and reported incidents that by most standards constituted severe bullying and harassment. This maltreatment began in his freshman year. In his junior year, Richard's tormentors pasted a photograph of his head onto the photograph of a young girl wearing underwear and then sent it in a text message to students in the school. Richard and his mother went to the principal and complained about harassment, but the principal took no action. Richard became increasingly depressed and his grades dropped. He no longer made the honor roll, an important prior source of self-esteem. He began thinking about suicide, at first tentatively, then with increasing commitment to the idea. His deceased father's handgun was in the home and the father had taught him how to use it. Richard set a date for his suicide and wrote a note, which his mother discovered. He had three sessions with a therapist and denied serious thoughts of killing himself. Richard's mother believed the crisis had past. However, he began thinking about shooting his tormentors before killing himself. This fantasy gave him a sense of mission that temporarily improved his feelings of helplessness and depression. He planned the attack for several months. Richard still had access to his father's handgun and ammunition. He planned to carry out the attack at the high school baseball game scheduled in the spring, an event he knew included most of the students he considered tormentors. He rehearsed the attack in his mind, then on paper, and then finally on the baseball field, where he "walked through the motions" of the attack. He aroused suspicion when he took photographs of the baseball field. Fortunately, a teacher discovered Richard's written plans for the attack in his desk. The teacher took the plans to the principal, who then requested an SBRA.

When information suggests that a student falls within Group D, school staff and/or the evaluator must consider alerting law enforcement officials. At this point, the practitioner conducting the SBRA takes a back seat to professionals with authority and training to conduct searches of person and place. Group D students require careful case management plans that address their motivation for violence and teach them alternative problem-solving strategies, along with restricted access to weapons and increased adult supervision.

A subset within Group D would be the "violent true believer" (Meloy, 2004), for whom a combination of homicidal and suicidal desires merge into an ideology or other strongly held conviction. The attack plan of the violent true believer would be labeled *terrorist*. A prototype is Timothy McVeigh, who bombed the Alfred P. Murrah Federal Building in Oklahoma City on April 19, 1995. At this time, there are no reports of a young person in the United States whose ideology formed an underlying motive for targeting a school and carrying out such a horrific and complex attack.

The classification of Group E (high risk—chronic aggression) moves into the realm of chronic violent behavior and impaired impulse control. Groups D and E are similar in that children in both categories are capable of violence. However, the risk for children in Group D is calculated, future oriented, and usually target specific. Children in Group E, by contrast, have a known history of conduct problems. For them, the critical incident is part of a larger pattern of inept and aggressive coping strategies. A discipline, special education, or mental health file often accompanies these children to the evaluation. Following the critical incident, they may find themselves in juvenile court as well as referred for the SBRA. They often require significant case management interventions and sometimes alternative education programs.

Sam, age 18, had been identified in second grade as having an "emotional disturbance" and a language-based learning disability. There was a family history of domestic violence and substance abuse. A child protection agency had removed Sam from the home when he was 11 years old, after his mother's boyfriend had attacked him and broken his arm. Sam was reportedly sexually abused by a foster father while in child protective custody. He received intensive special education and behavioral support from elementary to high school. He had a lengthy high school discipline file, including suspensions for fights, insubordination, and intimidation of students and faculty. He experienced two arrests: one for stealing, the other for an assault on a student at school. In his senior year Sam heard that a teacher had spoken negatively about him to his girlfriend. He was suspended after he told the teacher that he would slap her face if she ever "dissed" him again. At the time of the suspension, Sam was overheard saying that he would bring a gun to school and shoot the teacher.

A subset of Group E students display temperamental traits associated with predatory or instrumental aggression. Impulse control deficits and conduct problems often co-occur in this group (Lynam, 1996), along with a seeming absence of remorse for violating the rights of others. These children also lack empathy and use others for personal gain—behaviors that have been described as "callous-unemotional traits" (Frick et al., 2003; Kerig & Stellwagen, 2010). Sometimes these children are described as having "juvenile psychopathy," although this label is controversial (Seagrave & Grisso, 2002). However, males with an early and sustained history of aggression stand a high chance of becoming life-persistent offenders (Loeber et al., 1998; Broidy et al., 2003). Therefore, practitioners conducting SBRAs should recognize that an early-childhood-onset history of conduct problems portends less likelihood of remission without appropriate interventions.

SCHOOL-BASED RISK ASSESSMENT PROTOCOL AND FORMAT

The SBRA is an organized and deliberate protocol with specific questions, goals, and criteria. It contains several "gates" or "assessment stations" designed to assess risk for violence. This SBRA model is based on a prevention approach, not a predictive one. It is intended to provide relevant recommendations and case management strategies to reduce a student's risk for destructive behavior. The SBRA can be divided into seven stages, each with its own tasks and challenges: referral; review and organization of

> **The goal of SBRA is preventive: to provide recommendations and case management strategies to reduce a child's risk for destructive behavior.**

records; parental interview; collateral interviews; clinical interview of the child; psychological tests and checklists; and case formulation, findings, and recommendations. Each of these stages is discussed below.

Referral for a School-Based Risk Assessment

The SBRA begins when a school official makes the referral. The first task is to establish the nature and scope of the evaluation and the evaluator's ability to access corroborating information. An SBRA always involves scrutiny of the critical incident, a review of files, an interview with parents and collateral sources, and interviews with the child. If, at the referral stage, the evaluator determines that the school is unable to provide access to this information—for example, the school wants the evaluator only to interview the student—the information derived from the SBRA will be seriously compromised.

Schools seek SBRAs to ensure that a student is not dangerous or a threat to others. Sometimes the precipitating incident is worrisome (Group D or E); other times the critical incident may sound less troublesome (Group A or B). For example, a child who assaulted a teacher shows greater risk and elicits more concern than a child who drew a picture of a child with a gun. It is important to determine at the start of the assessment whether a child comes to the evaluation with a history of dangerous and aggressive behavior or has engaged in a relatively discrete act. It is also important to determine whether the child is so overwhelmed that immediate danger to self or other must be assessed. In the latter case, the evaluation should be considered a crisis intervention (Catenaccio, 1995; Newgass & Schonfeld, 2000), and the child should be referred to a crisis team or an organization that specializes in assessing imminent danger to self or others.

Given the ethical issues and the risk of professional conduct complaints in SBRAs and other coerced evaluations, practitioners who conduct such evaluations must carefully document their work (Committee on Ethical Guidelines for Forensic Psychologists, 1991; Drogin, Connell, Foote, & Sturm, 2010). This documentation begins at the referral stage when the practitioner obtains—or collaborates with staff to generate—a letter from the referral source requesting the evaluation, identifying its purpose, and specifying questions.

The evaluator must provide the student and his/her parents with an informed consent document that contains the terms, procedures, goals, possible outcomes, and limits of confidentiality for the evaluation (Foote & Shuman, 2006; Heilbrun, Marczyk, & Goldstein, 2008). Appendix 10.3 provides an example of an informed consent form. School-based practitioners will probably have to modify the usual evaluation consent form to apprise parents about the distinct nature of the SBRA. When the evaluation takes place as part of a special education process, manifestation determination, or FBA, the focus on violence risk assessment should be clearly identified. Then the evaluator should carefully go over the purposes and scope of the evaluation with the parents at or before the first meeting, answering questions and respectfully addressing their concerns and potential distress about the process.

Documents Related to the Critical Incident and Other Records

Early in the SBRA process, and before conducting interviews, evaluators should review the student's records. The most important of these are documents describing the critical incident that provoked the SBRA. For example, examine written threats and integrate these into clinical interviews with the student and others. Review any school-generated reports, such as a discipline file entry, about the critical incident. Also review the student's academic file, discipline history, and, if they exist, special education and mental health records. Special education or mental health records may contain crucial information for understanding a student's actions and formulating case management strategies.

In the SBRA, it is important to distinguish between *making* a threat and *posing* a threat (Borum et al., 1999; Reddy et al., 2001). Many people make threats but are not violent or dangerous; others, who *are* dangerous, do not make threats. A person who poses a threat usually displays behavior that suggests an underlying motive to damage a target. In cases of credible threats, the would-be attacker often leaves a trail of goal-directed acts. For example, in order to accomplish a serious attack a person must know details about a target, have access to and skill with specific weapons, avoid detection, consider possible escape routes, and manage security apparatus or personnel. In other words, a matrix of discrete thoughts and behaviors is necessary to accomplish an act as complex as a planned attack.

> It is important to distinguish between *making* and *posing* a threat. A person who poses a threat leaves a trail of goal-directed acts to damage a person.

The student's records may be extensive or relatively brief. In either case, the first step is to organize the history from this file. One approach is to replicate the record chronologically, creating an abstract or excerpts from it. In organizing the various documents by dates and content, a chronological history will emerge that will aid in understanding the child and assist with interviews and interpretations of findings. The next step is to cross-check and verify information. The organization of the file can be augmented later by interviews with collateral sources, parents, and the youth. Information from two or more sources is more credible than data from only one source. At the end of the assessment, the evaluator should have gathered sufficient information from multiple sources from which to seek convergent findings and to distinguish salient from rarefied data.

Interviews with Parents

The parental or caretaker interview is a critical aspect of the SBRA. Because of the power dynamics of an SBRA, it is important to speak to parents early in this process. Often parents are upset, resent the school's demands, and/or view the decision to have their child evaluated as capricious. To address these reactions, assure parents that they play a critical role in the evaluation and that their views are respected, and later try to elicit their cooperation with subsequent recommendations. Avoid acting judgmental about the alleged critical incident or the parents' distress about the evaluation. Remaining nonjudgmental increases the chances of joining with parents and collaborating on solutions to their child's problems. Ethical principles such as beneficence, responsibility, fairness, and respect also apply to interviews with parents (American Psychological Association, 2002). In addition, parents are stakeholders in the SBRA, even if they are not the identified client. The multiple constituents in the SBRA (school, child, parents) are not unlike multiple parties involved in other types of forensic evaluations (Halikias, 1994).

Appendix 10.4 provides a general outline of steps and questions for interviewing parents and children in the SBRA. After obtaining informed consent from parents, begin by addressing the critical incident and their understanding of the child's reported intimidating behavior. This phase involves reviewing details of the child's actions, reports about the incident, and the parents' understanding of the context that led to the child's actions. Also ask parents about the child's mental health and his/her developmental and social history, including any history of child abuse or other trauma, an impulse control disorder, a mood or thought disorder, and cognitive limitations.

Evaluators should then review with parents the core "risk-relevant" questions of the SBRA (Appendix 10.4, Section 6). These questions cover the child's interest in targeted violence, extremist groups, or gang affiliation; recent or anticipated loss; a loss of status; and any concern about the child's ability to harm self or others. Be sure to ask about weapons in the home or other locations accessible to the child and his/her ability to use those weapons. According to Vossekuil et al. (2002), many school shooters obtained firearms from home, even though parents thought those weapons were secure. Resist the temptation to gloss over questions about weapons or to accept superficial statements that guns are safe. Many locked gun cabinets have breakable glass doors so that owners can admire their weapons. Parents may report that the guns are locked in a chest-but the key is readily accessible.

> **It is important to ask parents about weapons in the home or other locations and the child's ability to access and use those weapons.**

Collateral Interviews

Collateral sources include other students, administrators, teachers, therapists, and community members who have relevant knowledge about the child. Unless two meetings are scheduled with the child, the collateral interviews should occur prior to interviewing the child. Otherwise, evaluators cannot incorporate these reports into the child interview. Here the school-based practitioner may have more flexibility than a consulting psychologist. For consulting psychologists, it is possible to make the SBRA a day-long event, and in that case, the collateral interviews should occur before seeing the child.

> **Interviews with students, administrators, teachers, therapists, and community members should be conducted prior to interviewing the referred child.**

Students may be the most difficult collateral group to access, but sometimes they are essential people to interview. In the SSI study, attackers rarely advertised their plans to the intended target or targets, but told friends or peers about it (Fein et al., 2002). Students have a unique culture that often excludes adults. They may know before a teacher that a student is in trouble, has been abused, feels bullied, is seeking weapons, or intimidates others. Fein et al. (2002) described a situation in which a planned attack was so well known among students that 24 had gathered at the school to witness it.

If a child has a history of violence, access to other students may not be as critical. Sufficient information may already exist in the student record or may be elicited from adults. It becomes critical to speak to students when they have witnessed threatening statements or behavior or experienced intimidation. When interviewing student witnesses is indicated, school administrators must balance privacy rights delineated in the Family Education Rights and Privacy Act (FERPA; 1974) with a mandate to ensure the safety of others (Safe and Drug Free Schools and Communities Act, 1994). For the consulting psychologist, or when policy directs the school psychologist in this area, a school administrator or the evaluator must obtain parental permission to interview other students. In addition, the evaluator should always obtain an informed consent from each student and others interviewed. Collateral sources should be told how the information they report will be used and the limits of privacy in this situation. Fein et al. (2002) caution that when a student or an adult is a possible attack target, he or she should be interviewed with "special sensitivity" (p. 54). In addition, psychologists have a duty to warn an intended victim or to inform police when there is reasonable suspicion that one person poses a danger to another (*Tarasoff v. Regents of the University of California*, 1976; Tolman, 2001).

From the collateral interviews, SBRA evaluators learn what others think or know about the referred child, including whether others fear him/her. Learning about people's fears will help to determine whether the referred child should stay at that school or faces an uphill battle to overcome negative attitudes. Learning the context surrounding people's fears is another reason for asking about these feelings. Hearing frightening gossip is different from experiencing intimidation or having firsthand information about an attack scheme. Two examples illustrate reports about such worrisome behavior. In one case, a child threatened to stick another student with a pin that he said contained a deadly virus. In another case, a child approached two students and asked them how to obtain guns. In the first instance, the child intimidated another student. In the second, the child revealed that he was thinking about a planned attack.

Clinical Interview with the Child

The results of various data collection methods prove invaluable when conducting clinical interviews with the child. Such investigatory techniques distinguish evaluations, such as SBRAs, from other mental health or educational assessments. For example, therapists have a different mandate from practitioners who evaluate risk. Because therapists see the child only in the therapeutic context, they may fail to consider that the child in their office may look different at school. Because therapists act as advocates or support persons, it may be inappropriate to ask them to jeopardize such a relationship by offering opinions about a child's risk level (Greenberg & Shuman, 2008). Crisis intervention is also different from an SBRA because crisis intervention attempts to determine whether a person is a danger to self or others within the next 24–48 hours. A crisis evaluation may miss high-functioning children who are not experiencing an acute crisis but who still need interventions to reduce their potential for violence.

Early tasks during the child interview include (1) helping the child understand the nature of the evaluation, (2) correcting any misunderstandings, and (3) informing him/her about the potential outcomes of the assessment. The next step is to ask the child to recount the reported statement or action that led to the SBRA. Often these children are afraid or guarded because restrictions may have been imposed on them by family members or other involved parties, and there may be police involvement, or they have a sense that they are in trouble. Denial or minimization is common under these circumstances. In this context, children's lies or distortions provide a window into their problem solving behavior or response style that may generalize beyond the evaluation. Deception is a complex human response (Rogers, 2008) that includes dimensions of self-deception versus deception of others, minimization or denial, and dissimulation attempts that are sophisticated or primitive. For example, a child who attempts to outsmart a psychologist is different from a child who uses distortion to avoid hurting an attachment figure.

The SBRA, although future oriented, is also retrospective because evaluators try to understand the past thoughts and actions leading to a critical incident. In this regard, the SBRA resembles the mental status at time of offense (MSO) evaluation in criminal cases. Melton, Petrila, Poythress, and Slobogin (2007) use a "spiraling approach" (p. 254) in the MSO interview, going from general to specific questions, and collecting more details from the subject over the course of the interview. With children, evaluators can designate a point in time before the critical event and, in a sequential manner, move toward the incident. Specifically, ask children about their routine on the day of the event, what they ate for lunch, the people they saw. Such questions help engender cooperation with more pertinent inquires such as, "When did you get the idea to write this threat?" or "What were you thinking before you slapped the principal?" Situational factors, such as alcohol or other drug use, peer influence, the illness or death of a significant other or a loss of status, should be explored during this discussion.

> **In the child interview for SBRA, evaluators can use a "spiraling approach" by moving from general to more specific questions about details of the incident.**

Like many forensic assessments, SBRAs seek details. If a student reports that he drank alcohol the night before an assault, the evaluator inquires about the type and amount of alcohol consumed. If an incident was prompted by a fight with a friend, the evaluator asks for details about that relationship. This information helps to deconstruct the seriousness and motivation for a destructive act, to understand if it was impulsive or planned, to explore possible contributing personal or environmental factors, and to consider how to prevent such behavior in the future.

Following Melton et al.'s (2007) MSO strategy, evaluators move from general to more probing questioning. Be sure to explore inconsistencies in the child's story and encourage him/her to address thoughts or feelings that he/she may have been reticent to discuss. With more direct and threatening questions, it is important to convey understanding and respect, for example, saying, "I know this is hard for you to talk about, but it's important that I understand it." Always convey a supportive rather than confrontational style. These approaches are especially important with adolescents who are hypervigilant to feeling manipulated or humiliated, and who withdraw or go on the offensive when upset. The evaluator walks a tightrope with many adolescents, balancing support with direction, acceptance with skepticism, and neutrality with probing questions, trying to build and sustain what has been called a "fragile alliance" (Meeks & Bernet, 2001).

Psychological Tests and Checklists

Although the SBRA does not rely as heavily on tests as do some other types of evaluations, certain instruments can and should be integrated into this process. The most important development since the last publication of this chapter (Halikias, 2005) has been a movement in risk assessment practice toward SPJ techniques. As discussed, SPJ is an attempt to reconcile actuarial and clinical approaches to risk assessment by identifying salient, empirical, and rationally derived factors. SPJ is consistent with the scientist-practitioner philosophy, facilitating an idiographic and narrative approach to individualizing intervention and case management strategies, while also attending to nomothetic and algorithmic rules.

One of the more important SPJ instruments to consider when conducting SBRA is the Structured Assessment of Violence Risk in Youth (SAVY; Borum et al., 2006). The SAVY was designed for clinicians attempting to assess risk for violence within educational settings. It follows a format developed by other well-established, adult-based risk assessment instruments, including the Historical Clinical Risk–20 (Webster, Douglas, Eaves, & Hart, 1997) and the Violence Risk Assessment Guide (Quinsey, Harris, Rice, & Cormier, 1998), although the SAVY distinguishes itself with the inclusion of 6 Protective Factors items. The core of the SAVY consists of 10 Historical Risk Factors items, 6 Social/Contextual Risk Factors items, and 8 Individual/Clinical Risk Factors items. The research thus far on the SAVY looks promising, and it appears to have good predictive accuracy in distinguishing between violent and nonviolent children (McGowan et al., 2011; Meyers & Schmidt, 2008; Welsh, Schmidt, McKinnon, Chattha, & Meyers, 2008). Other SPJ risk-focused instruments for youth include the Youth Level of Service/Case Management Inventory (Hoge & Andrews, 2002) and the Hare Psychopathy Checklist: Youth Version (PCL: YV; Forth, Kosson, & Hare, 2003), although the theory embedded in the PCL: YV (juvenile psychopathy) may prove too controversial for general use in schools settings. An SPJ instrument, along with the core questions discussed earlier (see Appendix 10.1), are best completed at the end of the SBRA, once all other data have been collected. An evaluator trained with SPJ instruments uses the professional manual to rank a condition (e.g., from the SAVY, Stress and Poor Coping) on a continuum of low, moderate, or high.

> One of several risk-focused instruments for youth, based on the SPJ approach, can be used in the SBRA as adjunct assessment methods.

Other psychological tests that may prove helpful in SBRAs are measures of mental health status. With these personality tests and checklists, the evaluator tries to establish if the child presents with any social, emotional, or behavioral problems that relate to the analysis of risk and case management strategies. Finally, the SBRA is sometimes integrated into a special education assessment and may require an evaluator to have expertise with cognitive as well as risk-for-violence instruments and procedures.

Case Formulation, Findings, and Recommendations

In the final stage of the SBRA, the evaluator formulates not only a child's level of risk for violence but also those circumstances and environments that may increase or decrease the chances of this behavior. Aggression is usually not a random act but is dependent on the interaction of circumstance and temperament.

In the formulation stage the evaluator answers the core questions relevant to violence potential, listed in Appendix 10.1. These questions concern a child's motivation for the critical incident, what he or she did or said, the fear that he or she engendered, and other issues pertinent to assessing risk for violence. Answering these questions helps evaluators formulate "thick" rather than "thin" one-dimensional or dichotomous (violent vs. not violent) descriptions. The answers to these questions should lead to reasonable, cost-effective case management strategies. Unlike a predictive approach, case management allows for postassessment control, such as observing and monitoring compliance, providing support, and reassessing the child, if necessary, over time (Borum, 2003; Heilbrun, 1997).

Recommendations and case management fall on a continuum from minimally invasive to more intrusive, intensive, and costly (see Appendix 10.2). As discussed earlier, for children who pose low to medium risk (Group A or B), a conference between the child and the principal, a restitution plan, or letter of apology might be indicated. A boy who joked about making a bomb could write a letter of apology or provide a service in recognition of his mistake. A Group C child who poses medium risk might benefit from support and problem-solving guidance, including (1) having the school administrator consider ways to improve a degrading school climate, (2) implementing individual therapy to manage feelings of helplessness or anger, and (3) providing opportunities to enhance status or self-esteem. Group D children require more careful and intensive case management, including contracting with each child for safety, removing weapons from the home, using therapeutic and anger management techniques, recruiting a supportive juvenile police officer to work with the youth, and addressing grievances or disabilities. Group E children, who are chronically aggressive, also need comprehensive and more intensive case management strategies. There is a very high incidence of language-based learning disabilities (Dionne, Tremblay, Boivin, Laplante, & Perusse, 2003) and co-occurring mental health problems in this population (Abram et al., 2007). Furthermore, Group E children comprise the majority of youth referred to mental health and other treatment centers (Loeber, Burke, Lahey, Winters, & Zera, 2000) and have a higher frequency of placement in special programs for emotionally disturbed students (Dodge & Pettit, 2003). Interventions might include removing weapons from the home and coordinating school, therapeutic, and community-based services. Alternative school programs, day treatment centers, or residential facilities become options when these children have injured others and continue to pose this risk.

The SBRA usually ends with an oral or written report of observations, findings, and recommendations. Reports should be free of jargon, so that parents, administrators, and other nonpsychologists will understand this information. The oral or written report should include a cautionary statement regarding the limitations of predicting violence and a rationale for suggested case management strategies. As an example, evaluators can introduce the conclusion section of the SBRA with the following statement:

> **The oral/written report should include a caution on the limitations for predicting violence and a rationale for suggested case management strategies.**

"School staff wanted this evaluation to help them understand Sam's threat potential, learn strategies to avert violence, and help assure that Sam and others remain safe. Given the rarity of this type of violence, a threat assessment, especially of calculated and planned school violence, cannot realistically predict such incidents. Rather, this evaluation attempted to identify risk factors for destructive behavior, and it offers recommendations for ways to help decrease the possibility of violence. In this regard, helping Sam to function more effectively holds the greatest promise for reducing destructive or violent behavior."

A critical skill of the evaluator at this juncture is collapsing data into meaningful and salient categories. This involves establishing convergent findings while minimizing the error associated with isolated or fragmented data.

SUMMARY

The SBRA is a complex and specialized evaluation that requires knowledge about child development, familiarity with the literature relevant to risk for violence assessments, an understanding of school systems and special education procedures, and the ability to conduct the required investigatory procedures. The SBRA also requires the ability to determine risk potential, along with an understanding of the limitations of that task. Crafting reasonable case management strategies is a key goal of the SBRA in order to mobilize adults on the child's behalf and reduce risk for violence. The SBRA requires the collection and integration of information across multiple informants and data sources (history, interviews, observations, tests, records) and the systematic organization of these data, seeking convergent sources and minimizing the error associated with isolated reports.

The majority of children referred for the SBRA will not pose a danger to others; only a small number fit a targeted violence profile or pose that high level of risk. Practitioners who perform SBRAs have the opportunity to reach a diverse group of students with special needs. With few exceptions, referred children benefit more from supportive services and good case management than from stereotyping and punishment.

School-based practitioners should adopt a pragmatic and case-focused approach to SBRAs, given the limitations of accurately predicting school violence. Instead of drawing "yes" or "no" conclusions about risk for violence, SBRA evaluators can help others understand the reasons for a child's destructive behavior and offer solution-focused recommendations to improve functional skills in school and the larger society.

School-Based Risk Assessment Worksheet

Child's name _____ Date of birth ___/___/___
First   Middle   Last   Month Day Year

Child's school _____

Informants _____

Evaluator _____ Dates of evaluation _____

Use this worksheet to conduct interviews with the referred child, parents, and collateral sources. When you have completed the school-based risk assessment, record a succinct answer for each question in the space below or write "nonapplicable" (n/a). Use this completed form when you conduct the feedback conference or write the report.

1. What was the motive for the behavior that brought the child to the evaluation?

2. What has the child said, written, or done that involved a risk for violence?

3. Does the child have pertinent information about a target, if one exists (e.g., the person's schedule, activities, home address)?

4. Does the child have an interest in targeted violence or extremist groups? Is there any gang affiliation or membership?

5. Are weapons available to the child, and does he/she know how to use them?

6. Has the child exhibited intimidating behaviors, such as stalking or harassing others?

(continued)

7. What is the child's mental condition and history of mental illness? Does he/she have delusions, hallucinations, or paranoid states?

8. Is there evidence of substance abuse or dependence?

9. Has there been a recent loss, including a loss of status, that produced feelings of despair?

10. If the child shows a history of past violence, does the violence appear to be calculated or impulsive?

11. Were the child's past aggressive actions done in concert with others, or were they solitary acts?

12. Were the child's aggressive actions rare, occasional, frequent, or ongoing?

13. Do people in the school or the community have fears about the child's potential for violence? Have others experienced intimidation because of the child's behavior?

14. Are there factors that might increase or decrease the risk of future violence? What are these factors?

Risk Assessment Groups and Case Management Strategies

Child's name _____ Date of birth ___/___/___
First   Middle   Last   Month Day   Year

Child's school _____

Informants _____

Evaluator _____ Dates of evaluation _____

Use this form to estimate the risk status of the child referred for a school-based risk assessment. Identifying a child's sense of membership in one or more groups can help you estimate his/her level of violence potential and the intensity of postassessment resources needed. There is no precise empirical method for classifying children referred for school-based risk assessments. However, you can use this form to assign a rough estimate of risk for violence, based on the critical incident and the child's motivation for threatening behavior. A child's apparent membership in a group can guide you in making specific recommendations for case management intervention. Consider that some children may fall between groups or may be assigned to more than one group. Check categories, descriptions, and sample recommendations that apply to this particular child.

☐ Group A. Low Risk	
Characteristics • Often they have done something that violated a zero tolerance policy. • Come to assessment with little or no history of psychological problems. • History and motivation for act make them appear to pose little risk.	*Case Management* • Conference with child. • Restitution plan. • Apology letter.

☐ Group B. Low to Medium Risk	
Characteristics • Nonviolent children who did something thoughtless and/or accidental. • Come to assessment with little or no history of psychological problems. • History and motivation for act make them appear to pose little risk to harm others, but they may be at risk for future behavior that places their status at school in jeopardy.	*Case Management* • Conference with child. • Restitution plan. • Apology letter. • Behavior contract. • Short-term counseling to address problem solving.

(continued)

☐ **Group C. Medium Risk**	
Characteristics	*Case Management*
• Critical incident is a distress signal. • May or may not come to the assessment with a history of psychological problems. • Inept problem-solving and/or social skills.	• Improve problem-solving skills. • Attend to possible problems reflecting a degrading school climate (e.g., sensitivity training for staff; bullying intervention and prevention programs). • Therapy for possible social–emotional problems (e.g., depression, anxiety, recent loss, family problems). • Designate an adult support person at school who will have daily contact with the child. • Provide anger management therapy when indicated. • Seek ways to enhance child's status or self-esteem at school or in the community.
☐ **Group D. High Risk—Specific Target**	
Characteristics	*Case Management*
• Referral and motivation reflect ongoing interest in injuring or having unwelcome contact with a target. • May or may not come to the assessment with a known history of psychological problems. • Evidence exists that they have considered or begun to implement a plan to injure others emotionally or physically. • Threatening behavior often evolved from a crisis (e.g., loss, harassment, suicidal feelings).	• Contract with child for safety. • Recommend that weapons be removed from the home and other locations to which the child has access (e.g., a friend or relative's home). • Notify law enforcement if a child's behavior or plans pose a threat to a target. • Employ family counseling or anger management techniques to address underlying crisis. • Consider if suicide prevention strategies are indicated. • Consider recruiting a supportive juvenile police officer, or other adult in authority, who has sensitivity to the child's problems to work with the child. • If the child returns to school, structure the school day to ensure regular adult check-ins (at a minimum: at the beginning and end of each school day) with the child. • Consider whether additional assessment is indicated (e.g., assessment for special education, mental health services, psychopharmacotherapy). • Address grievances at school.

(continued)

☐ **Group E. High Risk—Chronic Aggression**	
Characteristics • Come to evaluation with a known history of emotional, developmental, or conduct problems. • Critical incident is part of a larger pattern of problematic behaviors. • Has a discipline, special education, or mental health file. • Verbal and physical aggression look historical, and usually predate the critical incident by 1 or more years.	*Case Management* • Ascertain if child has received appropriate educational services (e.g., a suspected but not diagnosed language disability). • Incorporate vocational/technical curricula into child's school program, if these appear helpful. • Seek opportunities to expose child to extracurricular activities and prosocial experiences (e.g., clubs, sports, work opportunities). • Recommend that weapons be removed from the home or other locations to which the child has access (e.g., a friend's or relative's home). • Recommend needed mental health interventions (e.g., anger management training, substance abuse counseling, psychopharmacotherapy). • Recommend "wraparound" or other cross-discipline teams to help manage child's behavior. • Examine the need for family counseling or home-based family services. • Recommend ways to reduce abusive or chaotic features in the child's life. • If the child injured others and continues to pose this risk, consider alternative school programs, day treatment centers, or residential facilities. • If child returns to school, structure school day to ensure regular adult check-ins (at a minimum: at the beginning and end of each school day) with the child. • Adopt a "zero tolerance" policy around future aggression and threats of aggression. • Use restitution plans and apology letters when the child has injured another person.

Sample Informed Consent for a School-Based Risk Assessment

INFORMED CONSENT FOR RISK ASSESSMENT EVALUATION

Your child, _____, has been referred to me by the _____ School for a risk assessment evaluation. Specifically, this is an assessment of risk for dangerousness following incidents involving your child and the school. This evaluation may consist of interviews, observations, psychological tests, and a review of records. At the end of this evaluation I may write a report and/or conduct a verbal conference detailing my observations, conclusions, and recommendations. The school will pay for this evaluation.

You will allow me to interview school employees or family members, to review records about your child, or to obtain information from other professionals.

Because the school has referred your child to me and is paying for this service, you acknowledge that I will communicate with and send reports to staff at _____ School.

If you decide to withdraw from this evaluation, you may not retroactively revoke consent for me to communicate with the school about information already obtained from you, your child, significant others, or service providers. Once verbal or written reports are given to the school, I have no control over what they do with this information.

Examples of other circumstances when information from this evaluation may or must be shared with others include, but are not limited to, the following:

1) You may sign a release of information giving me permission to speak with, or send information to, another person or organization.
2) If you or your child present as a clear and present danger to self or other, I must release information in order to protect you, your child, or another person from harm.
3) If I have reasonable cause to believe that a child under the age of 18 years is suffering abuse or neglect, I am required by law to report this information to social services.

It is not possible for me to send you psychological test protocols (the test forms) or manuals because this information is protected by rules mandating test security. Should you wish to obtain this information, you agree to employ a licensed psychologist or certified school psychologist with expertise in test and measurement to review and interpret this information for you. I will, of course, provide you with the results and interpretation of psychological tests.

_____   _____
Parent/Guardian Signature   Date

_____   _____
Parent/Guardian Signature   Date

General Outline for SBRA Parent and Child Interviews

1. Present informed consent or, if it has already been read and signed, review this information with the subject or subjects.

2. Answer questions that parents or children have about the evaluation.

3. Determine whether service providers or service organizations exist for the child or parents (e.g., mental health counselors, past psychiatric hospitalizations). Ask parents and, if appropriate, the child to sign releases that allow the evaluator to speak to these sources. Ask about the existence of other important adult relationships that may serve as useful collateral sources (e.g., employer, minister, relative, coach).

4. Ask a general question about how the parents or child understand what it means to be evaluated for a school-based risk assessment. The answer to this question should result in an initial explanation of the reason for referral. Sometimes the response will be short; other times, it may entail a long discussion.

   a. Be certain that you explore with the parents and child what the child said, wrote, or did that others perceived as threatening.

   b. Ask the child to carefully recount his/her activities that led up to the critical incident, and obtain details about his/her thoughts and behavior around an alleged incident.

5. Present parents or child with documents related to the critical incident (e.g., written threat from the child, discipline log entry, affidavits or police reports, letter from school to parents) and ask for their responses.

6. Review risk-relevant questions:

   a. What contact has the child had with the identified target, and what is the nature of that relationship? How familiar is the child with that person's schedule, activities, and home address?

   b. What movies, books, computer Internet sites, and group affiliations is the child most interested in or involved with? Begin to explore questions relevant to an interest in targeted violence or extremist groups and any possible gang affiliation.

   c. Have the adults and child describe the exact weapon(s) (e.g., rifles, shotguns, handguns, hunting or military knives, bow and arrows, explosive devices or materials) that exist in the home or elsewhere, to which the youth has access. Obtain details about the security system in place with the weapon(s). Establish the youngster's knowledge about, and skill with, these weapons.

   d. Other than the reason for referral, do the parents or child know of incidents when people felt intimidated or harassed by the child, regardless of whether the parents or child thought that reaction justified? Do the parents worry about their child? Do the parents or child know of people who have expressed fear of the child or concern that he/she could injure themselves or others?

(continued)

e. Ask questions that will provide information about the child's mental health or any history of mental illness, including any attempts at therapy or previous psychiatric hospitalization. Ask if the youngster has experienced abuse (physical, emotional, sexual, neglect). Has there ever been suicidal talk, writings, or actions by the child?

f. Establish academic strengths and weaknesses; include information about, or evidence for, learning or cognitive delays.

g. Perform a focused inquiry about substance use and abuse with the youngster, his/her siblings, and the parents.

h. Ask if the child or family has any present or past involvement with a child protection agency, the police, or courts, and the reasons this involvement.

i. Has there been a recent loss that produced feelings of despair? This loss may include a death or severe, prolonged illness of an important attachment figure. Ask if the youth experienced any recent blows to his/her self-esteem. For example, was the child cut from a sports team? Has the child experienced the loss of a romantic or other important relationship?

j. Ask parents and the child to recount all incidents of physical violence on the part of the child, regardless of whether they view such acts as self-defense and justifiable or intended to harm another person. Establish any possible themes that appear to precipitate aggressive acts. The evaluator comes away from this part of the interview with a sense of how the parents and child describe and perceive past aggression: minimal to substantial, impulsive versus planned, intermittent versus chronic, done in concert with others or alone.

7. Obtain a developmental and social history from the parents. This history may begin with a description of the family's environment and lifestyle at the time of conception, move sequentially through the pregnancy, birth, infancy, preschool years, elementary school, and continue to the critical incident that resulted in the school-based risk assessment. Use the document generated from the file review (notes and excerpts from historical documents) to assist the parents with recall or to ask them to explain contradictions between their reports and information in the record. The history ends with a review of the extended family history, with an eye toward relatives suffering mental health problems, substance abuse issues, learning difficulties, or criminal involvement. This appendix cannot cover the complexities and skill required to obtain a good social and developmental history, and it is assumed the clinician comes to the school-based risk assessment with this knowledge and training.

8. Establish the child's strengths and productive interests in and outside of school.

9. At this point the interview with the parents may be near or past the 2-hour mark, or the 1-hour mark with the child. This is an opportunity to take a break, during which time the clinician can compare notes from the interview with the record and reports about the critical incident. Following the break, the clinician focuses more actively on contradictions between self-reports and reports obtained from the file and collateral sources.

10. Ask the parents and child for any additional information they wish to convey. Ask if they have any questions about the interview process and how they felt about being interviewed. Clarify with them what may happen next in this process.

References

Achenbach, T. M. (2001). *Youth Self-Report for Ages 11–18*. Burlington, VT: University of Vermont, Research Center for Children, Youth, and Families.

Achenbach, T. M., & McConaughy, S. H. (1997). *Empirically based assessment of child and adolescent psychopathology: Practical applications* (2nd ed.). Newbury Park, CA: Sage.

Achenbach, T. M., McConaughy, S. H., & Howell, C. T. (1987). Child/adolescent behavioral and emotional problems: Implications of cross-informant correlations for situational specificity. *Psychological Bulletin, 101*, 213–232.

Achenbach, T. M., Newhouse, P., & Rescorla, L. A. (2004). *Manual for the ASEBA Older Adult Forms & Profiles*. Burlington, VT: University of Vermont, Research Center for Children, Youth, and Families.

Achenbach, T. M., & Rescorla, L. A. (2000). *Manual for the ASEBA Preschool Forms & Profiles*. Burlington, VT: University of Vermont, Research Center for Children, Youth, and Families.

Achenbach, T. M., & Rescorla, L. A. (2001). *Manual for the ASEBA School-Age Forms & Profiles*. Burlington, VT: University of Vermont, Research Center for Children, Youth, and Families.

Achenbach, T. M., & Rescorla, L. A. (2003). *Manual for the ASEBA Adult Forms & Profiles*. Burlington, VT: University of Vermont, Research Center for Children, Youth, and Families.

Achenbach, T. M., & Rescorla, L. A. (2007). *Multicultural supplement to the Manual for the ASEBA School-Age Forms & Profiles*. Burlington, VT: University of Vermont, Research Center for Children, Youth, and Families.

Ambrosini, P. J. (2000). Historical development and present status of the Schedule for Affective Disorders and Schizophrenia for School-age Children (K-SADS). *Journal of the American Academy of Child and Adolescent Psychiatry, 39*, 49–58.

American Academy of Pediatrics. (2000). Diagnosis and evaluation of the child with attention deficit hyperactivity disorder (AC0002). *Pediatrics, 105*, 1158–1170.

American Education Research Association, American Psychological Association, and National Council on Measurement in Education. (1999). *Standards for educational and psychological assessment*. Washington, DC: Author.

American Psychiatric Association. (2000). *Diagnostic and statistical manual of mental disorders* (4th ed., text rev.). Washington, DC: Author.

American Psychiatric Association. (2012). *DSM-5*. Retrieved from *www.psychiatry.org/dsm5*.

American Psychiatric Association. (2013). *Diagnostic and statistical manual of mental disorders* (5th ed.). Washington, DC: Author.

American Psychological Association. (1993). *Violence in youth: Psychologists' response*. Washington, DC: Author.

American Psychological Association. (2002). Ethical principles of psychologists and code of conduct. *American Psychologist, 57*, 1060–1073.

American Psychological Association. (2010). Ethical principles of psychologists and code of conduct. 2010 Amendments. Retrieved from *www.apa.org/index.aspx*.

Americans with Disabilities Act. (1990). 42 U.S.C., §1201 et seq.

Angold, A., & Costello, J. (2000). The Child and Adolescent Psychiatric Assessment (CAPA). *Journal of the American Academy of Child and Adolescent Psychiatry, 39,* 39–48.

Barkley, R. A. (2006). *Attention-deficit/hyperactivity disorder: A handbook for diagnosis and treatment* (3rd ed.). New York: Guilford Press.

Barkley, R. A. (1997). *Defiant children: A clinician's manual for assessment and parent training* (2nd ed.). New York: Guilford Press.

Barkley, R. A., & Murphy, K. R. (2006). *Attention-deficit hyperactivity disorder: A clinical workbook* (3rd ed.). New York: Guilford Press.

Barrett, T. (1985). *Youth in crisis: Seeking solutions to self-destructive behavior.* Longmont, CO: Sopris West.

Beaver, R. B., & Busse, R. T. (2000). Informant reports: Conceptual and research bases of interviews with parents and teachers. In E. S. Shapiro & T. R. Kratochwill (Eds.), *Behavioral assessment in schools: Theory, research, and clinical foundations* (2nd ed., pp. 257–287). New York: Guilford Press.

Beck, A., & Steer, R. (1991). *Manual for the Beck Scale for Suicidal Ideation.* San Antonio, TX: Psychological Corporation.

Bergan, J. R., & Kratochwill, T. R. (1990). *Behavioral consultation and therapy.* New York: Plenum Press.

Berman, A. L. (2009). School-based suicide prevention: Research advances and practice implications. *School Psychology Review, 38,* 233–238.

Berman, A. L., Jobes, D. A., & Silverman, M. M. (2006). *Adolescent suicide: Assessment and intervention* (2nd ed.). Washington, DC: American Psychological Association.

Bierman, K. L. (2004). *Peer rejection: Developmental processes and intervention strategies.* New York: Guilford Press.

Bierman, K. L., Smoot, D. L., & Aumiller, K. (1993). Characteristics of aggressive–rejected, aggressive (nonrejected), and rejected (nonaggressive) boys. *Child Development, 64,* 139–151.

Bierman, K. L., & Welsh, J. A. (1997). Social relationship deficits. In E. J. Mash & L. G. Terdal (Eds.), *Assessment of childhood disorders* (3rd ed., pp. 328–365). New York: Guilford Press.

Borum, R. (2000). Assessing violence risk among youth. *Journal of Clinical Psychology, 56,* 1263–1288.

Borum, R. (2003). Managing at-risk juvenile offenders in the community: Putting evidence-based principles into practice. *Journal of Contemporary Criminal Justice, 19,* 114–137.

Borum, R., Bartel, P., & Forth, A. (2006). *Structured Assessment of Violence in Youth: Professional Manual.* Lutz, FL: Psychological Assessment Resources.

Borum, R., Fein, R., Vossekuil, B., & Berglund, J. (1999). Threat assessment: Defining an approach for evaluating risk of targeted violence. *Behavioral Sciences and the Law, 17,* 323–337.

Bradshaw, C. P., Sawyer, A. L., & O'Brennan, L. M. (2007). Bullying and peer victimization at school: Perceptual differences between students and school staff. *School Psychology Review, 36,* 361–382.

Brassard, M. A., Tyler, A., & Kehle, T. (1983). Sexually abused children: Identification and suggestions for intervention. *School Psychology Review, 12,* 93–97.

Brent, D. A. (1997). The aftercare of adolescents with deliberate self-harm. *Journal of Child Psychology and Psychiatry, 38,* 277–286.

Brock, S. E., & Sandoval, J. (1997). Suicidal ideation and behaviors. In G. C. Bear, K. M. Minke, & A. Thomas (Eds.), *Children's needs II: Development, problems and alternatives* (pp. 361–374). Bethesda, MD: National Association of School Psychologists.

Broidy, L. M., Nagin, D. S., Tremblay, R. E., Bates, J. E., Brame, B., Dodge, K. A., et al. (2003). Developmental trajectories of childhood disruptive behaviors and adolescent delinquency: A six-site, cross-national study. *Developmental Psychology, 39,* 222–245.

Brookmeyer, K. A., Fanti, K. A., & Henrich, C. C. (2006). School, parents, and youth violence: A multilevel, ecological analysis. *Journal of Clinical Child and Adolescent Psychology, 35,* 504–514.

Brown-Chidsey, R., & Steege, M. W. (2010). *Response to intervention: Principles and strategies for effective practice* (2nd ed.). New York: Guilford Press.

Buck, G. H., Bursuck, W. D., Polloway, E. A., Nelson, J., Jayanthi, M. J., & Whitehouse, F. A. (1996). Homework-related communication problems: Perspectives of special educators. *Journal of Emotional and Behavioral Disorders, 4,* 105–113.

Burns, R. C. (1982). *Self-growth in families: Kinetic Family Drawings (K-F-D) research and application.* New York: Brunner/Mazel.

Busse, R. T., & Beaver, B. R. (2000). Informant report: Parent and teacher interviews. In E. S. Shapiro & T. R. Kratochwill (Eds.), *Conducting school-based assessments of child and adolescent behavior* (pp. 235–273). New York: Guilford Press.

Butcher, J. N., Williams, C. L., Graham, J. R., Archer, R. P., Tellegen, A., Ben-Porath, Y. S., et al. (1992). *Minnesota Multiphasic Personality Inventory— Adolescent Version. Manual for administration and scoring.* San Antonio, TX: Pearson.

California Safe Schools Coalition & 4–H Center for Youth Development, University of California, Davis. (2004). *Consequences of harassment based on actual or perceived sexual orientation and gender nonconformity and steps to making schools safer.* San Francisco and Davis, CA: Authors.

Catenaccio, R. (1995). Crisis intervention with suicidal

adolescents: A view from the emergency room. In J. K. Zimmerman & G. M. Asnis (Eds.), *Treatment approaches with suicidal adolescents* (pp. 71–90). Oxford, UK: Wiley.

Centers for Disease Control and Prevention. (2002). Web-based injury statistics query and reporting system. *www.cdc.gov/ncipc/factsheets/suifacts.htm*.

Child Abuse Prevention and Treatment Act. (1974). Public Law 93–247; 42 U.S.C. §5106 et seq.

Chung, K. M., Organista, P. B., & Marin, G. (2003). *Acculturation: Advances in theory, measurement, and applied research.* Washington, DC: American Psychological Association.

Coie, J. D. (1990). Toward a theory of peer rejection. In S. R. Asher & J. D. Coie (Eds.), *Peer rejection in childhood* (pp. 365–401). Cambridge, UK: Cambridge University Press.

Coie, J. D., Dodge, K. A., & Kupersmidt, J. B. (1990). Peer group behavior and social status. In S. R. Asher & J. D. Coie (Eds.), *Peer rejection in childhood* (pp. 17–59). Cambridge, UK: Cambridge University Press.

Coie, J. D., & Kupersmidt, J. B. (1983). A behavior analysis of emerging social status in boys' groups. *Child Development, 54,* 1400–1416.

Committee on Ethical Guidelines for Forensic Psychologists. (1991). Specialty guidelines for forensic psychologists. *Law and Human Behavior, 15,* 655–665.

Confidentiality of Alcohol and Drug Abuse Patient Records. (1987, June 9). 52 Fed. Reg. 21796, 21797.

Conners, K. C. (2008). *Conners Comprehensive Behavior Rating Scales manual.* North Tonawanda, NY: MHS.

Cook, C. R., Williams, K. R., Guerra, N. G., Kim, T. E., & Sadek, S. (2010). Predictors of bullying and victimization in childhood and adolescence: A meta-analytic investigation. *School Psychology Quarterly, 25,* 65–83.

Cooper, H., Lindsay, J. J., Nye, B., & Greathouse, S. (1998). Relationships among attitudes about homework, amount of homework assigned and completed, and student achievement. *Journal of Educational Psychology, 90*(1), 70–83.

Costello, J., Egger, H., & Angold, A. (2005). 10–year research update review: The epidemiology of child and adolescent psychiatric disorders: I. Methods and public health burden. *Journal of the American Academy of Child and Adolescent Psychiatry, 44,* 972–986.

Crick, N. R. (1995). Relational aggression: The role of intent attributions, feelings of distress, and provocation type. *Development and Psychopathology, 7,* 313–322.

Crick, N. R., & Dodge, K. (1994). A review and reformulation of social information-processing mechanisms in children's social adjustment. *Psychological Bulletin, 115,* 74–101.

Crick, N. R., & Grotpeter, J. K. (1995). Relational aggression, gender, and social-psychological adjustment. *Child Development, 66,* 710–722.

Crick, N. R., Ostrov, J. M., & Kawabata, Y. (2007). Relational aggression and gender: An overview. In D. J. Flannery, A. T. Vazsonyi, & I. D. Waldman (Eds.), *The Cambridge handbook of violent behavior and aggression* (pp. 245–259). New York: Cambridge University Press.

Crone, D. A., Horner, R. H., & Hawken, L. S. (2004). *Responding to problem behavior in schools.* New York: Guilford Press.

Crooks, C. V., & Wolfe, D. A. (2007). Child abuse and neglect. In E. J. Mash & R. A. Barkley (Eds.), *Assessment of childhood disorders* (4th ed., pp. 639–684). New York: Guilford Press.

Cunningham, C. E., Cunningham, L. J., Ratcliffe, J., & Vaillancourt, T. (2010). A qualitative analysis of the bullying prevention and intervention recommendations of students in grades 5 to 8. *Journal of School Violence, 9,* 321–338.

Dahlberg, L. L. (1998). Youth violence in the United States: Major trends, risk factors, and prevention approaches. *American Journal of Preventive Medicine, 14,* 259–272.

Daniel, S., Power, T. J., Karustis, J. L., & Leff, S. S. (1999, November). *Parent-mediated homework intervention for children with ADHD: Its impact on parent–child relationships and parenting stress.* Poster session presented at the annual meeting of the Association for Advancement of Behavior Therapy, Toronto, Ontario, Canada.

D'Augelli, A. R. (2002). The cutting edges of lesbian and gay psychology. In A. Coyle & C. Kitzinger (Eds.), *Lesbian and gay psychology: New perspectives* (pp. xiii–xvi). London: British Psychological Society/Blackwell.

Debski, J., Spadafore, C. D., Jacob, S., Poole, D. A., & Hixson, M. D. (2007). Suicide intervention: Training, roles, and knowledge of school psychologists. *Psychology in the Schools, 44,* 157–170.

De Los Reyes, A. (2011). Introduction to the special section: More than measurement error: Discovering meaning behind informant discrepancies in clinical assessments of children and adolescents. *Journal of Child and Adolescent Psychology, 40,* 1–9.

Dionne, G., Tremblay, R., Boivin, M., Laplante, D., & Perusse, A. (2003). Physical aggression and expressed vocabulary in 19-month-old twins. *Developmental Psychology, 39,* 261–273.

Diperna, J. C., & Elliott, S. N. (2000). *Academic Competence Evaluation Scales.* San Antonio, TX: Pearson.

Dishion, T. J., McCord, J., & Poulin, F. (1999). When interventions harm: Peer groups and problem behavior. *American Psychologist, 54,* 755–764.

Dodge, K. A. (1991). The structure and function of reactive and proactive aggression. In D. J. Peper & K. H. Rubin (Eds.), *The development and treatment of childhood aggression* (pp. 201–216). Hillsdale, NJ: Erlbaum.

Dodge, K. A. (2008). Framing public policy and prevention of chronic violence in American youths. *American Psychologist, 63,* 573–590.

Dodge, K. A., & Pettit, G. S. (2003). A biopsychosocial model of the development of chronic conduct problems in adolescence. *Developmental Psychology, 39,* 349–371.

Doll, B. (1996). Prevalence of psychiatric disorders in children and youth: An agenda for advocacy by school psychology. *School Psychology Quarterly, 11,* 20–47.

Doll, B., & Cummings, J. (2007). *Transforming school mental health services: Population-based approaches to promoting the competency and wellness of children.* Thousand Oaks, CA: Corwin Press.

Douglas, K. S., Cox, D. N., & Webster, C. D. (1999). Violence risk assessment: Science and practice. *Legal and Criminological Psychology, 4,* 149–184.

Drach, K. M., Wientzen, J., & Ricci, L. R. (2001). The diagnostic utility of sexual behavior problems in diagnosing sexual abuse in a forensic child abuse evaluation clinic. *Child Abuse and Neglect, 25,* 489–503.

Drogin, E. Y., Connell, M., Foote, W. E., & Strum, C. A. (2010). The American Psychological Association's revised "Record Keeping Guidelines": Implications for the practitioner. *Professional Psychology: Research and Practice, 41,* 236–243.

Eaton, D. K., Kann, L., Kinchen, S., Shanklin, S., Ross, J., Hawkins, J., et al. (2010). Youth Risk Behavior Surveillance—United States, 2009. National Center for Chronic Disease Prevention and Health Promotion. *Morbidity and Mortality Weekly Report, 59,* 1–142. Retrieved from *www.cdc.gov/mmwr/pdf/ss/ss5905.pdf.*

Eckert, T. L., Miller, D. N., DuPaul, G. J., & Riley-Tillman, T. C. (2003). Adolescent suicide prevention: School psychologists' acceptability of school-based programs. *School Psychology Review, 32,* 57–76.

Eckert, T. L., Miller, D. N., Riley-Tillman, T. C., & DuPaul, G. J. (2006). Adolescent suicide prevention: Gender differences in students' perceptions of the acceptability and intrusiveness of school-based screening programs. *Journal of School Psychology, 44,* 271–285.

Elliott, D. S., Hamburg, B. A., & Williams, K. R. (1998). Violence in American schools: An overview. In D. Elliott, B. Hamburg, & K. Williams (Eds.), *Violence in American schools* (pp. 3–28). Cambridge, UK: Cambridge University Press.

Elliott, S. N., DiPerna, J. C., & Shapiro, E. (2001). *Academic Intervention Monitoring System guidebook.* San Antonio, TX: Psychological Corporation.

Epstein, M. H. (2004). *Behavioral and Emotional Rating Scale: A strength based approach to assessment* (2nd ed.). Austin, TX: PRO-ED.

Espelage, D. L., Aragon, S. R., Birkett, M., & Koening, B. W. (2008). Homophobic teasing, psychological outcomes, and sexual orientation among high school students: What influence do parents and schools have? *School Psychology Review, 37,* 202–216.

Espelage, D. L., & Swearer, S. M. (2003). Research on school bullying and victimization: What have we learned and where do we go from here? *School Psychology Review, 32,* 365–383.

Evans, T. M., & Meloy, J. R. (2011). Identifying and classifying juvenile stalking behavior. *Journal of Forensic Sciences, 56(S1),* S266–S270.

Family Education Rights and Privacy Act. (1974). Public Law 93–830. 20 U.S.C. §1232 et seq.

Farrington, D. P., Loeber, R., Elliott, D. S., Hawkins, J. D., Kandel, D., Klein, M., et al. (1990). Advancing knowledge about the onset of delinquency and crime. In B. Lahey & A. Kazdin (Eds.), *Advances in clinical and child psychology* (Vol. 13, pp. 231–342). New York: Plenum Press.

Favazza, A. (1998). The coming age of self-mutilation. *Journal of Nervous and Mental Disease, 186,* 259–268.

Favazza, A. (1999). Self-mutilation. In D. G. Jacobs (Ed.), *The Harvard Medical School guide to suicide assessment and intervention* (pp. 125–145). San Francisco: Jossey-Bass.

Fein, R. A., & Vossekuil, B. (1998). *Protective intelligence and threat assessment investigations: A guide for state and local law enforcement officials.* Washington, DC: U.S. Department of Justice.

Fein, R. A., & Vossekuil, B. (1999). Assassination in the United States: An operational study of recent assassins, attackers, and near-lethal approachers. *Journal of Forensic Sciences, 44,* 321–333.

Fein, R. A., Vossekuil, B., Pollack, W. S., Borum, R., Mozeleski, W., & Reddy, M. (2002). *Threat assessment in schools: A guide to managing threatening situations and to creating safe school climates.* Washington, DC: U.S. Secret Service & U.S. Department of Education.

Finkelhor, D. (1988). The trauma of sexual abuse: Two models. In G. Wyatt & G. Powell (Eds.), *Lasting effects of child sexual abuse* (pp. 61–82). Newbury Park, CA: Sage.

Fisher, T. A. (2003). Conducting functional behavioral assessments and designing behavior intervention plans for youth with emotional/behavioral disorders. In M. Breen & C. Fiedler (Eds.), *Behavioral approach to the assessment of youth with emotional/behavioral disorders: A handbook for school-based practitioners* (2nd ed., pp. 73–121). Austin, TX: PRO-ED.

Fishman, D. B. (1999). *The case for pragmatic psychology.* New York: New York University Press.

Fitzpatrick, K. (1999). Violent victimization among America's school children. *Journal of Interpersonal Violence, 14*, 1055–1069.

Fleischman, A., Bertolote, J. M., Belfer, M., & Beautrais, A. (2005). Completed suicide and psychiatric diagnoses in young people: Examination of the evidence. *American Journal of Orthopsychiatry, 75*, 676–683.

Foote, W. E., & Shuman, D. W. (2006). Consent, disclosure, and waiver for the forensic psychological evaluation: Rethinking roles of psychologist and lawyer. *Professional Psychology: Research and Practice, 37*, 437–445.

Forth, A. E., Kosson, D. S., & Hare, R. D. (2003). *Hare Psychopathy Checklist: Youth Version.* North Tonawanda, NY: MHS.

Fossey, R., & Zirkel, P. A. (2011). Student suicide case law in public schools. In D. N. Miller, *Child and adolescent suicidal behavior: School-based prevention, assessment, and intervention* (pp. 131–137). New York: Guilford Press.

Foster, S. L., & Robin, A. L. (1997). Family conflict and communication in adolescence. In E. J. Mash & L. G. Terdal (Eds.), *Assessment of childhood disorders* (3rd ed., pp. 627–682). New York: Guilford Press.

Frick, P. J. (2004). Developmental pathways to conduct disorder: Implications for serving youth who show severe aggressive and antisocial behavior. *Psychology in the Schools, 41*, 823–834.

Frick, P. J., Cornell, A. H., Bodin, S. D., Dane, H. E., Barry, C. T., & Loney, B. R. (2003). Callous unemotional traits and developmental pathways to severe conduct problems. *Developmental Psychology, 39*, 246–260.

Friedrich, W. N., & Grambsch, P. (1992). Child Sexual Behavior Inventory: Normative and clinical comparisons. *Psychological Assessment, 4*, 303–311.

Gadow, K. D., & Sprafkin, J. (1997). *Early Childhood Inventory–4—Teacher Checklist.* Stony Brook, NY: Checkmate Plus.

Gadow, K. D., & Sprafkin, J. (2005). *Child and Adolescent Symptom Inventory–4R.* Stony Brook, NY: Checkmate Plus.

Gadow, K. D., & Sprafkin, J. (2008). *Youth's Inventory–4R.* Stony Brook, NY: Checkmate Plus.

Gadow, K. D., & Sprafkin, J. (2010). *Early Childhood Inventory–4R—Parent Checklist.* Stony Brook, NY: Checkmate Plus.

Garbarino, J., & Scott, F. M. (1989). *What children can tell us.* San Francisco: Jossey-Bass.

Gellman, R. A., & Delucia-Waack, J. L. (2006). Predicting school violence: A comparison of violent and nonviolent male students on attitudes toward violence, exposure level to violence, and PTSD symptomatology. *Psychology in the Schools, 43*, 591–598.

Ginsburg, H., & Opper, S. (1969). *Piaget's theory of intellectual development: An introduction.* Englewood Cliffs, NJ: Prentice-Hall.

Goldstein, A. P., Glick, B., & Gibbs, J. (1998). *Aggression replacement training* (rev. ed.). Champaign, IL: Research Press.

Goldston, D. B. (2003). *Measuring suicidal behavior and risk in children and adolescents.* Washington, DC: American Psychological Association.

Goldston, D. B., Davis Molock, S., Whitbeck, L. B., Murakami, J. L., Zayas, L. H., & Nagayama Hall, G. C. (2008). Cultural considerations in adolescent suicide prevention and psychosocial treatment. *American Psychologist, 63*, 14–31.

Goleman, D. (1995). *Emotional intelligence.* New York: Bantam Books.

Gould, M. S., & Kramer, R. A. (2001). Youth suicide prevention. *Suicide and Life-Threatening Behavior, 31*(Suppl.), 6–31.

Gould, M. S., Marrocco, F. A., Kleinman, M., Thomas, J. G., Mostkoff, K., Kote, J., et al. (2005). Evaluating iatrogenic risk of youth suicide screening programs: A randomized control trial. *Journal of the American Medical Association, 293*, 1182–1189.

Greenberg, S. A., & Shuman, D. W. (2008). Irreconcilable conflict between therapeutic and forensic roles. In D. N. Bersoff (Ed.), *Ethical conflicts in psychology* (4th ed., pp. 492–498). Washington, DC: American Psychological Association.

Greenspan, S. I., & Greenspan, N. T. (2003). *The clinical interview of the child* (3rd ed.). Arlington, VA: American Psychiatric Publishing.

Gresham, F. M., & Elliott, S. N. (2008). *Social Skills Improvement System manual.* San Antonio, TX: Pearson.

Gresham, F. M., & Gansle, K. A. (1992). Misguided assumptions of the DSM-III-R: Implications for school psychological practice. *School Psychology Quarterly, 7*, 79–95.

Gudeman, R. (2003, July–September). Federal privacy protection for substance abuse treatment records: Protecting adolescents. *Youth Law News*, pp. 1–4.

Halikias, W. (1994). Forensic family evaluations: A comprehensive model for professional practice. *Journal of Clinical Psychology, 50*, 951–964.

Halikias, W. (2000). Forensic evaluations of adolescents: Psychosocial and clinical considerations. *Adolescence, 35*, 467–484.

Halikias, W. (2004). School-based risk assessment: A conceptual framework and model for professional practice. *Professional Psychology: Research and Practice, 35*, 598–607.

Halikias, W. (2005). Assessing youth violence and threats of violence in schools: School-based risk assessments. In S. H. McConaughy, *Clinical interviews for children and adolescents: Assessment to intervention* (pp. 200–215). New York: Guilford Press.

Hartmann, D. P., Roper, B. L., & Bradford, D. C. (1979). Some relationships between behavioral and traditional assessment. *Journal of Behavioral Assessment, 1*, 3–21.

Health Insurance Portability and Accountability Act. (1996). Public Law 104–191. 26 U.S.C. §294, 42 U.S.C. §§201, 1395b-5.

Heilbrun, K. (1997). Prediction versus management models relevant to risk assessment: The importance of legal decision-making context. *Law and Human Behavior, 21*, 447–359.

Heilbrun, K., Marczyk, G., & Goldstein, A. M. (2008). Standards of practice and care in forensic mental health assessment: Legal, professional, and principles-based considerations. *Psychology, Public Policy, and Law, 14*, 1–26.

Henggeler, S. W., & Schaeffer, C. (2010). Treating serious antisocial behavior using multisystemic therapy. In J. R. Weisz & A. E. Kazdin (Eds.), *Evidence-based psychotherapies for children and adolescents* (2nd ed., pp. 259–276). New York: Guilford Press.

Henker, B., Whalen, C. K., & O'Neil, R. (1995). Worldly and workaday worries: Contemporary concerns of children and young adolescents. *Journal of Abnormal Child Psychology, 23*, 685–702.

Hoffmann, J., Meloy, J. R., Guldimann, & Ermer, A. (2011). Attacks on German public figures, 1968–2004: Warning behaviors, potentially lethal and non-lethal acts, psychiatric status, and motivations. *Behavioral Sciences and the Law, 29*, 155–179.

Hoge, R., & Andrews, D. (2002). *The Youth Level of Service/CaseManagement Inventory manual and scoring key.* North Tonawanda, NY: MHS.

Horton, C. B., & Cruise, T. K. (2001). *Child abuse and neglect: The school's response.* New York: Guilford Press.

Hughes, J., & Baker, D. B. (1990). *The clinical child interview.* New York: Guilford Press.

Individuals with Disabilities Education Act. (1990). Public Law 101–476. 20 U.S.C. §1401 et seq. Amended by Public Law 105–17 (1997). 20 U.S.C. §1400 et seq. Amended by Individuals with Disabilities Education Improvement Act. (2004). Public Law 108–446. 20 U. S. C. §§ 1400 et seq.

Institute for Youth Development. (1999). Age of risk behavior debut: Trends and implications. Washington, DC: Author. Retrieved from *www.youthdevelopment.org/download/debut/pdf.*

Jackson, Y., Alberts, F. L., & Roberts, M. C. (2010). Clinical child psychology: A practice specialty serving children, adolescents, and their families. *Professional Psychology: Research and Practice, 41*, 75–81.

Jacob, S. (2002). Best practices in utilizing professional ethics. In A. Thomas & J. Grimes (Eds.), *Best practices in school psychology* (4th ed., pp. 77–90). Washington, DC: National Association of School Psychologists.

Jacob, S. (2009). Putting it all together: Implications for school psychology. *School Psychology Review, 38*, 239–243.

Jacob, S., Decker, D. M., & Hartshorne, T. S. (2011). *Ethics and law for school psychologists* (6th ed.) New York: Wiley.

Jacobson, C. M., & Gould, M. (2007). The epidemiology and phenomenology of non-suicidal self-injurious behavior among adolescents: A critical review of the literature. *Archives of Suicide Research, 11*, 129–147.

January, A. M., Casey, R. J., & Paulson, D. (2011). A meta-analysis of classroom-wide interventions to build social skills: Do they work? *School Psychology Review, 40*, 242–256.

Jenson, W. R., Rhode, G., & Hepworth, M. N. (2003). *The tough kid parent book.* Longmont, CO: Sopris West.

Jenson, W. R., Rhode, G., & Reavis, H. K. (1994). *The tough kid tool box.* Longmont, CO: Sopris West.

Jobes, D. A. (2003). *Manual for the collaborative assessment and management of suicidality—revised* (CAMS-R). Unpublished manuscript.

Jobes, D. A. (2006). *Managing suicidal risk: A collaborative approach.* New York: Guilford Press.

Johnston, L. D., O'Malley, P. M., Bachman, J. G., & Schulenberg, J. E. (2010). *Monitoring the Future national results on adolescent drug use: Overview of key findings, 2009* (NIH Publication No.10–7583). Bethesda, MD: National Institute on Drug Abuse.

Joiner, T. E. (2005). *Why people die by suicide.* Cambridge, MA: Harvard University Press.

Joiner, T. E. (2009). Suicide prevention in schools as viewed through the interpersonal- psychological theory of suicidal behavior. *School Psychology Review, 38*, 244–248.

Joiner, T. E., Van Orden, K. A., Witte, T. K., & Rudd, M. D. (2009). *The interpersonal theory of suicide:*

Guidance for working with suicidal clients. Washington, DC: American Psychological Association.

Kalafat, J., & Lazarus, P. J. (2002). Suicide prevention in schools. In S. E. Brock, P. J. Lazarus, & S. R. Jimerson (Eds.), *Best practices in school crisis prevention and intervention* (pp. 211–223). Bethesda, MD: National Association of School Psychologists.

Kamphuis, J. H., & Finn, S. E. (2002). Incorporating base rate information in daily clinical decision making. In J. E. Butcher (Ed.), *Clinical personality assessment: Practical approaches* (2nd ed., pp. 257–268). New York: Oxford University Press.

Kann, L., O'Malley Olsen, E., McManus, T., Kinchen, S., Chyen, D., Harris, W. A., et al. (2011). Sexual identity, sex of sexual contacts, and health-risk behaviors among students in grades 9–12: Youth Risk Behavior Surveillance, selected sites, United States, 2001–2009. National Center for Chronic Disease Prevention and Health Promotion, *Morbidity and Mortality Weekly Report, 60*, 1–133. Retrieved from *www.cdc.gov/mmwr/pdf/ss/ss60e0606.pdf*.

Katsiyannis, K., & Smith, C. R. (2003). Disciplining students with disabilities: Legal trends and the issue of interim alternative education settings. *Behavioral Disorders, 28*, 410–418.

Kay, P., Fitzgerald, M., & McConaughy, S. H. (2001). Building effective parent–teacher partnerships. In R. Algozzine & P. Kay (Eds.), *Preventing problem behaviors: A handbook of successful prevention practices* (pp. 104–125). Thousand Oaks, CA: Corwin Press.

Kazdin, A. E. (2010). Problem-solving skills training and parent management training for oppositional defiant disorder and conduct disorder. In J. R. Weisz & A. E. Kazdin (Eds.), *Evidence-based psychotherapies for children and adolescents* (2nd ed., pp. 211–226). New York: Guilford Press.

Keith, T. Z., & DeGraff, M. (1997). Homework. In G. G. Bear, K. M. Minke, & A. Thomas (Eds.), *Children's needs: II. Development, problems, and alternatives* (pp. 477–487). Bethesda, MD: National Association of School Psychologists.

Kelley, M. L. (1990). *School–home notes: Promoting children's classroom success*. New York: Guilford Press.

Kerig, P. K., & Stellwagen, K. K. (2010). Roles of callous–unemotional traits, narcissism, and Machiavellianism in childhood aggression. *Journal of Psychopathology and Behavioral Assessment, 32*, 343–352.

Kindler, A. L. (2002). *Survey of the states' limited English proficient students and available educational programs and services 1999–2000 summary report*. Washington, DC: National Clearinghouse for English Acquisition and Language Instruction Educational Programs.

Knoff, H. M. (2001). *The stop & think social skills program*. Longmont, CO: Sopris West.

Knoff, H. M. (2002). Best practices in personality assessment. In A. Thomas & J. Grimes (Eds.), *Best practices in school psychology* (4th ed., pp. 1281–1302). Bethesda, MD: National Association of School Psychologists.

Knoster, T. P. (2000). Understanding the difference and relationship between functional behavioral assessments and manifestation determinations. *Journal of Positive Behavior Interventions, 2*, 53–58.

Knowledge Networks. (2009). The Associated Press–MTV poll digital abuse survey. Retrieved from *http://surveys.ap.org/data/KnowledgeNetworks/AP_Digital_Abuse_Topline_092209.pdf*.

Kohlberg, L. (1976). Moral stages and moralization: The cognitive developmental approach. In T. Lickona (Ed.), *Moral development and moral behavior* (pp. 31–53). New York: Holt, Rinehart & Winston.

Kovacs, M. (2010). *Children's Depression Inventory 2*. North Tonawanda, NY: MHS.

Kratochwill, T. R., Elliott, S. N., & Callan-Stoiber, K. (2002). Best practices in problem-solving consultation. In A. Thomas & J. Grimes (Eds.), *Best practices in school psychology* (4th ed., pp. 583–608). Bethesda, MD: National Association of School Psychologists.

Kratochwill, T. R., & Shapiro, E. S. (2000). Conceptual foundations of behavioral assessment in schools. In E. S. Shapiro & T. R. Kratochwill (Eds.), *Behavioral assessment in schools: Theory, research, and clinical foundations* (2nd ed., pp. 3–15). New York: Guilford Press.

Lachar, D., & Gruber, C. P. (1995). *Personality Inventory for Youth*. Los Angeles: Western Psychological Services.

La Greca, A. M. (1990). *Through the eyes of the child*. Boston: Allyn & Bacon.

Lahey, B. B., & Loeber, R. (1994). Framework for a developmental model of oppositional defiant disorder and conduct disorder. In D. K. Routh (Ed.), *Disruptive behavior disorders in childhood* (pp. 139–180). New York: Plenum Press.

Lahey, B. B., Loeber, R., Burke, J., Rathouz, P. J., McBurnett, K. (2002). Waxing and waning in concert: Dynamic comorbidity of conduct disorder with other disruptive and emotional problems over 7 years among clinic-referred boys. *Journal of Abnormal Psychology, 111*, 556–567.

Lane, K. L., Kalberg, J. R., & Menzies, H. M. (2009). *Developing schoolwide programs to prevent and manage problem behaviors: A step-by-step approach*. New York: Guilford Press.

Lee, J. F., & Pruitt, K. W. (1979). Homework assignments: Classroom games or teaching tools? *Clearinghouse, 53,* 31–35.

Lenhart, A., Ling, R., Campbell, S., & Purcell, K. (2010). Teens and mobile phones. *Pew Research Center's Internet and American Life Project.* Retrieved from *http://pewinternet.org/Reports/2010/Teens-and-mobile-phones.aspx.*

Lenhart, A., Madden, M., Smith, A., Purcell, K., Zickuhr, K., & Rainie, L. (2011). Teens, kindness and cruelty on social network sites. *Pew Research Center's Internet and American Life Project.* Retrieved from *http://pewinternet.org/Reports/2011/Teens-and-social media.aspx.*

Lewis, L. M. (2007). No-harm contracts: A review of what we know. *Suicide Life-Threatening Behavior, 37,* 50–57.

Lieberman, R., & Poland, S. (2006). Self-mutilation. In G. G. Bear & K. M. Minke (Eds.), *Children's needs III: Development, prevention, and intervention* (pp. 965–976). Bethesda, MD: National Association of School Psychologists.

Linehan, M. M. (1993). *Cognitive-behavioral treatment of borderline personality disorder.* New York: Guilford Press.

Lockman, J. E., Boxmeyer, C. L., Powell, N. P., Barry, T. D., & Pardini, D. A. (2010). Anger control training for aggressive youth. In J. R. Weisz & A. E. Kazdin (Eds.), *Evidence-based psychotherapies for children and adolescents* (2nd ed., pp. 227–242). New York: Guilford Press.

Loeber, R., Burke, J. D., Lahey, B. B., Winters, A., & Zera, M. (2000). Oppositional defiant and conduct disorder: A review of the past 10 years, Part I. *Journal of the American Academy of Child and Adolescent Psychiatry, 39,* 1468–1484.

Loeber, R., Farrington, D. P., & Waschbusch, D. A. (1998). Serious and violent juvenile offenders. In R. Loeber & D. P. Farrington (Eds.), *Risk factors and successful interventions* (pp. 13–29). Thousand Oaks, CA: Sage.

Lynam, D. R. (1996). Early identification of chronic offenders: Who is the fledgling psychopath? *Psychological Bulletin, 120,* 209–234.

Mash, E. J., & Hunsley, J. (2007). Assessment of child and family disturbance: A developmental–systems approach. In E. J. Mash & R. A. Barkley, *Assessment of childhood disorders* (4th ed. pp. 3–50). New York: Guilford Press.

McClellan, J., McCurry, C., Ronnei, M., Adams, J., Eisner, A., & Storck, M. (1996). Age of onset of sexual abuse: Relationship to sexually inappropriate behaviors. *Journal of the American Academy of Child and Adolescent Psychiatry, 34,* 1375–1383.

McComas, J. J., Hoch, H., & Mace, F. C. (2000). Functional analysis. In E. S. Shapiro & T. R. Kratochwill (Eds.), *Conducting school-based assessments of child and adolescent behavior* (pp. 78–120). New York: Guilford Press.

McConaughy, S. H. (2000a). Self-report: Child clinical interviews. In E. S. Shapiro & T. R. Kratochwill (Eds.), *Conducting school-based assessments of child and adolescent behavior* (pp. 170–202). New York: Guilford Press.

McConaughy, S. H. (2000b). Self-reports: Theory and practice in interviewing children. In E. S. Shapiro & T. R. Kratochwill (Eds.), *Behavioral assessment in schools: Theory, research, and clinical foundations* (2nd ed., pp. 323–352). New York: Guilford Press.

McConaughy, S. H. (2003). Interviewing children, parents, and teachers. In M. Breen & C. Fiedler (Eds.), *Behavioral approach to the assessment of youth with emotional/behavioral disorders: A handbook for school-based practitioners* (2nd ed., pp. 123–169). Austin, TX: PRO-ED.

McConaughy, S. H. (2004a). *Semistructured Parent Interview.* Burlington, VT: University of Vermont, Research Center for Children, Youth, and Families.

McConaughy, S. H. (2004b). *Semistructured Teacher Interview.* Burlington, VT: University of Vermont, Research Center for Children, Youth, and Families.

McConaughy, S. H. (2005). *Clinical interviews for children and adolescents: Assessment to intervention.* New York: Guilford Press.

McConaughy, S. H. (2012). *Semistructured Student Interview.* Burlington, VT: University of Vermont, Research Center for Children, Youth, and Families.

McConaughy, S. H., & Achenbach, T. M. (1994). *Manual for the Semistructured Clinical Interview for Children and Adolescents.* Burlington, VT: University of Vermont, Research Center for Children, Youth, and Families.

McConaughy, S. H., & Achenbach, T. M. (2001). *Manual for the Semistructured Clinical Interview for Children and Adolescents* (2nd ed.). Burlington, VT: University of Vermont, Research Center for Children, Youth, and Families.

McConaughy, S. H., & Achenbach, T. M. (2004a). *Child and Family Information Form.* Burlington, VT: University of Vermont, Research Center for Children, Youth, and Families.

McConaughy, S. H., & Achenbach, T. M. (2004b). *Manual for the Test Observation Form for Ages 2–18.* Burlington, VT: University of Vermont, Research Center for Children, Youth, and Families.

McConaughy, S. H., & Achenbach, T. M. (2009). *Manual for the ASEBA Direct Observation Form.* Burlington, VT: University of Vermont, Research Center for Children, Youth, and Families.

McConaughy, S. H., Arnold, J., Jacobowitz, D., &

Achenbach, T. (1994). *Videotape training manual for the Semistructured Clinical Interview for Children and Adolescents (SCICA)*. Burlington, VT: University of Vermont, Research Center for Children, Youth, and Families.

McConaughy, S. H., Fitzhenry-Coor, I., & Howell, D. C. (1983). Developmental differences in story schemata. In K. Nelson (Ed.), *Children's language* (Vol. 4, pp. 385–421). New York: Erlbaum.

McConaughy, S. H., Kay, P. J., & Fitzgerald, M. (2000). The Achieving–Behaving–Caring Project for preventing ED: Two-year outcomes. *Journal of Emotional and Behavioral Disorders, 7,* 224–239.

McConaughy, S. H., Kay, P., Welkowitz, J., Hewitt, K., & Fitzgerald, M. (2008). *Collaborating with parents for early school success: The Achieving–Behaving–Caring Program*. New York: Guilford Press.

McConaughy, S. H., & Ritter, D. R. (in press). Best practices in multimethod assessment of emotional and behavioral disorders. In A. Thomas & J. Grimes (Eds.), *Best practices in school psychology* (6th ed.). Bethesda, MD: National Association of School Psychologists.

McConaughy, S. H., & Skiba, R. (1993). Comorbidity of externalizing and internalizing problems. *School Psychology Review, 22,* 421–436.

McConaughy, S. H., Volpe, R. J., Antshel, K. M., Gordon, M., & Eiraldi, R.B. (2011). Academic and social impairments of elementary school children with attention-deficit/hyperactivity disorder. *School Psychology Review, 40,* 200–225.

McGinnis, E. (2012). *Skillstreaming the elementary school child* (3rd ed.). Champaign, IL: Research Press.

McGinnis, E., Sprafkin, R. P., Gershaw, N. J., & Klein, P. (2012). *Skillstreaming the adolescent* (3rd ed.). Champaign, IL: Research Press.

McGowan, M. R., Horn, R. A., & Mellott, R. N. (2011). The predictive validity of the Structured Assessment of Violence Risk in Youth in secondary educational settings. *Psychological Assessment, 23,* 478–486.

McMahon, R. J., & Frick, P. J. (2007). Conduct and oppositional disorders. In E. J. Mash & R. A. Barkley (Eds.), *Assessment of childhood disorders* (4th ed., pp. 132–183). New York: Guilford Press.

McMahon, R. J., & Forehand, R. L. (2003). *Helping the noncompliant child: Family-based treatment for oppositional behavior*. New York: Guilford Press.

Meeks, J. E., & Bernet, W. (2001). *The fragile alliance* (5th ed.). Melbourne, FL: Krieger.

Meloy, J. R. (2004). Indirect personality assessment of the violent true believer. *Journal of Personality Assessment, 82,* 138–146.

Meloy, J. R., Hempel, A. G., Gray, T., Mohandie, K., Shiva, A., & Richards, T. C. (2004). A comparative analysis of North American adolescent and adult mass murderers. *Behavioral Sciences and the Law, 22,* 291–309.

Melton, G. B., Petrila, J., Poythress, N. G., & Slobogin, C. (2007). *Psychological evaluations for the courts: A handbook for mental health professionals and lawyers* (3rd ed.). New York: Guilford Press.

Merrell, K. W. (2002a). *Preschool and Kindergarten Behavioral Scales—Second Edition*. Austin, TX: PRO-ED.

Merrell, K. W. (2002b). *School Social Behavior Scales—Second Edition*. Eugene, OR: Assessment–Intervention Resources.

Merrell, K. W. (2008a). *Behavioral, social, and emotional assessment of children and adolescents* (3rd ed.). New York: Erlbaum.

Merrell, K. W. (2008b). *Helping children overcome depression and anxiety: A practical guide* (2nd ed.). New York: Guilford Press.

Merrell, K. W., & Caldarella, P. (2002). *Home and Community Social Behavior Scales*. Eugene, OR: Assessment–Intervention Resources.

Meyers, J. R., & Schmidt, F. (2008). Predictive validity of the Structured Assessment for Violence Risk in Youth (SAVY) with juvenile offenders. *Criminal Justice and Behavior, 35,* 344–355.

Miller, A. L., Rathus, J. H., & Linehan, M. M. (2007). *Dialectical behavior therapy with suicidal adolescents*. New York: Guilford Press.

Miller, D. N. (2010). Assessing internalizing problems and well-being. In G. Gimpel Peacock, R. A. Ervin, E. J. Daly, & K. W. Merrell (Eds.), *Practical handbook of school psychology: Effective practices for the 21st century* (pp. 175–191). New York: Guilford Press.

Miller, D. N. (2011). *Child and adolescent suicidal behavior: School-based prevention, assessment, and intervention*. New York: Guilford Press.

Miller, D. N., & Brock, S. E. (2010). *Identifying, assessing, and treating self-injury at school*. New York: Springer.

Miller, D. N., & Eckert, T. L. (2009). Youth suicidal behavior: An introduction and overview. *School Psychology Review, 38,* 153–167.

Miller, D. N., Eckert, T. L., DuPaul, G. J., & White, G. P. (1999). Adolescent suicide prevention: Acceptability of school-based programs among secondary school principals. *Suicide and Life-Threatening Behavior, 29,* 72–85.

Miller, D. N., Eckert, T. L., & Mazza, J. J. (2009). Suicide prevention programs in the schools: A review and public health perspective. *School Psychology Review, 38,* 168–188.

Miller, D. N., & Jome, L. M. (2008). School psychologists and the assessment of childhood internalizing disorders: Perceived knowledge, role preferences, and training needs. *School Psychology International, 29*, 500–510.

Miller, D. N., & Nickerson, A. B. (2006). Projective assessment and school psychology: Contemporary validity issues and implications for practice. *California School Psychologist, 11*, 73–84.

Miller, G. E., Arthur-Stanley, A., & Lines, C. (2012). Family–school collaboration services: Beliefs into action. *Communique, 40*(1), 12–14.

Millon, T. (1993). *Millon Adolescent Clinical Inventory*. San Antonio, TX: Pearson.

Moffitt, T. E. (1993). Adolescence-limited and life-course persistent antisocial behavior: A developmental taxonomy. *Psychological Review, 100*, 674–701.

Moffitt, T. E. (2003). Life-course persistent and adolescence—limited antisocial behavior: A ten-year research review and research agenda. In B. B. Lahey, T. E. Moffitt, & A. Caspi (Eds.), *Causes of conduct disorder and juvenile delinquency* (pp. 49–75). New York: Guilford Press.

Moffitt, T. E., Arseneault, L., Jaffee, S. R., Kim-Cohen, J., Koenen, K. C., Oders, C. L., et al. (2008). DSM-V conduct disorder: Research needs for an evidence base. *Journal of Child Psychology and Psychiatry, 49*, 3–33.

Monahan, J. (1981). *Predicting violent behavior: An assessment of clinical techniques*. Beverly Hills, CA: Sage.

Monahan, J., & Steadman, H. (2001). Violence risk assessment: A quarter century of research. In L. Frost & R. Bonnie (Eds.), *The evolution of mental health law* (pp. 195–211). Washington, DC: American Psychological Association.

Muehlenkamp, J. J., & Gutierrez, P. M. (2004). An investigation of differences between self-injurious behavior and suicide attempts in a sample of adolescents. *Suicide and Life-Threatening Behavior, 34*, 12–23.

Muehlenkamp, J. J., & Gutierrez, P. M. (2007). Risk for suicide attempts among adolescents who engage in non-suicidal self-injury. *Archives of Suicide Research, 11*, 69–82.

Mulvey, E. P., & Cauffman, E. (2001). The inherent limits of predicting school violence. *American Psychologist, 56*, 797–802.

Muris, P., Meesters, C., Merckelbach, H., Sermon, A., & Zwakhalen, S. (1998). Worry in normal children. *Journal of the American Academy of Child and Adolescent Psychiatry, 37*, 703–710.

Nagin, D. S., & Tremblay, R. (1999). Trajectories of boys' physical aggression and hyperactivity on the path to physically violent and nonviolent juvenile delinquency. *Child Development, 70*, 1181–1196.

Nagin, D. S., & Tremblay, R. (2001). Parental and early childhood predictors of persistent physical aggression in boys from kindergarten to high school. *Archives of General Psychiatry, 58*, 389–394.

Naglieri, J. A., LeBuff, P. A., & Pfeiffer, S. L. (1993). *Devereux Behavior Rating Scales School Form*. San Antonio, TX: Psychological Corporation.

Nansel, T. R., Overpeck, M., Pilla, R. S., Ruan, W. J., Simons-Morton, B., & Scheidt, P. (2001). Bullying behavior among U.S. youth: Prevalence and association with psychosocial adjustment. *Journal of the American Medical Association, 285*, 2094–2100.

Nastasi, B. K. (Ed.). (1998). Mini-series: Mental health programming in schools and communities. *School Psychology Review, 27*, 165–174.

National Association of School Psychologists. (2003a). *Position statement on student grade retention and social promotion*. Bethesda, MD: Author.

National Association of School Psychologists. (2003b). *Position statement on mental health services in the schools*. Bethesda, MD: Author.

National Association of School Psychologists. (2008). School violence: NASP position statements. In A. Thomas & J. Grimes (Eds.), *Best practices in school psychology* (5th ed., Vol. 1, pp. cxxxi–cxxxiv). Bethesda, MD: National Association of School Psychologists.

National Association of School Psychologists. (2010). *Principles of professional ethics*. Bethesda, MD: Author.

National Registry of Interpreters for the Deaf. (2002). *Code of ethics*. Alexandria, VA: Author.

National Survey on Drug Use and Health. (2010). *Violent behaviors and family income among adolescents*. Rockville, MD: Substance Abuse and Mental Health Services Administration, Office of Applied Studies.

Newgass, S., & Schonfeld, D. J. (2000). School crisis intervention, crisis prevention, and crisis response. In A. R. Roberts (Ed.), *Crisis intervention handbook: Assessment, treatment, and research* (2nd ed., pp. 209–228). London: Oxford University Press.

No Child Left Behind Act. (2001). Public Law No. 107–110. 20 U.S.C. 7801, §9101 (25).

Ochoa, S. H., Gonzalez, D., Galarza, A., & Guillemard, L. (1996). The training and use of interpreters in bilingual psycho-educational assessment: An alternative in need of study. *Diagnostique, 21*, 19–40.

Olweus, D. (1993). Bully/victim problems among school-children: Long-term consequences and an effective intervention program. In S. Hodgins (Ed.), *Mental disorder and crime* (pp. 317–349). Thousand Oaks, CA: Sage.

Olweus, D., Limber, S., & Milhalic, S. (1999). *Blueprints for violence prevention: Bullying prevention program*. Boulder, CO: Institute of Behavioral Science, Regents of the University of Colorado.

Parker, J. G., & Asher, S. R. (1993). Beyond group acceptance: Friendship adjustment and friendship quality as distinct dimensions of children's peer adjustment. In D. Perlman & W. H. Jones (Eds.), *Advances in personal relationships* (Vol. 4, pp. 261–294). London: Kingsley.

Parker, J. G., Rubin, K. H., Price, J. M., & DeRosier, M. E. (1995). Peer relationships, child development, and adjustment: A developmental psychopathology perspective. In D. Cicchetti & D. Cohen (Eds.), *Developmental psychopathology: Vol. 2. Risk, disorder and adaptation* (pp. 96–161). New York: Wiley.

Patterson, G. R. (1986). Performance models for antisocial boys. *American Psychologist, 41*, 432–444.

Patterson, G. R., Forgatch, M. S., Yoerger, K. L., & Stoolmiller, M. (1998). Variables that initiate and maintain an early-onset trajectory for juvenile offending. *Development and Psychopathology, 10*, 531–547.

Perry, D. G., Perry, L. C., & Kennedy, E. (1992). Conflict and the development of antisocial behavior. In C. Shantz & W. Hartup (Eds.), *Conflict in the child and adolescent development* (pp. 301–329). Cambridge, UK: Cambridge University Press.

Pfeffer, C. R. (2006). Assessing suicidal behavior in children and adolescents. In R. A. King & A. Apter (Eds.), *Suicide in children and adolescents* (pp. 211–226). New York: Cambridge University Press.

Piquero, A. R., & Buka, S. L. (2002). Linking juvenile and adult patterns of criminal activity in the Providence cohort of the National Collaborative Perinatal Project. *Journal of Criminal Justice, 30*, 259–272.

Poland, S. (1989). *Suicide intervention in the schools*. New York: Guilford Press.

Poland, S., & Lieberman, R. (2002). Best practices in suicide prevention. In A. Thomas & J. Grimes (Eds.), *Best practices in school psychology* (4th ed., pp. 1151–1165). Bethesda, MD: National Association of School Psychologists.

Power, T. J., Dombrowski, S. C., Watkins, M. W., Mautone, J. A., & Eagle, J. W. (2007). Assessing children's homework performance: Development of multi-dimensional, multi-informant rating scales. *Journal of School Psychology, 45*, 333–348.

Power, T. J., Karustis, J. L., & Habboushe, D. F. (2001). *Homework success for children with ADHD*. New York: Guilford Press.

Purcell, K. (2010). Teens, the Internet, and communication technology. *Pew Research Center's Internet & American Life Project*. Retrieved from *www.pewinternet.org/~/media/Files/Presentations/2010/Jun/Purcell%20YALSA%20pdf.pdf*.

Public Health Services Act. (1987). 42 U.S.C. §201 et seq.

Quinn, K. P., & Lee, V. (2007). The wraparound approach for students with emotional and behavioral disorders: Opportunities for school psychologists. *Psychology in the Schools, 44*, 101–111.

Quinsey, V. L., Harris, G. T., Rice, M. E., & Cormier, C. A. (1998). *Violent offenders: Appraising and managing risk*. Washington, DC: American Psychological Association.

Ramsey, A., & O'Day, J. (2010). *ESEA evaluation brief: The English language acquisition, language enhancement, and academic achievement act*. Washington, DC: U.S. Department of Education. Retrieved from *www.air.org/files/Title_III_State_of_the_States_043010_r1.pdf*.

Reddy, M., Borum, R., Berglund, J., Vossekuil, B., Fein, R., & Modzeleski, W. (2001). Evaluating risk for targeted violence in schools: Comparing risk assessment, threat assessment, and other approaches. *Psychology in the Schools, 38*, 157–172.

Rehabilitation Act. (1973). Section 504. 29 U.S.C. §794 et seq.

Reich, W. (2000). Diagnostic Interview for Children and Adolescents. *Journal of the American Academy of Child and Adolescent Psychiatry, 39*, 59–66.

Reich, W., Welner, Z., Herjanic, B., & MHS Staff. (1999). *Diagnostic Interview for Children and Adolescents–IV*. North Tonawanda, NY: MHS.

Reynolds, C. R., & Kamphaus, R. W. (2004). *Behavior Assessment System for Children manual* (2nd ed.). San Antonio, TX: Pearson.

Reynolds, W. M. (1988). *Suicidal Ideation Questionnaire manual*. Odessa, FL: Psychological Assessment Resources.

Reynolds, W. M. (1991). A school-based procedure for the identification of adolescents at risk for suicidal behaviors. *Family Community Health, 14*, 64–75.

Reynolds, W. M. (1998). *Adolescent Psychopathology Scale psychometric and technical manual*. Odessa, FL: Psychological Assessment Resources.

Reynolds, W. M. (2002). *Reynolds Adolescent Depression Scale manual* (2nd ed.). Odessa, FL: Psychological Assessment Resources.

Reynolds, W. M. (2010). *Reynolds Child Depression Scale manual* (2nd ed.) Odessa, FL: Psychological Assessment Resources.

Reynolds, W. M., & Mazza, J. J. (1994). Suicide and suicidal behaviors in children and adolescents. In W. M. Reynolds & H. F. Johnston (Eds.), *Handbook of depression in children and adolescents* (pp. 525–580). New York: Plenum Press.

Rhode, G., Jenson, W. R., & Reavis, H. K. (1993). *The tough kid book: Practical classroom management strategies*. Longmont, CO: Sopris West.

Rhodes, R. L., Ochoa, S. H., & Ortiz, S. O. (2005). *Assessing culturally and linguistically diverse students: A practical guide*. New York: Guilford Press.

Rivers, I. (2001). The bullying of sexual minorities at school: Its nature and long-term correlates. *Educational and Child Psychology, 18,* 33–46.

Rivers, I., & Noret, N. (2008). Well-being among same-sex- and opposite-sex-attracted youth at school. *School Psychology Review, 37,* 174–187.

Roberts, S., Zhang, J., & Truman, J. (2010). *Indicators of school crime and safety: 2010.* Washington, DC. National Center for Education Statistics, U.S. Department of Education & Bureau of Justice Statistics, U.S. Department of Justice.

Rogers, R. (2008). An introduction to response styles. In R. Rogers (Ed.), *Clinical assessment of malingering and deception* (3rd ed., pp. 1–13). New York: Guilford Press.

Rorty, R. (1982). *Consequences of pragmatism.* Minneapolis: University of Minneapolis Press.

Ross, S., & Heath, N. (2002). A study of the frequency of self-mutilation in a community sample of adolescents. *Journal of Youth and Adolescence, 31,* 67–77.

Rubin, K. H., & Stewart, S. L. (1996). Social withdrawal. In E. J. Mash & R. A. Barkley (Eds.), *Child psychopathology* (pp. 277–310). New York: Guilford Press.

Rudd, M. D. (2006). *The assessment and management of suicidality.* Sarasota, FL: Professional Resource Press.

Rudd, M. D., Mandrusiak, M., & Joiner, T. E. (2006). The case against no-suicide contracts: The commitment to treatment statement as a practice alternative. *Journal of Clinical Psychology, 62,* 243–251.

Ryan-Arredondo, K., Renouf, K., Egyed, C., Doxely, M., Dobbins, M., Sanchez, S., et al. (2001). Threats of violence in schools: The Dallas Independent School District's response. *Psychology in the Schools, 38,* 185–196.

Safe and Drug Free Schools and Community Act. (1994). 20 U.S.C. § 7101 et seq.

Saigh, P. A. (1992). Structured clinical interviews and the inferential process. *Journal of School Psychology, 30,* 141–149.

Sameroff, A. (2010). A unified theory of development: A dialectic integration of nature and nurture. *Child Development, 81,* 6–22.

Sattler, J. M. (1998). *Clinical and forensic interviewing of children and families.* San Diego: Author.

Scherff, A., Eckert, T. L., & Miller, D. N. (2005). Youth suicide prevention: A survey of public school superintendents' acceptability of school-based programs. *Suicide and Life-Threatening Behavior, 35,* 154–169.

Seagrave, D., & Grisso, T. (2002). Adolescent development and the measurement of juvenile psychopathy. *Law and Human Behavior, 26,* 219–239.

Segool, N., & Crespi, T. D. (2011). Sexting in the schoolyard. *Communique, 39,* 30–31.

Sewell, K. W., & Mendelsohn, M. (2000). Profiling potentially violent youth: Statistical and conceptual problems. *Children's Services: Social, Policy, Research, and Practice, 3,* 147–169.

Shaffer, D., & Craft, L. (1999). Methods of adolescent suicide prevention. *Journal of Clinical Psychiatry, 60,* 70–74.

Shaffer, D., Fisher, P., Lucas, C. P., Dulcan, M., & Schwab-Stone, M. E. (2000). NIMH Diagnostic Interview Schedule for Children—Version IV (NIMH DISC-IV): Description, differences from previous versions and reliability of some common diagnoses. *Journal of the American Academy of Child and Adolescent Psychiatry, 39,* 28–38.

Shapiro, E. S. (2011). *Academic skills problems: Direct assessment and intervention* (4th ed.). New York: Guilford Press.

Shapiro, E. S., & Kratochwill, T. R. (Eds.). (2000). Introduction: Conducting a multidimensional behavioral assessment. In E. S. Shapiro & T. R. Kratochwill (Eds.), *Conducting school-based assessments of child and adolescent behavior* (pp. 1–20). New York: Guilford Press.

Shea, S. C. (2002). *The practical art of suicide assessment.* Hoboken, NJ: Wiley.

Sheridan, S. M. (1997). *The tough kid social skills book.* Longmont, CO: Sopris West.

Sheridan, S. M., Kratochwill, T. R., & Bergan, J. R. (1996). *Conjoint behavioral consultation: A procedural manual.* New York: Plenum Press.

Skiba, R., & Grizzle, K. (1991). The social maladjustment exclusion: Issues of definition and assessment. *School Psychology Review, 20,* 577–595.

Skiba, R., & Grizzle, K. (1992). Qualifications vs. logic and data: Excluding conduct disorders from the SED definition. *School Psychology Review, 21,* 23–28.

Smetana, J. G., Campione-Barr, N., & Metzger, A. (2006). Adolescent development in interpersonal and societal contexts. *Annual Review of Psychology, 57,* 255–284.

Smith, T. E. (2005). IDEA 2004: Another round in the reauthorization process. *Remedial and Special Education, 26,* 314–319.

Stanger, C. (2003). Behavioral assessment: An overview. In M. J. Breen & C. R. Fiedler (Eds.), *Behavioral approach to assessment of youth with emotional/behavioral disorders: A handbook for school-based practitioners* (pp. 3–20). Austin, TX: PRO-ED.

Stanger, C., Achenbach, T. M., & Verhulst, F. C. (1997). Accelerated longitudinal comparison of aggressive versus delinquent syndromes. *Development and Psychopathology, 9,* 43–58.

Steege, M. W. & Watson, T. S. (2009). *Conducting school-based functional behavioral assessments: A practitioner's guide.* (2nd ed.). New York: Guilford Press.

Steinberg, L., & Morris, A. S. (2001). Adolescent development. *Annual Review of Psychology, 52,* 83–110.

Stinnett, T. A., Havey, J. M., & Oehler-Stinnett, J. (1994). Current test usage by practicing school psychologists: A national survey. *Journal of Psychoeducational Assessment, 12,* 331–350.

Stricker, G. (2002). What is a scientist–practitioner anyway? *Journal of Clinical Psychology, 58,* 1277–1283.

Stricker, G., & Trierweiler, S. J. (1995). The local clinical scientist: A bridge between science and practice. *American Psychologist, 12,* 995–1002.

Sue, D. W., & Sue, S. (1999). *Counseling the culturally different* (3rd ed.). New York: Wiley.

Swearer, S. M., Espelage, D. L., & Napolitano, S. A. (2009). *Bullying prevention and intervention: Realistic strategies for schools.* New York: Guilford Press.

Tarasoff v. Board of Regents of the University of California, 551 P. 2d 334 (Cal. Sup. Ct. 1976).

Tolman, A. O. (2001). Clinical training and the duty to protect. *Behavioral Sciences and the Law, 19,* 387–404.

Tremblay, R. E., Japel, C., Perusse, D., Boivin, M., Zocolillo, M., Montplaisir, J., et al. (1999). The search for the age of "onset" of physical aggression: Rousseau and Bandura revisited. *Criminal Behavior and Mental Health, 9,* 8–23.

Turnbull, H. R. (2005). Individuals with Disabilities Education Act reauthorization: Accountability and personal responsibility. *Remedial and Special Education, 26,* 320–326.

U.S. Census Bureau. (2010). *State and county quick facts.* Washington, DC: U.S. Department of Commerce. Retrieved from *http://quickfacts.census.gov/qfd/states/00000.htlm.*

U.S. Department of Education. (2008). *Thirtieth annual report to Congress on the implementation of the Individuals with Disabilities Education Act.* Washington, DC: Author. Retrieved from *www2.ed.gov/about/reports/annual/osep/index.html.*

U.S. Department of Education and United States Department of Justice. (1999). *1999 annual report on school safety.* Washington, DC: Author.

U.S. Department of Health and Human Services. (2010). Administration for Children and Families, Administration on Children, Youth and Families, Children's Bureau. *Child Maltreatment 2009.* Retrieved from *www.acf.hhs.gov/programs/cb/stats_research/index.htm#can.*

Vasey, M. W., & Daleiden, E. (1994). Worry in childhood. In G. Davey & F. Tallis (Eds.), *Worrying: Perspectives on theory, assessment, and treatment* (pp. 185–207). New York: Wiley.

Vasquez-Nuttall, I. V., Li, C., Sanchez, W., Nuttall, R. L., & Mathisen, L. (2003). Assessing culturally and linguistically different children with emotional and behavioral problems. In M. Breen & C. Fiedler (Eds.), *Behavioral approach to the assessment of youth with emotional/behavioral disorders: A handbook for school-based practitioners* (2nd ed., pp. 463–496). Austin, TX: PRO-ED.

Vossekuil, B., Fein, R., Reddy, M., Borum, R., & Modzeleski, W. (2002). *The final report and findings of the Safe School Initiative: Implications for the prevention of school attacks in the United States.* Washington, DC: U.S. Secret Service and U.S. Department of Education.

Walsh, B. W. (2012). *Treating self-injury: A practical guide* (2nd ed.). New York: Guilford Press.

Watkins, C. E., Campbell, V. L., Nieberding, R., & Hallmark, R. (1995). Contemporary practice of psychological assessment by clinical psychologists. *Professional Psychology Research and Practice, 26,* 54–60.

Watson, T. S., & Steege, M. W. (2003). *Conducting school-based functional behavioral assessments: A practitioner's guide.* New York: Guilford Press.

Webster, C. D., Douglas, K. S., Eaves, S. D., & Hart, S. D. (1997). *HCR-20: Assessing risk for violence* (Version 2). Vancouver, Canada: Mental Health Law & Policy Institute, Simon Fraser University.

Welsh, J. L., Schmidt, F., McKinnon, L., Chattha, H. K., & Meyers, J. R. (2008). A comparative study of adolescent risk assessment instruments: Predictive and incremental validity. *Assessment, 15,* 104–115.

Williams, K. R., & Guerra, N. G. (2007). Prevalence and predictors of Internet bullying. *Journal of Adolescent Health, 41,* S14–S21.

Wissow, L. S. (1995). Child abuse and neglect. *New England Journal of Medicine, 332,* 1425–1431.

Wolfe, V. V. (2007). Child sexual abuse. In E. J. Mash & R. A. Barkley (Eds.), *Assessment of childhood disorders* (4th ed., pp. 685–748). New York: Guilford Press.

Ybarba, M. L., & Mitchell, K. J. (2004). Online aggressors/targets, aggressors, and targets. A comparison of associated youth characteristics. *Journal of Child Psychology and Psychiatry, 45,* 1308–1316.

Zins, J. E., & Erchul, W. P. (2002). Best practices in school consultation. In A. Thomas & J. Grimes (Eds.), *Best practices in school psychology* (4th ed., pp. 625–643). Bethesda, MD: National Association of School Psychologists.

Index